American

Physicians dedicate

MW00412759

A Physician's

Guide

to Return *to* Work

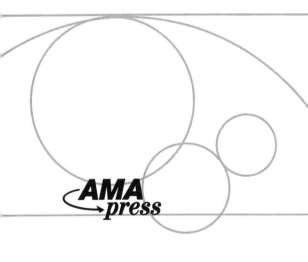

AMA *press*

Editors

James B. Talmage, MD

J. Mark Melhorn, MD

AMA Press

Vice President, Business Products: Anthony J. Frankos
Publisher: Michael Desposito
Director, Production and Manufacturing: Jean Roberts
Senior Acquisitions Editor: Barry Bowlus
Developmental Editor: Katharine Dvorak
Copy Editor: Nicole Netter
Director, Marketing: J. D. Kinney
Marketing Manager: Erica Duke
Senior Production Coordinator: Rosalyn Carlton
Senior Print Coordinator: Ronnie Summers

© 2005 by the American Medical Association
Printed in the United States of America.
All rights reserved.

Internet address: www.ama-assn.org

Additional copies of this book may be ordered by calling 800 621-8335 or from the secure AMA Press Web site at www.amapress.org. Refer to product number OP324005.

Library of Congress Cataloging-in-Publication Data

A physician's guide to return to work / edited by James B. Talmage, J. Mark Melhorn.
   p. ; cm.
  Includes bibliographical references and index.
  ISBN 1-57947-628-7 (alk. paper)
  1. Work capacity evaluation—United States. 2. Disability evaluation—United States.
3. Vocational rehabilitation—United States. 4. Workers' compensation—United States.
5. Work—Psychological aspects. 6. Convalescence—Psychological aspects. I. Talmage,
James B. II. Melhorn, J. Mark.
  [DNLM: 1. Rehabilitation—psychology. 2. Convalescence—psychology. 3. Disability
Evaluation. 4. Employment—psychology. WB 320 P5803 2005]
  RC963.4.P48 2005
  616.07'5—dc22

                   2004028168

The authors, editors, and publisher of this work have checked with sources believed to be reliable in their efforts to confirm the accuracy and completeness of the information presented herein and that the information is in accordance with the standard practices accepted at the time of publication. However, neither the authors nor the publisher nor any party involved in the creation and publication of this work warrant that the information is in every respect accurate and complete, and they are not responsible for any errors or omissions or for any consequences from application of the information in this book.

Although we believe the authors to be experts in their fields, the ideas and opinions expressed in this book do not reflect the views or official policy of the American Medical Association (unless otherwise specifically indicated). The ideas and opinions provided in this book are intended to provide guidance only and should not be used as a substitute for independent medical judgment. It is the responsibility of the attending physician or other healthcare professional, relying on independent experience and knowledge of the patient, to determine the best treatment course for the patient. The American Medical Association does not assume any responsibility for any injury and/or damage to persons or property arising out of or related to any use of the material contained in this book.

ISBN 1-57947-628-7
BP05:04-P-034-R:01/10

This book is dedicated to my parents, George and Helen Talmage, who taught me the importance of a strong work ethic, and to my wife, Jill, and daughter, Heidi, who love me despite it.

—JBT

This book is dedicated to my patients and to my family, who taught me the benefits and value of work and gave me the opportunity to share this knowledge with others.

—JMM

Contents

Preface

Work. For most individuals, work is part of what gives life meaning and purpose, as well as what provides the income for life's necessities—food, shelter, clothing, and medical care. *A Physician's Guide to Return to Work* is designed to help employees (ill and injured workers), employers, administrative staff, legal and legislative bodies, and healthcare providers understand the importance of staying at work or appropriate early return to work.

A Physician's Guide to Return to Work approaches return-to-work issues from the healthcare provider's point of view, because the healthcare provider is often looked to by the other parties for guidance. Science is the standard to which the healthcare provider looks for answers. This book is based on the science but also provides insight into the art of medicine as it applies to the dilemmas encountered when patients ask, "Can I work despite my [*fill in the blank*]?"

An etymological analysis of several of the languages of Europe reveals that *work* means "worry, trouble, and/or toil." The French word, *travailler,* was derived from the Latin, *tripotium,* or "feared instrument of torture."[1] Yet, work for man is necessary (see Chapter 1). If the reader is a believer in the theory of evolution, man has evolved while working over eons. Work is part of the environment to which man has adapted. Taking work away from man is thus like placing penguins at the equator. If the reader is a creationist, man was created to work, or perhaps work was created for man by a benevolent God.[2,3] Thus, either way, man has been intertwined with work since the beginning of time.

The editors and authors of this text have the firm belief, supported by science and consensus, that work is good for man,[1] and that it is the physician's role to encourage work and return to work, as part of treatment.[4–7]

Many brief work absences occur due to minor illness or minor injury. On a daily basis physicians deal with requests for work-absence certification for such events. According to Canadian Medical Association policy, absences for five or fewer days should not need physician certification of disability, and such certification is inappropriate retrospectively (the physician must have attended to the patient for the illness or have satisfactory knowledge of such illness).[8]

This book is not about minor, brief illness or injury. This is a text dedicated to the problem of long-term medical certification of disability by physicians.

Despite the fact that work in developed nations is getting progressively easier due to automation, ergonomics, and labor legislation, and despite the disappearance of diseases such as polio and improvements in medical care, the rate of medical disability certification in working-age adults is increasing dramatically, and faster than the population is increasing.[9,10] This book is about how physicians can help patients by thinking through the issues of "risk," "capacity," and "tolerance" when return-to-work decision making occurs in the context of persistent problems from illness or injury.

Disability can be viewed in many ways. These include at least a biomedical model, a biopsychosocial model, and a naturalistic sociolegal model.[11] Less than severe illness or injury with alleged disability conforms much better to the biopsychosocial model than to the biomedical model. However, employers, disability insurers, and the United States Social Security Administration all utilize a biomedical model for disability assessment, assuming that impairment or pathology equates to work capacity and risk. Thus far Hadler[12] has been the clearest voice calling for logic and compassion to change the current Western way of thinking about disability. Until Western society changes the "system," physicians caring for patients will be forced to use the biomedical model. As such, this book uses the biomedical model to think through return-to-work issues based on this current general acceptance of the biomedical model.

Return to work is not a subject about which physicians have received extensive training in their medical educations. Patients, employers, and disability insurers believe physicians have the necessary knowledge and experience to scientifically answer disability certification questions. The employers and insurers who have developed forms for physician documentation of disability certification may not realize that few physicians have had any formal training in such certification. There are organizations teaching these principles at physician Continuing Medical Education (CME) meetings.

The authors of the chapters in this book are all practicing physicians (except Chapter 8, which was written by lawyers) who face these issues on a frequent basis. Many are involved in teaching disability evaluation to physicians in CME conferences. Some chapter authors think and write with a "workers' compensation mindset," while others think and write with a "long term disability insurance mindset." While the term they use for the patient may differ (either *injured worker, patient,* or *disability applicant*), the approach they advocate is consistent.

A Physician's Guide to Return to Work is a text, and not a systematic review. On many disability certification issues, there is little pertinent scientific literature. Wherever possible, the authors have included and cited relevant medical literature.

This book does not cover all body systems. Each chapter on a body system discusses only a few common problems to teach the thought process of assessing risk, capacity, and tolerance. Examples of consensus-defined disability durations are included. There are more extensive texts on appropriate disability durations for individual illnesses and injuries.[13–15] Of the three most commonly used texts, the editors[*] chose to include data from *The Medical Disability Advisor*, based on the fact that the MDA includes data from physician-coded *International Classification of Diseases, Ninth Revision, Clinical Modification* (ICD-9-CM) diagnoses, and based on the need to keep this text brief. For help with the many conditions not discussed in this text, the reader is referred to these three excellent texts.[13–15]

A Physician's Guide to Return to Work attempts to describe a methodology for physicians to use to think through return-to-work issues based on risk, capacity, and tolerance. Relevant scientific literature, consensus documents, and "common sense" are the tools available. This text is meant to be read "cover to cover," as the material in the later chapters assumes the reader has read the beginning chapters.

Every patient is unique, and must be evaluated by a physician intimately familiar with that patient's condition and co-morbidities. Medicine is both an art and a science. There is no guarantee that an individual will not be re-injured or sustain a new injury if he or she chooses to return to work with, or despite, physician recommendations.

In the final analysis, return-to-work decisions are always those of the patient and his or her employer. The physician's role is merely one of advisor. The advice for a particular patient must come from the physician who knows intimately the unique aspects of the patient's illness or injury, co-morbidities, and personality.

In light of ongoing research and changes in clinical experience and in governmental regulations, readers are encouraged to confirm the information contained herein with additional sources.

---

[*]James B. Talmage, MD, was a paid contributor to *The Medical Disability Advisor*, 3rd and 4th editions and is currently on the Advisory Board of the Official Disability Guidelines (ODG). J. Mark Melhorn, MD, is on the Advisory Board of the ODG, and will be involved in future editions of *The Medical Disability Advisor*. Neither was involved in the *American College of Occupational and Environmental Medicine's Occupational Medicine Practice Guidelines, 2nd Edition*.

References

1. Nordin M. 2000 International society for the study of the lumbar spine presidential address: back to work—some reflections. *Spine.* 2001;26:851–856.

2. Genesis 2:15.

3. Genesis 3:17.

4. Canadian Medical Association. *CMA Policy: The Physician's Role in Helping Patients Return to Work After an Illness or Injury (Update 2000).* Available at: www.cma.ca/multimedia/staticContent/HTML/N0/l2/where_we_stand/return_to_work.pdf. Accessed May 21, 2004.

5. American College of Occupational and Environmental Medicine. *ACOEM Consensus Opinion Statement: The Attending Physician's Role in Helping Patients Return to Work after an Illness or Injury.* Available at: www.acoem.org/guidelines/pdf/Return-to-Work-04-02.pdf. Accessed May 21, 2004.

6. American Academy of Orthopaedic Surgeons. *AAOS Position Statement: Early Return to Work Programs.* Available at: www.aaos.org/wordhtml/papers/position/1150.htm. Accessed May 21, 2004.

7. American Medical Association. *Report 12 of the Council on Scientfic Affairs (A-04) Full Text.* Available at: www.ama-assn.org/ama/pub/article/print/2036-8668.html. Accessed May 24, 2004.

8. Canadian Medical Association. *CMA Policy: Certificate of Disability.* Available at: www.cma.ca/index.cfm/ci_id/3212/la_id/1.htm. Accessed May 24, 2004.

9. Waddell G, Aylward M, Sawney P. *Back Pain, Incapacity for Work and Social Security Benefits: An International Literature Review and Analysis.* London, England: The Royal Society of Medicine Press, Ltd; 2002.

10. Leopold RS. *A Year in the Life of a Million American Workers.* New York, NY: Metropolitan Life Insurance Company; 2003.

11. Halligan PW, Bass C, Oakley DA. Willful deception as illness behavior. In: Halligan PW, Bass C, Oakley DA. *Malingering and Illness Deception.* New York, NY: Oxford University Press, Inc; 2003.

12. Hadler NM. *Occupational Musculoskeletal Disorders.* 2nd Ed. Philadelphia, Pa: Lippincott, Williams, & Wilkins; 1999.

13. Reed P. *The Medical Disability Advisor: Workplace Guidelines for Disability Duration.* 5th ed. Westminster, Colo: Reed Group, Ltd; 2005.

14. Denniston P, ed. *Official Disability Guidelines.* 9th ed. Encinitas, Calif: Work Loss Data Institute; 2004.

15. Glass L, ed. *American College of Occupational and Environmental Medicine: Occupational Medicine Practice Guidelines.* 2nd ed. Beverly Farms, Mass; 2004.

Acknowledgments

For help in the creation of this book I would like to thank Richard A. Hoffmeister, MD, and Sam T. Barnes, MD, who taught me how to think "like an orthopedist"; John LoCasio, MD, who first introduced me to the concepts of risk, capacity, and tolerance; Amy Sullivan, Medical Librarian at the Cookeville Regional Medical Center, who obtained countless reference articles for me; and my patients over the past 32 years, who taught me about the human experiences of life and work. —JBT

For help in the creation of this book I would like to thank Henry O. Marsh, MD, and Herbert H. Stark, MD, who contributed to my development as an occupational orthopaedic hand surgeon; Peggy Gardner, PhD, who nurtured my interest in researching the prevention of work-related musculoskeletal pain; the medical librarians at Via Christi Regional Medical and Wesley Medical Center, who continue to obtain references for me; and my office staff at The Hand Center who help to communicate the message to my patients about the benefits of staying at work and early return to work. —JMM

We would also like to thank Barry Bowlus, Senior Acquisitions Editor at AMA Press, who proposed this book project; Katharine Dvorak, Developmental Editor, who shepherded this book through the publishing process; and Catherine Weldon at The Reed Group, who hepled us to include the most up-to-date disability duration tables.

About the Editors

James B. Talmage, MD, is an old man who has wandered through medicine for years in search of the perfect job. He remembers very little of his infancy. However, throughout childhood, he enjoyed school. He went to college to become a college professor in math and physics. Unfortunately, he took a part-time job in a hospital, and was kidnapped by the medical staff. After extensive brainwashing, he went to medical school. He is thus a graduate of Ohio State University, where he received his undergraduate degree and doctor of medicine degree. His orthopedic surgery training was in the United States Army.

Dr Talmage began a civilian orthopedic practice in Cookeville, Tennessee. Yet, he liked to sleep nights, which is not possible for an orthopedic surgeon in a trauma practice. So he left active orthopedic practice and for four years practiced full time as an emergency room physician. He became board certified in both orthopedic surgery and emergency medicine. However, emergency physicians work half of their shifts at night, so he still wasn't sleeping well. He therefore moved into an internal medicine group. After five years of internal medicine practice, he opened an occupational medicine practice in 1991.

Dr Talmage has been a Fellow of the American Academy of Disability Evaluating Physicians since 1987. He has served on the Continuing Education Committee, the Nominating Committee, and the Fibromyalgia Position Paper Committee of the Academy. He has been the Course Director of two Overview courses; the Advanced Clinical courses in 2001, 2002, 2003; and for the Scientific Session of the Annual Meeting in Nashville in 1997. In 1998, and again in 2001, he received the "President's Award" for Distinguished Service to AADEP. He served on the Board of Directors of the Academy from 1999 to 2001.

Dr Talmage is one of the original Examination Committee members for the American Board of Independent Medical Examiners. He was on the Board of Directors for the Tennessee College of Occupational and Environmental Medicine from 1998 to 2001 and served as Secretary/Treasurer in 2001, Vice President in 2002/2003, President Elect in 2003/2004, and President in 2004/2005.

Dr Talmage is the Associate Editor of *The Guides Newsletter* and was an associate editor of *The Guides Casebook*, published by AMA Press.

In addition, Dr Talmage was a reviewer for the AMA's *Guides to the Evaluation of Permanent Impairment, 5th Edition.*

Dr Talmage is a member of the Impairment Rating Committee of the International Association of Industrial Accident Boards and Commissions. He has chaired the Musculoskeletal Advisory Board for the *Medical Disability Advisor, Third Edition* published by the Reed Group, and he was Associate Chair for the *Fourth Edition* of that text. He served on the Editorial Board from 1999 to 2000 of the journal, *Disability*, published by the American Academy of Disability Evaluating Physicians and beginning in 2001, he has served on the Editorial Board of *Tennessee Medicine*, the journal of the Tennessee Medical Association.

Dr Talmage teaches regularly for the American Academy of Orthopaedic Surgeons, the American Academy of Disability Evaluating Physicians, the American Board of Independent Medical Examiners, and the American College of Occupational and Environmental Medicine.

In his spare time, he is an avid hiker. He enjoys climbing the Tennessee mountains where he can sit and ponder questions such as "What is truth?" and "What do I want to be when I grow up?"

J. Mark Melhorn, MD, is an occupational orthopedic physician who specializes in the hands and upper extremities. He received his undergraduate degree from McPherson College and his doctor of medicine degree from the University of Kansas.

Dr Melhorn is board certified in orthopedic surgery with added qualifications in surgery of the hand. In addition to his practice of orthopedics at The Hand Center in Wichita, Kansas, Dr Melhorn is a Clinical Assistant Professor in the Department of Surgery at the University of Kansas School of Medicine.

He has authored over 220 articles, book chapters, and other publications about his research of workplace injuries and illnesses, return-to-work options, impairment and disability, and prevention of musculoskeletal pain in the workplace. He has lectured extensively to physicians, employers, insurers, administrators, and legislators on industrial musculoskeletal, upper extremity disorders, and prevention of musculoskeletal pain in the workplace.

Dr Melhorn is currently the chairman of the American Academy of Orthopaedic Surgeons continuing education course on "Occupational Orthopaedics and Workers' Compensation: A Multidisciplinary Perspective."

He serves on the board of directors for the American Academy of Disability
Evaluating Physicians, and on the Committee for Occupational Health and
Continuing Medical Education for the American Academy of Orthopaedic
Surgeons, the Industrial Injuries and Prevention Committee for the American
Society for Surgery of the Hand, and the Return to Work Committee for the
American College of Occupational and Environmental Medicine.

Dr Melhorn reviewed the Upper Extremities chapter for the AMA's *Guides
to the Evaluation of Permanent Impairment, 5th Edition* and is a member of
the Medical Advisory Board for the Official Disabilities Guidelines of the
Work Loss Data Institute, a previous member of the Ergonomic Committee
for the American College of Occupational and Environmental Medicine,
a faculty member and 2004 co-chairperson for the American Academy of
Disability Evaluating Physician's Annual Continuing Education Meeting,
and past president of the Kansas Orthopedic Society.

Contributors

Gerald M. Aronoff, MD
Chairman, Department of Pain Medicine
Presbyterian & Presbyterian Orthopedic Hospitals
Charlotte, North Carolina

Michael Erdil, MD
Medical Director, Eastern Rehabilitation Network
    Affiliate of Hartford Hospital, Hartford, Connecticut
Medical Director, Health Direct
    Farmington, Connecticut

Elizabeth Genovese, MD, MBA
Bala Cynwyd, Pennsylvania

Robert H. Haralson III, MD, MBA
Executive Director, Medical Affairs
American Academy of Orthopaedic Surgeons
Rosemont, Illinois

Natalie P. Hartenbaum, MD, MPH
President and Chief Medical Officer
OccuMedix, Inc
Dresher, Pennsylvania

Edward B. Holmes, MD, MPH
Chief Medical Consultant
    Disability Determination Services for Social Security
    State of Utah
Assistant Professor Occupational Medicine
    University of Utah
    Salt Lake City, Utah

Lezzlie E. Hornsby, JD
Vickery & Waldner, LLP
Houston, Texas

Mark H. Hyman, MD
Associate Clinical Professor of Medicine
University of California, Los Angeles
Los Angeles, California

Edwin H. Klimek, MD
St. Catharines
Ontario, Canada

John L. LoCascio, MD
Unum Provident
Portland, Maine

Trang H. Nguyen, MD
University of Cincinnati
Department of Environmental Health
Cincinnati, Ohio

Phillip Osborne, MD
Healthsouth Evaluation Center
Occupational Medicine
Dallas, Texas

Mark D. Pilley, MD
Medical Director
IntegriGuard, LLC
Omaha, Nebraska

John D. Pro, MD
Research Medical Center
Kansas City, Kansas

David C. Randolph, MD, MPH
Midwest Occupational Health Management
Milford, Ohio

Yvonne Smallwood Sherrer, MD
Fort Lauderdale, Florida

Paul F. Waldner, JD
Vickery & Waldner, LLP
Houston, Texas

Why Staying at Work or Returning to Work Is in the Patient's Best Interest

James B. Talmage, MD, and J. Mark Melhorn, MD

> *No other technique for the conduct of life attaches the individual so firmly to reality as laying emphasis on work; for his work at least gives him a secure place in a portion of reality, in the human community.*
>
> —Sigmund Freud[1]

> *An unemployed existence is a worse negation of life than death itself. Because to live means to have something definite to do—a mission to fulfill—and in the measure in which we avoid setting our life to something, we make it empty. . . . Human life, by its very nature, has to be dedicated to something.*
>
> —Josè Ortega y Gasset[1]

> *Without work all life goes rotten.*
>
> —Albert Camus[1]

Philosophers and psychiatrists have grasped the central importance of work to human existence. This book will help the reader think through helping patients with return-to-work decisions when persisting symptoms and problems from illness or injury make work difficult. This chapter is devoted to why physicians should encourage early and ultimate return to work whenever possible. Simply stated: *because it is usually in the patient's best interest to remain in the workforce.*

There are serious injuries and illnesses that clearly leave patients unable to engage in any meaningful work activity. In this circumstance, the severity of the impairments is objectively obvious, and Western society has provided the protection of a "social security disability" safety net. The chapters that deal with specific body systems refer to the US Social Security Administration's criteria for such severe and disabling conditions.

This book focuses on the less obvious and less severe illness and injury situations in which many patients with similar problems work, and yet some patients consult with physicians, seeking disability certification. In these cases the disability is not obvious, and patients, employers, and disability insurers may request information from treating physicians and from "second opinion" physicians or independent medical examiners. In cases in which there are neither obvious severe disability nor obvious minor pathology (and thus returning to work is clearly indicated), what weight should be given to the benefits of patients returning to work?

Consensus Statements

In the introduction to this book, the consensus statements of the Canadian Medical Association,[2] the American College of Occupational and Environmental Medicine,[3] and the American Academy of Orthopaedic Surgeons[4] were introduced. All three documents strongly recommend that physicians return patients to their usual work roles as soon as possible:

> Prolonged absence from one's normal roles, including absence from the workplace, is *detrimental to a person's mental, physical, and social well-being* [italics added]. Physicians should therefore encourage a patient's return to function and work as soon as possible after an illness or injury. . . .[2]

> Prolonged absence from one's normal roles, including absence from the workplace, is detrimental to a person's mental, physical, and social well being. . . .[3]

The American Academy of Orthopaedic Surgeons and the American Association of Orthopaedic Surgeons (AAOS) support safe, early return-to-work programs that help injured workers improve their performance, regain functionality, and enhance their quality of life. . . . As patient advocates, physicians realize that early return to work results in many benefits for the injured worker, including the prevention of de-conditioning and the psychological sequels of prolonged time off work.[4]

At its summer 2004 meeting, the American Medical Association (AMA) adopted its version of this policy statement:

The AMA encourages physicians everywhere to advise their patients to return to work at the earliest date compatible with health and safety and recognizes that physicians can, through their care, facilitate patients' return to work.[5]

Physicians are familiar with prescribing medications for patients. If a physician looked up a drug in the *Physician's Desk Reference*[6] and found a "black box" warning required by the Food and Drug Administration (FDA) like this one:

> **Warning: This drug is detrimental to your patient's mental, physical, and social well-being!**

would physicians prescribe that medication?

What is the science behind the consensus statements by these organizations? Is it really true that being out of work is hazardous to one's health?

A Review of the Literature

The Australian Faculty of Occupational Medicine conference report on the health outcomes of compensable injuries was published with medical, legal, insurance, and government representation.[7] The report concluded that compensable injuries have a worse prognosis than the same injury would if it were not compensable. This was felt to be due to a complex interaction of factors. The medical review concluded that "unemployment is, in itself, a risk factor for poor health."

A 1995 review from Canada of 46 original articles concluded that, on an epidemiologic basis, unemployment has a strong positive association with many adverse health outcomes.[8] Despite a reduction in mortality from motor vehicle accidents, unemployment was positively associated with increased overall mortality, and with mortality from cardiovascular disease and suicide. Workers laid off because of factory closure have more symptoms and objectively validated illnesses, and are more likely to take medication and be hospitalized.

A 1996 review concluded that unemployment is pathogenic, with increased mortality and decreased physical and mental health.[9] The most common documented disorders were emotional and cardiopulmonary disease. A 1998 review from Australia concluded that unemployment itself is detrimental to health, and that it is associated with increasing mortality rates, causes physical and mental illness, and results in a greater use of health services.[10]

Three recent large studies add to the certainty of these conclusions. Nylen and Floderus[11] reported in 2001 from the Swedish Twin Registry data on all-cause mortality in 9,500 women and 11,132 men followed up from 1973 to 1996. Unemployment was associated with a relative risk of mortality of 1.98 (95% confidence interval [CI] 1.16–3.38) for women and of 1.43 (95% CI 0.91–2.25) for men, even when controlled for potential social, behavioral, work, and health-related confounders.

Quaade et al[12] reported in 2002 on the effect of early retirement. Some retire early because they are ill with serious disease(s), but what is the subsequent health status of those who are financially able to retire early while apparently healthy? This study utilized the Danish population-based registers of individuals born between 1926 and 1936 who were evaluated from 1986 to 1996. Those who continued to work had the lowest mortality. Those who were retired because of disease or injury disability had the highest mortality. Those who were well, but were able to choose an "early" retirement, had an intermediate mortality rate, consistent with an adverse effect on health of retirement itself.

In 2003, Gerdtham and Johannesson[13] described the mortality experience of 30,000 Swedes followed up for 10 to 17 years, concluding that unemployment increased the risk of death by nearly 50% (from 5.36% to 7.83%).

There are also reviews showing the effects of unemployment on specific diseases such as cancer and heart disease.[14–16] A recent study of 24,036 Swedes with complete employment records from biennial national Swedish Work Environment Surveys from 1989 to 1999 confirmed that unemployment due to employer downsizing was associated with health risks.[17] In addition, Barth and Roth[18] published a review of some of the pertinent articles on the mental health effects of unemployment.

Thus, there is sound science indicating that unemployment is hazardous to a patient's physical, mental, and social well-being. As patient advocates, physicians therefore should strongly urge patients to return to work or to stay at work, and should decline to certify disability unless it is obvious. Ethically, in these cases, beneficence trumps autonomy.

References

1. Peter LJ. *Peter's Quotations: Ideas for Our Time*. New York, NY: Bantam Books; 1977.

2. Canadian Medical Association. *CMA Policy: The Physician's Role in Helping Patients Return to Work After an Illness or Injury (Update 2000)*. Available at: www.cma.ca/multimedia/staticContent/HTML/N0/l2/where_we_stand/return_to_work.pdf. Accessed May 21, 2004.

3. American College of Occupational and Environmental Medicine. *ACOEM Consensus Opinion Statement: The Attending Physician's Role in Helping Patients Return to Work After an Illness or Injury*. Available at: www.acoem.org/guidelines/pdf/Return-to-Work-04-02.pdf. Accessed May 21, 2004.

4. American Academy of Orthopaedic Surgeons. *AAOS Position Statement: Early Return to Work Programs*. Available at: www.aaos.org/wordhtml/papers/position/1150.htm. Accessed May 21, 2004.

5. American Medical Association. *Report 12 of the Council on Scientific Affairs (A-04) Full Text: Physician's Guidelines for Return to Work After Injury or Illness*. Available at: www.ama-assn.org/ama/pub/article/print/2036-8668.html. Accessed June 24, 2004.

6. *Physician's Desk Reference*. 58th ed. Montvale, NJ: Medical Economics Co, Inc; 2004.

7. The Royal Australasian College of Physicians. *Compensable Injuries and Health Outcomes*. Available at: www.racp.edu.au/afom/compensable/index.htm. Accessed May 21,2004.

8. Jin RL, Shah CP, Svoboda TJ. The impact of unemployment on health: a review of the evidence. *CMAJ*. 1995;153:529–540.

9. Shortt SE. Is unemployment pathogenic? A review of current concepts with lessons for policy planners. *Int J Health Serv*. 1996;26:569–589.

10. Mathers CD, Schofield DJ. The health consequences of unemployment: the evidence. *Med J Aust*. 1998;168:178–182.

11. Nylen L, Floderus B. Mortality among women and men relative to unemployment, part time work, overtime work, and extra work: a study based on data from the Swedish Twin Registry. *Occup Environ Med*. 2001;58:52–57.

12. Quaade T, Enghlom G, Johansen AM, et al. Mortality in relation to early retirement: a population-based study. *Scand J Public Health*. 2002;30:216–222.

13. Gerdtham UG, Johannesson M. A note on the effect of unemployment on mortality. *J Health Econ*. 2003;22:505–518.

14. Lynge EI. Unemployment and cancer: a literature review. In: Kogavinas M, Oearce N, Boffetta P, eds. *Social Inequalities and Cancer*. Lyon, France: International Agency for Research on Cancer; 1997. IARC Scientific Publications No. 138.

15. Brenner MH. Heart disease mortality and economic changes; including unemployment; in Western Germany 1951–1989. *Acta Physiol Scand Suppl.* 1997;640:149–152.

16. Gallo WT, Bradley EH, Falba TA, et al. Involuntary job loss as a risk factor for subsequent myocardial infarction and stroke: findings from the Health and Retirement Survey. *Am J Indust Med.* 2004;45:408–416.

17. Westerlund H, Ferrie J, Hagbert J, et al. Workplace expansion, long-term sickness, absence, and hospital admission. *Lancet.* 2004;363:1193–1197.

18. Barth RJ, Roth VS. Health benefits of returning to work: review of the literature. *Occup Environ Med Rep.* 2003;17:13–17.

How to Think About Work Ability and Work Restrictions: Risk, Capacity, and Tolerance

James B. Talmage, MD, and J. Mark Melhorn, MD

C hapter 1 reviewed the consensus documents and scientific literature indicating that it is generally in the patient's best interest to remain at work or to return to work. For this to happen, physicians are usually asked for medical information and work status certification. They are often asked to fill out forms describing what patients can do at work, and thus to certify either that they are capable of returning to a specific job, or that they are not capable of that particular work. While physicians are well trained in diagnosis and treatment, most have received little or no training in how to evaluate their patient's ability to do work. Whenever asked about a patient's work ability, physicians should think through the issues by considering three terms: *risk*, *capacity*, and *tolerance*.

Risk

Risk refers to the chance of harm to the patient, or to the general public, if the patient engages in specific work activities. Familiar examples are that the Department of Transportation medical certification processes require examining physicians to disqualify individuals with uncontrolled seizure disorders from working as aircraft pilots and as commercial motor vehicle drivers. When patients should *not* attempt certain work activities because of known risk, this is clearly a basis for physician-imposed "work restrictions." A *work restriction* is something a patient can do, but should not do, as opposed to a *work limitation*, which is defined later in this chapter (under "capacity") as something the patient cannot physically do. The terms *work restriction* and *work limitation* are frequently seen on work status certification forms.

Unfortunately, there is little scientific literature on the real-world observed risks of working despite known medical conditions. Ideally, this would be the type of information on which to base work restrictions. Where generally accepted sound scientific evidence exists, there should logically be universal agreement among physicians about the issue in question. Sometimes, there are consensus documents that are helpful in assigning work restrictions based on risk. One example is the American College of Cardiology guidelines for physicians in approving participation in competitive sports.[1] While this is a consensus document, and thus not scientifically proven, following these guidelines is our best approach to achieve consistency among physicians. In the chapters in this book that deal with specific organ systems (Chapters 12–18), each author discusses the existing scientific studies on the risk of working as they relate to that organ system.

If a patient or examinee is applying for work, the US physician performing the pre-placement medical examination for the employer must remember that the Americans with Disabilities Act of 1990 permits the employer to deny the tentatively offered employment *only if,* on the basis of objective information, the work activities of the "essential job functions" pose a substantial risk of significant harm to self or others that is imminent. Under this law, these criteria would be the basis for physician-imposed work restrictions that would disqualify an applicant from working.

Substantial harm means an objectively verifiable worsening in the patient-examinee's condition, and not merely an increase in previously present symptoms, like pain or fatigue. This US law says that individuals may choose to work despite pain or fatigue. While physicians in pre-placement examinations generally remember and adhere to the maxim that "if there is not objective evidence of substantial risk of significant harm, the patient may choose whether or not to work despite symptoms," many times the obverse of this principle is forgotten when physicians are asked by patients to certify work disability based on subjective symptoms (tolerance) without evidence of risk of harm. If the decision to do or not to do work one is capable of doing with no significant risk, and despite symptoms, is the patient's decision (and not the physician's decision) when the patient is a willing job applicant, logically *the decision is still the patient's* when the patient is requesting disability certification.

There are recurring situations in which physicians have historically restricted patients on the basis of medically plausible risk assessment. Examples include heavy overhead lifting after shoulder rotator cuff repair, and heavy lifting, carrying, and jumping with combined anterior and medial instability in a knee. In these cases it is plausible to argue that recurrent cuff rupture and progressive osteoarthritis may occur, despite the lack of prospective human studies to prove that these risks are real. Until studies disprove these risks, they will be "generally accepted" and noted by consensus groups.

For decades, spine surgeons placed permanent lifting and other activity restrictions on patients who had good results after a first-operation lumbar diskectomy. Recently, studies have shown that those with good results can return quickly to full work with no increase in the incidence of disk re-rupture.[2,3]

Capacity

Capacity refers to concepts such as strength, flexibility, and endurance. These are measurable with a fair degree of scientific precision. Actually, "capacity" indicates that the individual is already maximally trained and fully acclimated to the job or activity in question. Thus, an athlete trained and ready to run a marathon and a worker accustomed to a heavy construction labor job may function at near "capacity." This current level of fitness can be quantified.

Physicians most often deal with an individual's *current ability*. Current ability can increase with exercise and activity, or it can decrease with inactivity. The aphorism "use it or lose it" summarizes the concept that the cardiopulmonary and musculoskeletal systems are affected by activity level. Current ability may increase up to capacity with exercise. This exercise may be rehabilitative exercise, recreational exercise, or even progressively more difficult work activity. Current ability may decrease with inactivity (deconditioning), and the effects of a sedentary lifestyle on exercise ability are well known.

Examples of lack of capacity are the individual with a rotator cuff tear in the shoulder who can not raise his arm high enough to reach the overhead controls of a factory press, and the individual who can exercise only to 4 MET (metabolic equivalent) on a treadmill before she reaches her maximal predicted heart rate, and who thus cannot return to a job that requires frequent 6 MET exertion. While physicians *impose* work restrictions (proscribe certain activities), physicians *describe* work limitations (what the patient is not physically able to do).

There are situations in which a patient lacks the "current ability" for specific work activities. If lifting 100 pounds is required, a significant percentage of the population will not have this ability. However, many, but not all, can acquire this ability with an exercise training program. Physicians are often asked to certify whether a patient has the "current ability" to perform certain work tasks (or perhaps the misnomer "capacity" appears on the form). Sometimes it is objectively obvious whether or not the patient has the ability in question. Many times the physician has no objective way to decide whether the patient does or does not have the current ability to do a task. This is the scenario in which a functional capacity evaluation (FCE) test is frequently ordered. (Chapter 7 reviews the reliability and validity of this testing in detail.) The term *functional capacity evaluation* is a misnomer in that it tells the physician whether or not, on the day of testing, the patient was or was not willing to demonstrate the "current ability" to do a job or job tasks. Unless the individual is already trained to maximal ability, it does not measure capacity. It usually reflects tolerance for symptoms, and not necessarily current ability.

If there are no scientific data on risk, and if it is not objectively obvious that the patient lacks the current ability to do certain job tasks, whether he or she will work is usually a question of tolerance.

Tolerance

Background

Tolerance is a psychophysiologic concept. It is the ability to tolerate sustained work or activity at a given level. Symptoms such as pain and/or fatigue are what limit the ability to do the task(s) in question. The patient may have the ability to do a certain task (no work limitation), but not the ability to do it comfortably. Thus, tolerance is not scientifically measurable or verifiable. Tolerance is frequently less than either capacity or current ability.

Tolerance is dependent on the rewards available for doing the activity in question. Tolerance is exemplified when an individual chooses, because of pain, not to work for minimum wage at a job he dislikes, but, when offered a much more physically demanding job at three or four times minimum wage, he happily works and endures (tolerates) even greater pain. This confirms that tolerance is not scientifically measurable, and explains why physicians will never all agree on questions of tolerance.

When a patient describes his or her activity tolerances, a physician may feel that this should be the basis for physician-imposed activity restrictions. However, on a medical certification form, the term *work restrictions* means what the patient *should not* do on the basis of risk of harm; symptoms are not harm, so "work restrictions" are not appropriate. The term *work limitations* describes what the patient lacks the current ability to do. In this example, work limitations are not appropriate as clearly this patient can do what he dislikes doing, as it causes symptoms.

If multiple physicians see the same patient in a contested work ability/ disability case, the physicians are likely to agree on questions of risk and capacity. Serious "risk of harm" situations are rare, and easily analyzed with common sense. Most often there is no scientific study that can clearly be generalized to the specific patient's work risk questions.

On questions of tolerance, when multiple physicians each offer strongly held opinions on work tolerance, but phrased as *work ability* or *restrictions*, the physicians appear to patients, employers, insurers, judges, and juries to be either unscientific, or biased, or "paid for." This obviously reflects poorly on medicine as a profession. Yet, many times, two equally well-qualified and honest physicians will testify in contested cases to exactly opposite conclusions about whether a given patient can do a specific job. This sort of grossly contradictory testimony does not tend to occur on questions of appropriate diagnostic criteria or treatment options, because there is a generally accepted scientific answer to each of those questions.

Tolerance, however, is not a scientifically verifiable concept. When two physicians offer strongly held but contradictory testimony on work ability in which both claim to be scientific ("reasonable medical probability"), not recognizing that they are arguing about the nonscientific concept of tolerance, they confuse the legal system and damage the medical profession.

When objective pathology is dramatic, physicians generally agree that working despite pain or fatigue the patient considers to be intolerable is not reasonable, and thus physicians generally agree that this patient has believable "problems" based on tolerance. For example, if severe osteoarthritis of the hip is present radiographically, and the patient describes severe pain when attempting work that requires prolonged heavy lifting and carrying (proving that he has the current ability to do this task), a work problem is "believable," and physicians agree on the pathology and the problem it causes. In this example, the patient would meet the criteria for total hip replacement surgery on the basis of believable pain and radiographic severe hip arthritis. This patient may also meet the Social Security Administration (SSA) "listing" of an impairment severe enough to qualify for social security disability.[4]

When there is no objective pathology, but rather only symptoms that are clearly out of proportion to the physical examination and test results, most physicians agree that working despite symptoms poses no major risk, and the patient is free to work if he or she wishes. Thus, a patient with no objective findings who alleges intolerable pain when attempting to lift a postage stamp would clearly have an issue of tolerance, and not an issue of risk or current ability. Most physicians would certify that this patient can work. In this case the tolerance is not believable, although there are conditions such as fibromyalgia in which some physicians (perhaps inappropriately) impose severe activity restrictions solely on the basis of tolerance. (See Chapter 19 for more information about working with functional syndromes.)

Models

Almost all Western societies use a "biomedical model" to determine disability. This is a "severe objective impairment equals disability" model in which objective medical fact is all that is considered. A "biopsychosocial model" is much better at explaining and dealing with disability in problematic cases.[5] Thus, third parties (employers, disability insurers, etc) inquire of physicians about "work restrictions" (based on risk) and "work limitations" (based on capacity) expecting scientific answers based on the biomedical model of severe impairment-based disability. When some physicians answer these requests on the basis of the patient's tolerance of symptoms by using the biopsychosocial model, and inappropriately state answers as "work restrictions" that are not confirmed by second-opinion examinations, all physicians involved appear to be either biased and unscientific, or influenced by financial considerations. Physicians may feel strongly about the biopsychosocial model for disability, and they may feel that employers and insurers who ask about disability in terms of the biomedical model are asking the wrong question, but "there is no right answer to the wrong question."[6] As long as Western society asks questions phrased in the biomedical model of disability, physicians will be expected to answer using the biomedical model.

There is a continuum from no objective pathology to severe objective pathology. Where in this continuum physicians should logically accept a patient's report of intolerable symptoms and advise the patient to pursue a different job or even to pursue disability status based only on tolerance can not be answered scientifically. In contested disability cases the scenario frequently is similar to the following:

Dr A: "I usually declare patients like Joe fit to work despite his symptoms. They usually remain at work in this type job and do fine, so I must be correct."

Dr B: "I usually declare patients like Joe to require work limitations. They usually can not tolerate staying at work in this type job, so I must be correct."

Both physicians are honest, well trained, and experienced, yet they have diametrically opposed answers to the question, "Can Joe do this job?" This is because there is no scientific answer to the question, and both physicians are answering on the basis of either anecdotal experience with similar patients or personal bias. When these two physicians fill out forms, write reports, and testify under oath with these contradictory answers to what seems to be a simple question, they again give the appearance to patients, employers, insurers, judges, and juries of being either unscientific, or biased, or "paid for."

Faced with this predicament, physicians have three choices:

1. "Play secretary" and write down on return-to-work forms what work activities the patient is willing to do
2. Try to assess tolerance
3. Abstain, and leave the tolerance decision to the patient.

If society wants the physician to merely ask the patient what activity he or she can tolerate, there is in reality no need for a physician to be involved in filling out work ability forms. In this scenario the physician functions as a secretary taking dictation, and the patient could logically fill out the form without the aid, or expense, of a physician.

Testing

Functional capacity evaluation (FCE) is an attempt to assess tolerance, although, as is discussed in Chapter 7, it is far from a perfect tool. It lacks proven reliability and validity.[7-9] In the only published study in which an FCE was performed on patients with back pain and the FCE result was then ignored, when patients were sent back to full duty even though the FCE frequently said that the patients were not capable of full duty, ignoring the FCE findings improved the treatment results.[10]

Because pain cannot be measured, how does a physician assess a patient's tolerance for work? Can any two physicians come to the same conclusion?

If physicians will never be able to agree on what activity a given patient with less than dramatic objective pathology should be able to tolerate in terms of symptoms like pain and fatigue, it is best that physicians not pretend there is a medical answer to this question. Recalling the discussion in Chapter 1, that remaining at work has clear benefit for the individual and thus is in his or her long-term best interest, the best answer a physician can give to such a patient may be the following:

> You do not appear to meet the Social Security Administration's criteria for total disability. Thus, in our society, there is some job you're expected to be able to do. Because there is no medical evidence that you are at high risk of significant harm by working, I can not certify that you're disabled for this job. There is no basis for work restrictions based on risk. I realize that you have pain (or fatigue, etc), but you have the ability to do many things despite your pain. Whether the rewards of working are sufficient for you to choose to remain at work, or whether the pain you feel is sufficient for you to choose a different type of work, or not to work at all, is a question only you can answer. I can record on this form what you feel to be your current activity tolerances, but not as "work restrictions" or as "work limitations." These tolerances are not scientific, and they may change in the future.

If this type of statement is included in a medical report or work ability form, it should be on the line for "comments" and the "work guides" should be clearly labeled as based only on patient-described tolerance. The physician should include a disclaimer that medicine is both a science and an art, and that the future is not foreseeable. (See Chapter 8 for more information about disclaimers and legal considerations in return-to-work decisions.)

Unfortunately, physicians have not done a good job of educating patients, employers, insurers, and judges that there is some science on risk assessment, but that tolerance for symptoms is the usual problem in contested disability cases, and tolerance is *not* scientifically measurable.

How to Evaluate Work Ability: A Seven-Step Process

By using an organized approach, a physician can determine appropriate work guides for an individual. Understanding the principles discussed in this chapter permits such an approach:

1. What is the job in question? Do I have an adequate job description? Do I have information from both the individual and the employer as to what this patient is expected to do at work? If "no," request such information before answering.
2. What is this patient's medical problem? What are the objective signs of pathology? What are the symptoms? Is this permanent or temporary?

Is this problem improvable with time, or medical treatment, or exercise (which includes work)? If the condition is temporary or improvable, record this fact.

3. Does this patient have severe pathophysiology that appears to meet the Social Security Administration's criteria for total disability? If "yes," tell this fact to the patient and support his or her disability application if he or she chooses to apply for disability. If not, consider risk.

4. Is there significant risk of substantial harm with work activity (not merely an increase in subjective symptoms)? If "yes" on the basis of sound science or a major consensus document, certify that work *restrictions* are appropriate on the basis of risk. If "no," consider current ability.

5. Is this patient actually able to physically do the task in question (not considering symptoms, but ability)? If "no," state the reason as a *limitation* ("lacks shoulder range of motion to reach overhead machine controls"). If "yes," consider tolerance.

6. If the patient has the ability to do the work task, at acceptable risk, and wants to do the job, certify that he or she is medically able.

7. If the patient has the ability to do the work task, at acceptable risk, and does not like doing the job based on tolerance for symptoms like pain and fatigue, is there severe objective pathology present that makes physician agreement on work problems based on tolerance likely? If "yes," certify that work "problems" are present "on the basis of believable symptoms and severe objective pathology," but certify that the patient may work despite the symptoms if he or she wishes. (Note that there will usually not be a line or box on the work ability form for "work problems" but there frequently is a line for "comments.") If "no," and the objective pathology is only mild or moderate, certify that the patient may work at the job in question, but that he or she describes symptoms at a certain level of work activity. This scenario represents a "medically unanswerable question," and should be labeled as such by physicians. The decision whether or not to work despite symptoms is *ultimately the patient's*, and not the physician's.

Summary

Most physicians have not been trained in work ability assessment. Multiple physicians often give contradictory answers to questions of work ability if tolerance of symptoms is what limits work performance. There is little good science on work risk assessment. There are some consensus documents that give useful information. Significant risk should justify work restrictions.

Few individuals function at capacity. Current ability can be measured, but is capable of increasing with activity or decreasing with inactivity. If individuals lack the current ability to do a work task, this is a work limitation.

Tolerance of symptoms such as pain and fatigue is what in most cases gives patients work problems. Multiple physicians will not agree on work limitations based on tolerance unless there is severe objective pathology. This level of impairment usually means the individual meets the Social Security Administration's "listing" of conditions severe enough to qualify for total disability, and or major reconstructive surgery.

If there is no medical answer to when a condition with mild or moderate pathology is significant enough that the individual should choose to pursue a different career, or to stop work entirely, physicians should not pretend there is a medical answer, and thus physicians should decline to certify such individuals as disabled. This is ultimately the patient's decision. Employers and insurers ask about work restrictions and work limitations, phrasing the questions in the biomedical model in which severe impairment equals disability. Physicians should not try to answer based on tolerance using the biopsychosocial model (despite its superiority). "There is no right answer to the wrong question." A suggested wording for discussing with patients why they are not eligible for disability certification is offered, and a seven-step process to think through specific work ability questions is recommended.

References

1. Maron BJ, Mitchell JH. Twenty-sixth Bethesda conference recommendations for determining eligibility for competition in athletes with cardiovascular abnormalities. *J Am Coll Cardiol.* 1994;24:845–899.

2. Carragee EJ, Han MY, Yang B, et al. Activity restrictions after posterior discectomy: a prospective study of outcomes in 152 cases with no postoperative restrictions. *Spine.* 1999;24:2346–2351.

3. Carragee EJ, Helms E, O'Sullivan GS. Are postoperative activity restrictions necessary after posterior lumbar discectomy? A prospective study of outcomes in 50 consecutive cases. *Spine.* 1996;21:1893–1897.

4. *Disability Evaluation Under Social Security.* Baltimore, MD: Social Security Administration; January 2003. SSA publication 64-039.

5. Waddell G. The biopsychosocial model. In: Waddell G, ed. *The Back Pain Revolution.* 2nd ed. London, England: Churchill Livingstone; 2004.

6. Carolyn Acuff, personal communication with the author (JBT).

7. King PM, Tuckwell N, Barrett TE. A critical review of functional capacity evaluations. *Phys Ther.* 1998;78:852–866.

8. Gross DP, Battie MC, Cassidy JD. The prognostic value of functional capacity evaluation in patients with chronic low back pain, part 1: timely return to work. *Spine*. 2004;29:914–919.

9. Gross DP, Battie MC. The prognostic value of functional capacity evaluation in patients with chronic low back pain, part 2: sustained recovery. *Spine*. 2004;29:920–924.

10. Hall H, McIntosh G, Melles T, Holowachuk B, Wai E. Effect of discharge recommendations on outcome. *Spine*. 1994;19:2033–2037.

Chapter 2

How to Negotiate Return to Work

J. Mark Melhorn, MD

"I can't go back to work. I still hurt!" This statement reflects the three elements of the return-to-work decision—risk, capacity, and tolerance—from the individual worker's point of view. As discussed in Chapter 2, *risk* is the possibility of reinjury or worsening of the medical condition, *capacity* is the physical ability based on the injury and the current medical condition, and *tolerance* is the decision by the patient to endure symptoms such as pain or fatigue in exchange for the benefits of returning to work.

The ability to return to work is dependent on the injury, the individual, the physician, the employer, and the support services. Each may have a different agenda with different goals. This chapter focuses on the predictive factors and impact of returning to work or being off work and how the physician should approach the patient about the return-to-work decision.

The Return-to-Work Decision Makers

There are four groups involved in making return-to-work decisions: the patient, the employer, the physician, and supplementary players, who can include administrators, attorneys, benefit adjudicators, case managers, consultants, insurers, judicial or physician reviewers, rehabilitation managers, unions, and the state-specific workers' compensation system.[1] Misunderstanding is common, communication is often poor, and unnecessary time off work often occurs.[2–5]

After an injury, a negative point of view is common for the employee and employer. They focus on incapacity rather than on retained ability. The common analogy is: Is the glass half empty or half full? By focusing on ability rather than incapacity, employers will be more likely to get injured or disabled employees back to work sooner. For the employee, this means a restoration of at least partial earnings and benefits. It also means that the employee is back in the running for any advancement or lateral job opportunities that may arise. A return to work, even in a light-duty position or with accommodation, also means the transition from incapacitated patient to productive employee, thus enhancing recovery and reducing disability.[4] Also, under current workers' compensation systems, unless an employee's medical condition precludes travel to and from work, being at work, or being able to perform assigned appropriate tasks and duties, the employer is not legally required to approve the employee's absence and the linked workers' compensation benefits. Conversely, prolonged absence from one's normal roles, including absence from the workplace, may be seen as detrimental to a person's mental, physical, and social well-being.[4] In addition, one study has shown that being unemployed results in an increased mortality for men and their families.[6] (See Chapter 1 for more information about the health consequences of being unemployed.)

For employers, the early and appropriate return to work of injured or disabled employees means a reduction in workers' compensation benefits and disability payments, and a halt to rising workers' compensation and health insurance premiums that are based on usage or experience. Thus, by directing employees to return to work when it is appropriate to do so, employers may see an overall decrease in the cost of benefits. Conversely, in some cases, especially when there were employee-relations problems before the injury, the employer may take the position that the employee may not return to work until classified as "100%." This is invariably a costly mistake. Foremost, it delays the employee's return to work, increases workers' compensation costs, and forces additional wage replacement costs. Beyond this, the effect of such an approach is to emphasize the employee's lost abilities and to define employees by their impairments. Eventually, this kind of approach causes employees to feel much less capable than they really are. This approach may also violate the Americans with Disabilities Act of 1990 for covered disabilities, under which employers are required to make reasonable accommodations that enable employees to perform the essential functions of their jobs.[7] (See Chapter 8 for more information about legal considerations in return-to-work decisions.) Therefore, the goal is to get the employee back to appropriate work in the shortest period of time.

Of the groups involved in making return-to-work decisions, physicians have the first opportunity to encourage a patient's return to function and work after an illness or injury.[4] Assuming the employer is willing and able to accommodate and the supplementary players are supportive, the task becomes an interaction (negotiation) between the patient-employee and the physician–care provider. Unfortunately, the return-to-work system often fails, because many factors influence the employee's decision-making process to stay at work or return early to work (tolerance).

Defining Negotiation and Agreement

Negotiation is defined as coming to terms; a dialogue, talk, or discussion intended to produce an agreement.[8] *Agreement* is defined as a compatibility of observations.[8] Synonyms include accord, arrangement, concord, correspondence, and understanding.[8] Because the patient and the physician have the same goal—maximum restoration of function with the least pain—reaching an understanding on work guides should be easy. Unfortunately, this interaction often results in the patient feeling that the physician is pushing him or her back to work. This perspective is the result of lack of knowledge and therefore a lack of understanding of the benefits of work. As a patient advocate, the physician will need to take more time to transfer knowledge, which will enable the physician to negotiate a successful return to work based on the science of capacity and an appreciation for the patient's tolerance (psychosocial issues).

Whether physicians realize it or not, they are in the middle of a negotiation every time they are asked to do something for their patient. So why are we not more successful in providing appropriate return-to-work guides?

The Five Steps From Injury to Resolution

Return to work is only one part of injury and restoration of function. The injured worker must move through five steps from injury to resolution in order to allow closure of the workers' compensation claim and to allow the individual to reach maximum medical improvement. These steps are:

1. Injury and relationship to the workplace
2. Diagnosis and treatment
3. Time off work and return to work
4. Impairment and disability
5. Settlement and resolution.

Injury and Relationship to the Workplace

The injury or illness is the event that triggers the workers' compensation claim. *Occupational injuries* result from a work-related event or from a single instantaneous exposure in the work environment as defined by the Occupational Safety and Health Administration (OSHA), while *occupational illness* is any abnormal condition or disorder (other than one resulting from an occupational injury) caused by exposure to a factor(s) associated with employment.[9]

Injuries are easy to understand. The individual usually has a cut, break, or strain. The relationship to the workplace is easy to understand, with a specific event, a specific injury, and a specific diagnosis.

Illnesses, as discussed in this chapter, are limited to musculoskeletal disorders, such as tendinitis, nerve entrapments, and musculoskeletal pain or disorders, which are sometimes called *cumulative trauma disorders*. With the longer onset of symptoms and lack of a specific event, it is sometimes difficult to demonstrate the work-relatedness, although physicians are often asked to do so. This requires an understanding of the symptoms (what hurts), the signs (the clinical examination), supporting tests (such as nerve conduction studies or x-rays), the diagnosis, and the natural disease process based on the diagnosis. This opinion is often given to a reasonable degree of medical probability (likely to occur 51% of the time), which is a legal, not a medical, definition of probability.

Diagnosis and Treatment

The diagnosis is based on collecting the information from symptoms, signs, and tests that are analyzed for a conclusion. The diagnosis may be easy or difficult, depending on the information available and the physician's experience and skills. Treatment is traditionally based on the diagnosis. For example, a simple fractured wrist is treated with a cast because medical outcome studies have demonstrated a reasonable outcome with casting. Treatment protocol or guides have been developed for many diagnoses. When a specific diagnosis is not available, the treatment becomes less specific and less effective.

Time Off Work and Return to Work

"I can't go back to work. I still hurt!"

As discussed at the beginning of this chapter, this statement reflects the three elements of return to work from the individual worker's point of view: risk, capacity, and tolerance. From an epidemiologic standpoint, this statement translates into 16 million upper-extremity injuries occurring yearly, resulting in more than 16 million days lost from work.[10]

Injuries, defined as events that occur from specific trauma events, are decreasing; *illnesses*, defined as events that do not occur from specific trauma events, are increasing.[11] Both are reportable by the employer on the Occupational Safety and Health Administration (OSHA) form 300 if they result in lost work time; if they require medical treatment (other than first aid); or if the worker experiences loss of consciousness, has restriction of work activities or motion, or is transferred to another job.[9]

As mentioned earlier in this chapter, musculoskeletal pain (also labeled *cumulative trauma disorders*, *musculoskeletal disorders*, or *nontraumatic soft-tissue musculoskeletal disorders*[12]) is defined as any pain that may involve the muscles, nerves, tendons, ligaments, bones, or joints and is the fastest growing category within the illness group.[13] Musculoskeletal pain is often separated into two categories: work related and non–work related. For the pain to be compensable under workers' compensation, the pain must be considered work related and meet specific legislated criteria as established by each state government.[14]

Workplace injuries and illnesses that result in lost time from work can have considerable financial repercussions for employer and employee alike, not to mention their physical and emotional impact on the employee. In 1997, direct health costs for both injuries and illnesses for the nation's work force were more than $418 billion, with estimated indirect costs of $837 billion.[15] Private industry reported 6.1 million injuries and illnesses, with a case rate of 7.1 cases per 100 equivalent full-time workers.[16] Reducing the total costs of more than $1.25 trillion has clearly become a priority for the American public and the American business community.

Many consider modified work as the cornerstone in job rehabilitation. A systematic review of the 2,345 articles in the scientific literature on return-to-work issues published since 1985 supported the following findings: modified work programs facilitate early return to work for the temporarily and permanently disabled worker; the likelihood of continued employment is increased by twofold for early return to work; individual physical impairments and costs for the employer are often decreased; and the quality of life for the employee is improved with early return to work.[17]

Impairment and Disability

Impairment is defined by the American Medical Association's (AMA's) *Guides to the Evaluation of Permanent Impairment (Guides)* as the loss, loss of use, or derangement of any body part, system, or function.[18] The physician's tasks are to identify impairments that could affect performance, to determine whether the impairments are permanent, and to identify impairments that could lead to sudden or gradual incapacitation, further impairment, injury, transmission of a communicable disease, or other adverse occurrence.

Disability is defined by the AMA *Guides* as a decrease in, or the loss or absence of, the capacity of an individual to meet personal, social, or occupational demands, or to meet statutory or regulatory requirements because of an impairment.[18] The Americans with Disabilities Act of 1990 uses the term *disability* to represent a concept that is similar to the concept of impairment used in the AMA *Guides*. It is important to note that under the Americans with Disabilities Act, identification of an individual with a "disability" does not depend on the results of a medical evaluation. An individual may be identified as having a disability if there is a record of an impairment that has substantially limited one or more major life activities or, of greater concern, if the individual is regarded as having a disability. *Disability* is also sometimes used to describe the time away from work due to a loss of full physical capacity, whether minor or major, temporary or permanent, as a result of a work-related injury or illness.

Settlement and Resolution

After injury, diagnosis, treatment, and return to work or time off work, the physician is often asked to provide an impairment rating, which is converted to a disability by the legal system to offer a settlement and provide for resolution of the process. The workers' compensation system represents a compromise for both employers and employees and is designed to be a no-fault and exclusive remedy. The workers and their dependents are not required to prove fault for personal injuries, diseases, or deaths arising out of and in the course of employment. The employer agrees to provide rapid payment to the injured worker for lost wages and medical care costs in exchange for limiting or eliminating the employer's potential liability for said occupational illness, injuries, and death and, thereby, the possibility of large tort verdicts. Although described as a system, each state, each US territory, and the US federal government have state-, territory-, and federal-specific workers' compensation laws and regulations. Although not specifically part of the workers' compensation system, Title XIV of the federal Social Security Disability Program provides benefits to disabled workers younger than 65 years who are expected to be totally disabled for at least 12 months.

The four objectives of the workers' compensation system are listed here:

- Provide prompt and reasonable income and medical benefits to injured workers, or income benefits to the dependents of injured workers, regardless of fault
- Provide a single and exclusive remedy for work-related injuries
- Reduce court delays, costs, and workloads arising out of personal injury litigation and eliminate attorney and witness fees
- Encourage employers to be interested in safety and rehabilitation through appropriate experience-rating mechanisms.

The Time Off Work and Return-to-Work Issue: Lost Work Days

Within the current workers' compensation system, physicians can improve the quality of life for the injured worker through medical care, return to work, and prevention. Early return to work can result in a win-win situation. Employers, patients, lawyers, and the courts often assume that time away from work after an illness or injury is necessary. They typically remain unquestioning as long as a physician makes a medical diagnosis or verifies that there is ongoing treatment.

However, they neglect to inquire whether the patient is actually unable to do any productive work safely. Lost work days may or may not be medically necessary. Certain injuries or illnesses will require that the employee-patient be off work. Other injuries or illnesses may allow the employee-patient back to work with restrictions, accommodations, or modifications. These lost work days would be considered medically necessary days. Lost work days because of poor or slow communication between the physician and the employer, inadequate information, litigation over benefits, disputes over other matters, lack of cooperation by any party, administrative delays, or lack of desire on the part of the individual-employee are medically unnecessary.

Unnecessary lost work days mean lost dollars in workers' compensation and benefits. The national average lost time claim costs more than $19,000 in medical and indemnity payments, compared with the average medical-only claim that costs less than $400.[19] Christian[20] surveyed occupational health physicians on their clinical experience regarding medically necessary days off work after injury. The majority said that less than 10% of the employees-patients would require a few days off work. Almost half of the physicians surveyed placed the percentage at 5%. The actual national average is 24%. Using this range of 5% to 10% would suggest that 60% to 80% of the lost work days involve medically unnecessary time off from work.

More than two thirds of the physicians surveyed gave the following reasons for the medically unnecessary time off work: the treating physician is unwilling to force a reluctant patient back to work (the most common reason cited), the treating physician is not equipped to determine the right restriction and limitations on work activity, the employer has a policy against light-duty work, the employer cannot find a way to temporarily modify a job, the treating physician feels caught between the employer's and the employee's version of events, the treating physician has been given too little information about the physical demands of the job to issue a work release for the patient, and a conflict exists between the opinions of two physicians.

Chapter 3

Arnetz et al[21] found that the use of case managers and ergonomists in workplace adaptation meetings resulted in a direct benefit–to–cost savings ratio of 6.8. Abramson et al[22] found that employee satisfaction with the job was the best predictor of returning to work. Anema et al[23] discussed medical management by treating physicians as an obstacle to early return to work. Bednar et al[24] reported that state-specific law for workers' compensation benefits had a significant effect on the results of medical treatment, return-to-work status, and the cost of medical care. Burdorf et al[25] found that workers with absences due to pain from back, neck or shoulder, upper extremity, or lower extremity conditions were at higher risk of subsequent absence because of sickness in the next year.

Return-to-Work Guides

Chapters 12 to 19 expand on determining capacity, understanding tolerance, and assessing risk for return-to-work guides. This section provides a general overview to assist in understanding how to negotiate return-to-work decisions.

Who is able to return to work depends as much on the injury as it does on the individual employee and employer. When two individuals with the same injury are considered, predictive factors for return to work as outlined in Table 3-1 should be used. In general, as age increases, return to work is more difficult.[26,27] Women have a lower rate of return to work than men.[28] As biosocial or psychosocial issues increase, return to work is more difficult.[29] Predictive factors for the job include task demands, organizational structure, and the physical work environment.[30,31] Some examples of how these factors impact return to work follow.

Job satisfaction is the foremost factor correlating with an early return to work.[32,33] Persons with high levels of discretion are more than two times as likely to be working as those with less autonomy. Those with high demands and little autonomy to deal with them are far less likely to return to work after what should be a temporarily disabling injury. An unpleasant

Table 3-1 Predictive Factors for Return to Work

Individual Risk	Job Risk
Age	Job or task demands
Gender	Organizational structure
Biosocial issues	Physical work environment

and stressful work environment will greatly reduce the probability of return to work. The individual employer has the greatest opportunity to reduce losses in the workers' compensation system and to return the injured employee to work. A single supportive telephone call from the employer to the injured worker would be a strong force in motivating the patient to return to work, especially if the patient is experiencing depression or has a need for emotional support. Unfortunately, some employers respond angrily to the injured worker and refuse to file an initial report of injury. Thus, not even the insurer has the opportunity to deal with the injured worker.

Occasionally, the employer is simply happy to be rid of the injured worker and does as little as possible to promote his or her return to work. Considering the prevalence of psychiatric comorbidity, it is possible to understand that attitude. Depressed, anxious, or substance-abusing people do not make the most desirable and productive employees.

In addition, unions with rigid seniority policies may assign the easier jobs to workers with more seniority instead of to those with limited abilities. This practice also hampers return-to-work efforts. Unions with strict rules prohibiting a worker from crossing trades can also hinder return to work. The physician must be actively involved in addressing these issues to facilitate the transitional work, which requires a partnership between the patient, the family, the health care provider, the employer, and the insurer. The overriding objective is a safe, speedy return to work with the interests of the patient being the primary responsibility.

Early identification and early intervention are the most helpful factors in returning the injured worker to the workplace. A treating physician can look for and respond to the "five D's" as described by Brena et al[34]: dramatization (vague, diffused nonanatomic pain complaints), drugs (misuse of habit-forming pain medications), dysfunction (unwillingness to function in various personal, social, and occupational roles), dependency (passivity, depression, and helplessness), and disability (unwillingness to return to work). The physician must realize that these psychosocial issues can impact recovery and the individual's willingness to return to work. This recognition can improve communication between the patient and the physician, which can reduce the impact of the workers' compensation system on the individual while improving the individual's ability to cope.[35]

Appropriate work guides require an understanding of the injury, the patient, and the job. Fortunately, physicians can make a fair estimate of the time required for healing based on empiric knowledge of specific injuries. The patient must be an active participant in the return-to-work guides. Patients possess unique knowledge of their jobs and their ability to perform their jobs. The physician must blend the patient's information with the employer's information. The National Institute for Occupational Safety and Health has been encouraging employers to develop job descriptions that outline the essential functions of a job. Essential functions are those parts of the job that must be performed and cannot be easily modified.[36–39] The US Department of Labor has provided guidelines for work by weight lifted or handled. By combining these elements, safe and reasonable work guides can be provided that will allow the injured employee to return to the appropriate work while using the workplace as an integral part of the therapy program, thus providing for cost-effective rehabilitation. Physicians who treat work-related injuries realize that there is no easy table for developing work guides. The process is slow, time consuming, and often frustrating for both the patient and the physician. The benefits to the employee-patient are significant and worthy of the effort.[40]

Why Physicians May Feel Uncomfortable Recommending Early Return to Work

Often physicians feel uncomfortable recommending early return to work because of the medical issues surrounding the decision. For example:

- Recommending a patient return to work early is outside the realm of the traditional medical model that focuses on anatomy, physiology, and pathology.
- Each individual and their work situation is unique. This makes translation of academic generalities difficult to apply to each individual.
- Standards for defining work capacities for injured workers are limited.
- Often the physician's position on return to work reflects his or her attitudes as much as scientific knowledge.[41]

Patient and physician relationship issues may also prevent physicians from recommending early return to work. For example:

- There may be a significant difference between physicians' opinions and those of the patient, the family, the case manager, the employer, the insurer, or even other health care providers.
- The normal partnership between the physician and patient may be disrupted by this difference.
- If differences in opinions exist, then negotiations must take place. These take time and are emotionally uncomfortable. This time is unusually not "codable" or "reimbursable."

Negotiation Strategies for Return to Work

Negotiations require strategies; strategies require understanding; understanding requires knowledge; knowledge requires communication; and communication results in understanding. Because many injured workers have little knowledge of the workers' compensation system, it is important for the physician to communicate that he or she is first a patient advocate, and that appropriate early return to work is in the patient's best interests. A general discussion of the four objectives of workers' compensation as listed earlier (providing prompt and reasonable income and benefits, providing a single remedy for work-related injuries, reducing court delays and costs, and encouraging employer interest in safety and rehabilitation) is helpful. The physician should acknowledge that, on occasion, the workers' compensation system does not run smoothly and delays may occur. Patients should be encouraged to communicate these occurrences and their other concerns. The physician will work with them to assist in the process, but patients must also take responsibility for their part and actively participate. Together, many of the obstacles to successful return to work can be overcome. This builds a relationship for successful negotiations to occur.

Like other capabilities learned by physicians, negotiation is both a skill and an art form. The key to negotiation is to be firm on the science (capacity and risk) and soft on the patient (tolerance) while making recommendations that the physician believes are in the patient's best interest for improving recovery and restoring function with the least amount of pain.[42]

A commonsense approach is outlined by the word *SUCCESS*:

> *S*et the stage
> *U*ncover the issues
> *C*onfine the issues
> *C*onfirm intent and authority
> *E*valuate the issues
> *S*olve the problem
> *S*atisfaction check

As with other skills, the more the physician practices, the better his or her ability to negotiate.[43] Studies suggest that the best way to begin learning negotiation skills is by examples.[44,45] The following are several examples of negotiation strategies between the physician and the injured worker.[14]

1. Judging Negotiation	
Must produce a wise agreement	
Should be efficient	
Should not damage relationships between physician and patient	
Physician	**Injured Worker**
It's time for you to go back to work.	I don't think that I am ready yet.
How much more time do you think you need?	I don't know. I don't seem any better.

2. Positional Bargaining	
Each side takes a position, argues over it, and makes concessions to reach a compromise	
Results are based on willpower	
Physician	**Injured Worker**
How about by the end of this month?	It seems you're only worried about my work and not my pain. I don't see how I can get better by then.

This combination can produce an agreement, though not always a wise one. This approach can be inefficient and stressful on the physician-patient relationship, especially if the physician holds his or her ground.[44]

3. Alternative Approach
Focus on basic interests, mutually satisfying options, and fair standards
Separate the *people* from the *problem*
Go hard on the problem, soft on the people
Separate the relationship from the substance
Recognize that human emotions are involved and try not to react to them
Focus on *interest*, not *positions*
Translate the patient's position into his or her interest (concern about injury, restoring normal lifestyle, financial security, etc)
In most situations, patient's and physician's interests are similar
Talk about interests
Develop *options* for mutual gain
Be open to options that solve the problem

3. Alternative Approach (*Continued*)

Insist on using *objective (medical)* criteria

Commit to making recommendations based on medical principles

Develop objective criteria

Respond to principles, not pressure

Statement/Question	Approach
Physician: By law I am required to define work capacities that are reasonable for a person with your injury.	Focus on problem, not people
Injured Worker: I don't feel that I am ready to go back to work yet.	
Physician: I understand your concern. I too am interested in your full recovery and we will continue to work toward that goal. I also know that you must be interested in returning to your job as quickly as you are able. From a medical viewpoint, you do not fulfill the necessary criteria for being totally disabled. Don't you agree that you are able to safely perform many useful activities at this point?	Identify mutual interests Begin to move to medical criteria Look for consensus on principles
Injured Worker: Such as what?	Remain open to explore options
Physician: Let's first look at hours of work per day. You are still in therapy three times per week and your workplace must accommodate that.	Address mutual medical interests
Injured Worker: I don't feel that I could work a full day!	State position
Physician: At this time there is no medical justification for rest, and these work recommendations must be based on medical criteria. What is the reason that you feel that you cannot work a full day?	Move to medical criteria Address concern

Chapter 3

Useful Responses to Three Common Attacks

Examples of three common responses by the injured worker will help physicians develop better negotiation skills.

Help Me Against My Big, Bad Employer	Approach
Injured Worker: You don't know my boss, he won't follow these restrictions.	
Physician: I am sorry to hear that your boss may be unreasonable. You might want to bring this concern to your personnel manager or his boss. As your doctor, my recommendations must be based solely on the medical issues related to your injury.	Separate the people from the problem Move to medical criteria

The Threat	Approach
Injured Worker: If I hurt myself, I'll hold you responsible.	
Physician: My responsibility is to continue to help you recover from your current injury, and to help you return to your normal lifestyle including work. It is a fact of life that all of us face a risk of future illness and injury. No one can alter that. The work recommendations that we have agreed upon today are based on your current situation. If something dramatically changes, please call me, as I am here to help you. Regardless, let's see each other again in a month to see how you're doing.	Recast an attack on you as an attack on the problem Move to medical criteria Reinforce your commitment to the physician-patient relationship

You Are a Bad Doctor	Approach
Injured Worker: You said I would be fine after the surgery, but I don't feel any better. And now I'm supposed to go back to work!	
Physician: It is unfortunate that surgery did not eliminate all of your symptoms. This possibility was explained to you before the surgery. I am committed to continue to work with you to improve your symptoms. However, at this time we are legally required to define work capacities that are reasonable for you. Let's review the criteria we use to do this.	Reinforce your commitment to the physician-patient relationship Move to medical criteria

Summary

For early return to work to be successful and to reduce unnecessary work disability, a partnership between the patient, the family, the health care provider, the employer, and the insurer is required.[4] Communication and education are key issues. The work guides must be safe and allow for speedy return to work, with the interests of the patient being the primary responsibility. Early return to work has been demonstrated to be in the patient's best interest.[40,46–62] Examples of these benefits include better self-image,[63] improved ability to cope,[64] improved work survivability,[40] and improved ability to be self-sufficient.[53] These benefits result in a win-win situation for employee and employer.[52,56,65,66]

Conversely, prolonged time away from work makes recovery and return to work progressively less likely.[67] Prevention of disability is challenging. Physicians cannot prove or disprove the existence of pain clinically. A person complaining of pain may or may not have nociception, suffering, pain behavior, impairment, or disability. When diagnostic evaluation has ruled out treatable nociception, and when impairment has been addressed, targets for intervention include the suffering component (emotional distress), pain behaviors, and disability issues.

The scientific benefits of early return to work will eventually change physicians' opinions and their application of early return-to-work approaches. However, the real question is whether we as physicians can convert the mind-set and motivational level of an injured worker who has comorbidity and overt barriers to behavioral change. Although the focus of this chapter has been on how the physician should approach the patient, change is only possible if motivation abounds. Overcoming this comorbidity is critical in promoting a degree of motivation to change that will allow the injured worker to create long-term behavioral changes and coping strategies to successful return to society.

Traumatic injuries occur at a rate of 7.1 per 100 equivalent full-time employees in the private business sector at an estimated cost of more than $1.25 trillion; therefore, the need for better management of work-related injuries has clearly become a priority for the American public and the American business community. Work-related injuries require complex decision making and require the physician to draw on an understanding of basic medical and surgical principles, prior experiences, and familiarity with the literature to formulate a reasonable diagnosis, an appropriate treatment plan, and consideration for reasonable return-to-work guides. In today's environment, where outcomes are important and economics matter greatly, the physician is in a unique position to provide better management of work-related injuries. Improved outcomes are possible when the physician treats the whole patient. This whole-patient approach requires an understanding of the factors that contribute to the poorer outcomes, medical treatment plans that include options to address the psychosocial issues, and early return-to-work guides. These inclusive medical treatment plans aid in the patient's recovery and rehabilitation while avoiding many of the pitfalls of the workers' compensation system. This approach requires a team effort on the part of the patient, physician, employer, insurer, and government, but the benefits are significant and well worth the additional effort.

References

1. Zeppieri JP. The physician, the illness, and the workers' compensation system. In: Beaty JH, ed. *Orthopaedic Knowledge Update 6*. Rosemont, Ill: American Academy of Orthopaedic Surgeons; 1999:131–137.

2. Melhorn JM. *Reducing Unnecessary Workplace Disability: Treating More Than the Injury*. Sacramento, Calif: California Industrial Medicine Council; 2003.

3. Melhorn JM. Occupational orthopaedics. *J Bone Joint Surg Am*. 2000;82A: 902–904.

4. Melhorn JM. Workers' compensation: avoiding the work-related disability. *J Bone Joint Surg Am*. 2000;82A:1490–1493.

5. Melhorn JM. Treating more than the injury—reducing disability with early return to work. In: Mandell PJ, ed. *Occupational Health at the Dawn of the New Millennium*. Sacramento, Calif: California Orthopaedic Association; 2000:1–15.

6. Wilson SH, Walker GM. Unemployment and health: a review. *Public Health*. 1993;107:153–162.

7. Americans with Disabilities Act, 42 USC 12101 (1991).

8. Mish FC, Gilman EW. *Webster's Ninth New Collegiate Dictionary*. Springfield, Mass: Merriam-Webster Inc; 1991.

9. Bureau of Labor Statistics. *Occupational Injuries and Illnesses: Counts, Rates, and Characteristics, 1994*. Washington, DC: US Department of Labor; 1997.

10. Kelsey JL, Pastides H, Kreiger N. *Upper Extremity Disorders: A Survey of Their Frequency and Cost in the United States*. St Louis, Mo: CV Mosby Co; 1980.

11. Bureau of Labor Statistics. *Workplace Injuries and Illnesses in 2002*. Washington, DC: US Department of Labor; 2003.

12. Melhorn JM. *Work-Related Injuries to the Upper Extremities*. Topeka, Kan: Kansas Department of Human Resources, Division of Workers Compensation; 2000.

13. Melhorn JM. Work injuries: the history of CTD/RSI in the workplace. In: Melhorn JM, Zeppieri JP, eds. *Workers' Compensation Case Management: A Multidisciplinary Perspective*. Rosemont, Ill: American Academy of Orthopaedic Surgeons; 1999:221–250.

14. Melhorn JM. Getting to yes: negotiating successful return to work. In: Melhorn JM, Spengler DM, eds. *Occupational Orthopaedics and Workers' Compensation: A Multidisciplinary Perspective*. Rosemont, Ill: American Academy of Orthopaedic Surgeons; 2003:517–534.

15. Brady W, Bass J, Royce M, et al. Defining total corporate health and safety costs: significance and impact. *J Occup Environ Med*. 1997;39:224–231.

16. Bureau of Labor and Statistics. *Workplace Injuries and Illnesses in 1997*. Washington, DC: US Department of Labor; 1999.

17. Melhorn JM. The benefits of returning the injured worker to work early: a review of the research. *J Workers Comp*. 2000;10:60–75.

18. American Medical Association. *Guides to the Evaluation of Permanent Impairment*. 5th ed. Chicago, Ill: American Medical Association; 2001.

19. Macher A. *Annual Statistical Bulletin*. Boca Raton, Fla: National Council on Compensation Insurance Inc; 1998.

20. Christian J. Reducing disability days: healing more than the injury. *J Workers Comp*. 2000;9:30–55.

21. Arnetz BB, Sjogren B, Rydehn B, Meisel R. Early workplace intervention for employees with musculoskeletal-related absenteeism: a prospective controlled intervention study. *J Occup Environ Med*. 2003;45:499–506.

22. Abramson JH, Gofin J, Habib J. Work satisfaction and health in the middle-aged and elderly. *J Epidemiol*. 1994;23:98–104.

23. Anema JR, Van Der Giezen AM, Buijs PC, Van Mechelen W. Ineffective disability management by doctors is an obstacle for return-to-work: a cohort study on low back pain patients sicklisted for 3-4 months. *Occup Environ Med*. 2002;59:729–733.

24. Bednar JM, Baesher-Griffith P, Osterman AL. Workers compensation effect of state law on treatment cost and work status. *Clin Orthop*. 1998;351: 74–77.

25. Burdorf A, Naaktgeboren B, Post W. Prognostic factors for musculoskeletal sickness absence and return to work among welders and metal workers. *J Occup Environ Med*. 1998;55:490–495.

26. Melhorn JM. Return to work issues: arm pain. In: Melhorn JM, Strain RE Jr, eds. *Occupational Orthopaedics and Workers' Compensation: A Multidisciplinary Perspective*. Rosemont, Ill: American Academy of Orthopaedic Surgeons; 2002.

27. Melhorn JM. Evidence to support early return to work: how to write appropriate return to work guides. In: *Annual Meeting 2003*. Sacramento, Calif: California Orthopaedic Association; 2002:75–98.

28. Melhorn JM. Upper extremities: return to work issues. In: Melhorn JM, Spengler DM, eds. *5th Annual Occupational Orthopaedics and Workers' Compensation: A Multidisciplinary Perspective*. Rosemont, Ill: American Academy of Orthopaedic Surgeons; 2003:256–285.

29. Melhorn JM. Return to work: the employer's point of view. In: *2003 Safety and Health Conference*. Topeka, Kan: Kansas Department of Human Resources; 2003.

Chapter 3

30. Melhorn JM. Return to work: workplace guides. In: Melhorn JM, Zeppieri JP, eds. *Workers' Compensation Case Management: A Multidisciplinary Perspective*. Rosemont, Ill: American Academy of Orthopaedic Surgeons; 1999:451–458.

31. Melhorn JM. Work restrictions for return to work. In: Zeppieri JP, Spengler DM, eds. *Workers' Compensation Case Management: A Multidisciplinary Perspective*. Rosemont, Ill: American Academy of Orthopaedic Surgeons; 1997:249–266.

32. Bigos SJ, Battie MC, Spengler DM, et al. A longitudinal, prospective study of industrial back injury reporting. *Clin Orthop*. 1992;279:21–34.

33. Fordyce WE, Bigos SJ, Battie MC, Fisher LD. MMPI Scale 3 as a predictor of back injury report: what does it tell us? *Clin J Pain*. 1992;8:222–226.

34. Brena SF, Chapman SL, Stegall PG, Chyatte, SB. Chronic pain states: their relationship to impairment and disability. *Arch Phys Med Rehabil*. 1979;60:387–389.

35. Melhorn JM. The advantages of early return to work. *IAIABC J*. 2003;41:128–147.

36. American College of Occupational and Environmental Medicine. *ACOEM's Eight Best Ideas for Workers' Compensation Reform*. In: *American College of Occupational and Environmental Medicine Conference*. Chicago, Ill: American College of Occupational and Environmental Medicine. 1997;4.

37. Colledge AL, Johns RE Jr, Thomas MH. Functional ability assessment: guidelines for the workplace. *J Occup Environ Med*. 1999;41:172–180.

38. Equal Employment Opportunity Commission. *Job Advertising and Pre-Employment Inquiries Under the Age Discrimination in Employment Act*. Washington, DC: Equal Employment Opportunity Commission; 1989.

39. Equal Employment Opportunity Commission. Equal Employment Opportunity Commission issues final enforcement guidance on preemployment disability-related questions and medical examinations under the Americans with Disabilities Act. *Equal Employment Opportunity Commission News*. 1995;95:1–5.

40. Melhorn JM. CTD injuries: an outcome study for work survivability. *J Workers Comp*. 1996;5:18–30.

41. Rainville J, Carlson N, Polatin P, Gatchel RJ, Indahl A. Exploration of physicians' recommendations for activities in chronic back pain. *Spine*. 2000;25:2210–2220.

42. Melhorn JM. Negotiating return to work: strategies to deal with the dreaded moment. In: Melhorn JM, Barr JS Jr, eds. *Occupational Orthopaedics and Workers' Compensation: A Multidisciplinary Perspective*. Rosemont, Ill: American Academy of Orthopaedic Surgeons; 2001.

43. Di Guida AW. Negotiating a successful return to work program. *AAOHN J*. 1995;43:101–106.

44. Fisher R, Ury W. *Getting to Yes: Negotiating Agreement Without Giving In*. New York, NY: Penguin Books; 1981.

45. Linney BJ. The successful physician negotiator. *Physician Exec*. 1999;25:62–65.

46. Cook AC, Birkholz S, King EF, Szabo RM. Early mobilization following carpal tunnel release: a prospective randomized study. *J Hand Surg.* 1995;20B:228–230.

47. Melhorn JM, Wilkinson LK. *CTD Solutions for the 90's: A Comprehensive Guide to Managing CTD in the Workplace.* Wichita, Kan: Via Christi Health Systems; 1996.

48. Melhorn JM. CTD solutions for the 90's: prevention. In: *Seventeenth Annual Workers' Compensation and Occupational Medicine Seminar.* Boston, Mass: Seak Inc; 1997:234–245.

49. Melhorn JM. Identification of individuals at risk for developing CTD. In: Spengler DM, Zeppieri JP, eds. *Workers' Compensation Case Management: A Multidisciplinary Perspective.* Rosemont, Ill: American Academy of Orthopaedic Surgeons; 1997:41–51.

50. Melhorn JM. Physician support and employer options for reducing risk of CTD. In: Spengler DM, Zeppieri JP, eds. *Workers' Compensation Case Management: A Multidisciplinary Perspective.* Rosemont, Ill: American Academy of Orthopaedic Surgeons; 1997:26–34.

51. Ballard M, Baxter P, Bruening L, Fried S. Work therapy and return to work. *Hand Clin.* 1986;2:247–258.

52. Bruce WC, Bruce RS. Return-to-work programs in the unionized company. *J Workers Comp.* 1996;38:9–17.

53. Burke SA, Harms-Constas CK, Aden PS. Return to work/work retention outcomes of a functional restoration program: a multi-center, prospective study with a comparison group. *Spine.* 1994;19:1880–1885.

54. Centineo J. Return-to-work programs: cut costs and employee turnover. *Risk Manage.* 1986;33:44–48.

55. Day CS, McCabe SJ, Alexander G. Return to work as an outcome measure in hand surgery. Paper presented at: Annual Meeting of the American Society for Surgery of the Hand; September 15, 1993; Baltimore, Md.

56. Devlin M, O'Neill P, MacBride R. Position paper in support of timely return to work programs and the role of the primary care physician. *Ont Med Assoc.* 1994;61:1–45.

57. Gice JH, Tompkins K. Cutting costs with return-to-work programs. *Risk Manage.* 1988;35:62–65.

58. Goodman RC. An aggressive return-to-work program in surgical treatment of carpal tunnel syndrome: a comparison of costs. *Plast Reconstr Surg.* 1989;89:715–717.

59. Groves FB, Gallagher LA. What the hand surgeon should know about workers' compensation. *Hand Clin.* 193;9:369–372.

60. Grunet BK, Devine CA, Smith CJ, et al. Graded work exposure to promote work return after severe hand trauma: a replicated study. *Ann Plast Surg.* 1992;29:532–536.

61. Kasdan ML, June LA. Returning to work after a unilateral hand fracture. *J Occup Environ Med.* 1993;35:132–135.

62. Nathan PA, Meadows KD, Keniston RC. Rehabilitation of carpal tunnel surgery patients using a short surgical incision and an early program of physical therapy. *J Hand Surg.* 1993;18A:1044–1050.

63. Bernacki EJ, Tsai SP. Managed care for workers' compensation: three years of experience in an "employee choice" state. *J Occup Environ Med.* 1996;38:1091–1097.

64. Bigos SJ, Spengler DM, Martin NA, et al. Back injuries in industry: a retrospective study. III. Employee related factors. *Spine.* 1986;11:252–256.

65. Dworkin RH, Handlin DS, Richlin DM, Rrand L, Vannucci C. Unraveling the effects of compensation, litigation, and employment on treatment response in chronic pain. *Pain.* 1985;23:49–59.

66. Hall H, McIntosh G, Melles T, Holowachuk B, Wai E. Effect of discharge recommendations on outcome. *Spine.* 1994;19:2033–2037.

67. Strang JP. The chronic disability syndrome. In: Aronoff GM, ed. *Evaluation and Treatment of Chronic Pain.* Baltimore, Md: Urban & Schwarzenberg; 1985:247–258.

Chapter 4

Return to Work: Forms, Records, and Disclaimers

J. Mark Melhorn, MD

Return to work is only one part of the life history of an accident. The injured worker must move through five steps: injury and the determination of a relationship to the workplace; diagnosis and treatment; time off work, if any, and return to work; determination of impairment and disability; and resolution of disputes and settlement of the claim. (See Chapter 3 for more information about each of these steps.) Within the current workers' compensation system, the physician can improve the quality of life for the injured worker through medical care, facilitation of return to work, and assistance with accident prevention.[1] As an advocate for patients and in the best interest of society, physicians should encourage appropriate early return to work and rehabilitation, not disability. Early intervention by the physician and a rehabilitation counselor after injury can facilitate a positive attitude and empower the worker to resist the negative effect of the system reinforcers that discourage early return to work.[2]

Many consider modified work to be the cornerstone of disability management.[3–5] Returning the injured employee to work is often challenging. Many obstacles develop that involve the employee, physician, and employer. Assuming the employee is willing to return to work and the employer is willing to provide modified work, the critical element becomes the physician's ability to communicate the appropriate physical capacity guides. Work guides are commonly referred to as "work restrictions."[6,7] As reviewed in Chapter 2, work restrictions should mean what the patient *can do* but *should not* do on the basis of risk. Physicians impose work restrictions for patient safety. Work limitations are what the patient lacks the current ability or capacity to do (cannot do). Physicians describe what patients are not capable of doing on the basis of capacity. The concepts of restrictions and capacity tend to focus on the loss, rather than on the retained ability of the employee.

Tolerance is whether patients are *willing to tolerate* symptoms such as pain or fatigue. Temporary work guides (or suggestions for modified duty) during the initial phases of recovery from injury or illness are frequently appropriate on the basis of symptom tolerance, but these should not become permanent. If incomplete recovery occurs, ultimately the employee-patient must decide whether the rewards of work outweigh the symptoms. The term *work guides* allows a physician to suggest appropriate levels of activity without having to specify whether the "guides" are restrictions, limitations, or statements about a believable tolerance for activity. As time for healing passes and the patient reaches maximum medical improvement, a physician should clarify for all concerned whether at this point in time the "guides" are work restrictions (based on risk), work limitations (based on capacity), or suggestions, but the issue of tolerance is the basis, and, ultimately the decision to work at jobs that exceed the "guides" is the patient's. Unfortunately, the term *work restrictions* wrongly applied to restriction, capacity, and tolerance is so ingrained into the workers' compensation system that it is unlikely to be changed, but it is important for all parties to understand and focus on the concept of retained ability.

Although a physician must consider all three parts of the return-to-work formula (risk, capacity, and tolerance) from the individual worker's point of view, perhaps the greatest amount of guesswork expected of the physician is in the determination of capacity. At the same time, this decision also has the greatest impact on the patient. Appropriate capacity or work guides require an understanding of the injury, the patient, and the job. Fortunately, physicians can make a fair estimate of the time required for healing on the basis of empiric knowledge of specific injuries. Also, patients possess unique knowledge of their job and their ability to perform their job and therefore need to actively participate in the functional capacity guides. The physician must then blend the patient's information with the employer's information while factoring in the science of the injury.

Employers often request detailed charts of "restrictions" based on ability to lift, push, pull, climb, bend, stoop, crawl, kneel, and other similar activities. When presented in a form, it is often difficult for the physician to differentiate what a normal healthy person of similar age, sex, education, and body build would be capable of doing. Standards created by the US Department of Labor, *The Dictionary of Occupational Titles*, Physical Demands of Work (Table 4-1), and *The Dictionary of Occupational Titles*, Physical Demand Characteristics of Work (Table 4-2), are a helpful starting point.[8] Millender and Conlon[9] expanded on these guides by matching possible additional job activities to eight general job categories (Table 4-3).

Table 4-1 Physical Demands of Work[8]

Physical Demand Level	Lb Lifting (Frequent/ Occasional)	Lb Carry (Frequent/ Occasional)	Lb Push/ Pull	Climbing	Bend, Stoop, Twist/h	Sit/Stand (min)	Walk (h/d)
Sedentary	0/10	0/10	100	None	0	30	1
Sedentary-light	5/15	5/15	125	Ramp	<10	30	2
Light	10/20	15/20	150	Stairs	15	45	3
Light-medium	20/35	20/35	200	Stairs	20	60	3+
Medium	20/50	25/50	250	Ladder	30	90	4
Medium-heavy	35/50	40/75	300	Ladder	40	120/120	4+
Heavy	50/100	50/100	350	Scaffold	50	180/150	5
Very heavy	50/100+	75/100+	400+	Pole/Rope	60+	210/180+	7

Table 4-2 Physical Demand Characteristics of Work[8]

Physical Demand Level	Occasional (0% to 33% of Workday)	Frequent (34% to 66% of Workday)	Constant (67% to 100% of Workday)	Typical Energy Required (Metabolic Equivalents)
Sedentary	10 lb	Negligible	Negligible	1.5–2.1
Light	20 lb	10 lb	Negligible	2.2–3.5
Light-medium	35 lb	20 lb	5 lb	3.6–4.5
Medium	50 lb	20 lb	10 lb	4.6–6.3
Medium-heavy	75 lb	35 lb	15 lb	6.4–7.0
Heavy	100 lb	50 lb	20 lb	7.1–7.5
Very heavy	>100 lb	>50 lb	>20 lb	>7.5

Communication: The Issues That Should Be Documented in Physician Records

In workers' compensation cases, and in non–workers' compensation cases in which private disability insurance or social security disability are likely to be involved, copies of the physician's records are likely to end up in the legal system. There should be a database in the records to support return-to-work decision making.

Chapter 4

Table 4-3 Guidelines for Tasks by Job Categories

Job Category	Job Description	Weight Lifted, lb*	Weight Pushed or Pulled, lb*	Weight Carried, lb*	Climbing†	Body Motion‡	Sitting-Standing Transition§	Walking (% of Day)
1	Sedentary	10/0	150/0	≤10/0	Ramp/none	<10	30 min	10
2	Sedentary-light	15/≤5	200/100–125	15/≤5	None/ramp	<10	30 min	20
3	Light	20/≤10	250/125–150	20/10–15	Stairs/none	10–15	30–45 min	30
4	Light-medium	35/≤20	300/200–250	35/20	None/stairs	15–20	45 to 60 min	40
5	Medium	50/≤35	350/250–300	50/25–30	Ladder/stairs	20–30	1–1.5 h	50
6	Medium-heavy	75/≤50	400/300–350	75/30–40	Scaffold/ladder	30–40	1.5–2 h	60
7	Heavy	100/≤50	450/350–400	100/40–50	Poles/scaffold	40–60	2–2.5 h	70
8	Very heavy	>100/>50	>450/>400	>100/>60	Rope/poles	>60	>2.5 h	80

* Values are expressed as weight infrequently (0%–33% of time)/weight frequently (67%–100% of time).
† Descriptions are expressed as type of climbing infrequently/frequently.
‡ Values are number of instances of body motion (bending, kneeling, squatting, or reaching) per hour.
§ Values are time spent in continuous transition between sitting and standing positions.
Reproduced with permission from Millender and Conlon.[9]

Initial Medical Record

The physician's initial medical record should include the following traditional medical information:

- The chief complaint
- History of present illness
- Review of systems
- History of previous illnesses
- Family and social history
- Physical examination, which should include:
  — general constitutional items
  — specific findings from pertinent organ system examination
- A working diagnosis
- Plans for further testing
- A medical treatment plan
- Administrative issues, which should include:
  — a description of the onset of symptoms and their relationship to the workplace
  — a statement establishing causation, aggravation, or exacerbation and any relationship to the workplace injury or illness
  — details of the job at the time of onset of symptoms; interval jobs and work capacity guides; current job and current work capacity guides; and a list of what job activities the employee currently can do without symptoms plus a list of jobs the employee believes he or she could perform without symptoms
  — suggestions for workplace modifications, accommodations, or ergonomic issues
- Functional capacity guides, which should include:
  — current ability to work, regular or modified, full-time or part-time
  — estimated time to maximum medical improvement (MMI)
  — specific functional capacity guides as listed in the next section.

Interval Report

Each follow-up office visit note should contain the interval history, including the following:

- The response to treatment (have symptoms and findings improved?)
- Any administrative and legal actions or conflicts that are of medical importance (employer refuses to accept causation, a lawyer has been retained, medical referrals, worker not receiving benefits)
- Treatment options, treatment changes, and medical testing decisions
- Work guides (these may be restrictions, limitations, or suggestions to minimize symptoms).

Chapter 4

Final Report

When the patient has reached MMI, the physician's record should include the following:

- A summary of treatment and the response to treatment
- A declaration of MMI, in the form of a statement that the patient has reached a medical end result and that no significant change in physical findings or activity levels is expected in the foreseeable future. No significant further treatment changes or diagnostic testing should be anticipated; maintenance treatment may be ongoing, but there is no plan for a future trial of a treatment that might decrease the impairment or increase the patient's function. This means that the work status is no longer temporary, but is now permanent. A need for vocational rehabilitation may be mentioned if appropriate
- An administrative progress statement detailing the ability to work and giving final work guides, but clearly stating whether the "guides" are work restrictions (based on risk), work limitations (based on capacity), or suggestions about the level of symptoms the patient is likely to tolerate to facilitate return to work
- A determination of permanent impairment, expressed as a percentage, if required (the American Medical Association's *Guides to the Evaluation of Permanent Impairment*[10] is the most frequently used reference)

Physicians should address these issues in patient records. Having a template or outline for dictation or recording of the visit may be helpful.

Four Screening Tests for Establishing Functional Capacity Guides

Four questions have been developed by Christian[3] to help the physician understand return to work, accommodations for the workplace, and the likelihood of successful return to work. Christian used these questions to develop a physicians' training course for work fitness and disability.

Question 1: Return to Work

The patient is asked the following questions in relation to his or her job:

- Is your injury going to make it hard for you to do your usual job the regular way?

- Are you going to have any problems with your boss or coworkers about your injury?
- Have you figured out a way to work despite your injury while you recover?

If the answers are "yes," "yes," and "no," returning to work will be difficult.

Question 2: The Grocery Store

If the patient owned his or her own grocery store, would he or she be able to find a way to work safely? If the answer is "yes," then absence from work is probably not medically required. Therefore, a nonmedical aspect (or psychosocial issue) of the injury to this individual, and *not* the medical condition, is creating the disability.

Question 3: The Molehill Sign

Is the patient making a mountain out of a molehill, or is an apparently minor health condition having a major effect on the individual's daily life and functions? This assessment requires the physician to mentally compare this patient to other patients with similar injuries or illnesses by objective disease or injury criteria. If the answer is "yes," motivation is the issue creating disability, and the physician's job is to find the source: worker, supervisor, employer, etc.

Question 4: The Obstacle

What is the specific obstacle preventing the individual from working today? This question may uncover situational or environmental obstacles to returning to work.

Establishing Reasonable Functional Capacity Guides or Work Guides

Physicians who treat work-related injuries realize that there is no easy reference for developing work guides. By combining the elements of the injury, the patient, and the job, safe and reasonable functional capacity guides can be provided that will allow the injured employee an opportunity to return to appropriate work while using the workplace as an integral part of the therapy program, thus providing cost-effective rehabilitation.

It may be useful to consult published disability durations such as those in *The Medical Disability Advisor* by the Reed Group,[11] the *Official Disability Guides* by the Work Loss Data Institute,[12] and the *Occupational Medicine*

Practice Guidelines by OEM Press and the American College of Occupational and Environmental Medicine.[13] If the individual has exceeded the recommended maximal disability duration for the illness or injury in question, that fact can be shared with the patient and used to support written decisions by the physician encouraging a prompt return to work.

Work characteristics, including frequency of task performance and weight, should be discussed. Weight guides are based on the US Department of Labor *Dictionary of Occupational Titles* (Tables 4-1 and 4-2).[8]

Total activities should be considered next. These may include lift, push-pull, carry, climb, body motion, sitting, standing, and walking (Table 4-3). Total activities occur in three domains: activities of daily living, therapy (occupational and physical), and workplace activities. After arriving at a general range for total activities, the physician should apportion a percentage to home, therapy, and work.

The graph in Figure 4-1 shows how to balance the amount of time and activities for therapy and work, because home usually remains fairly constant. As each patient is unique, the general approach to balancing activities is to gradually increase work while gradually decreasing therapy. Some individuals may be able to tolerate therapy and a regular work day. Others may require work guides that limit work activities, especially work hours, on therapy days. These individuals may benefit from a more frequent and active therapy program. As endurance for work activities improves, the frequency and level of activity of the therapy program can be decreased. Each individual will start this graph at a different location.

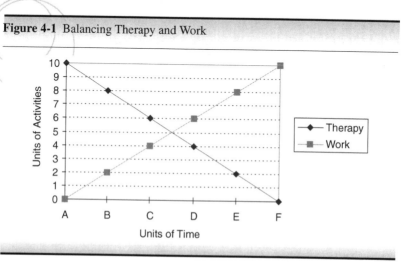

Figure 4-1 Balancing Therapy and Work

Work characteristics can be provided in both frequency ("limited" at 0% to 12% of the work day, "occasional" at 0% to 33%, "frequent" at 34% to 66%, and "constant" at 67% to 100%) and time (0, 2, 4, 6, or 8 hours per work day). The activities that can be performed, eg, repetitive grasping, pushing, pulling, fine manipulation, vibratory tools, power tools, and hand over shoulder, should be stated.

On follow-up visits, it is important to record the patient's current working status. The medical status can simply be "yes" or "no" for presently working. If not working, why is the patient not working? It could be that no work is available from the employer, or the patient does not want to work, or the patient or employer is uncertain as to work guides. Expected future changes in work guides should be discussed. For example, the physician might say: "Today you are available for light work; if you continue to do well, we might consider light to medium work at your next follow-up visit." This communication allows the patient time to consider the physician's recommendations; the patient may even try this weight level a few times to see if he or she can do it before the next visit, allowing time to build confidence, and the physician has emphasized the plan of continued improvement, not continued disability. By using the same work guides form, the physician has developed a communication tool, a record of the improvement, and the successful transition from alternative work to regular work. In addition, the last work guide can be used to complete information contained in the permanent physical impairment report.

Another example of the communication in advance is the section for patients undergoing elective surgery. This section encourages discussion about early return to work and includes the following:

> Before surgery—same work pattern. After surgery—you may return to modified light work the day after surgery (maximum 20 lb or less lift/carry; frequent at 10 lb for both arms, possible cast or dressing on, no large power or vibratory tools, limit extremity use on operated side). Your work production may initially be decreased in the postoperative period. In general, you should gradually increase your activities at home and at work. Please provide these guides to your employer prior to surgery. These workplace guides have been reviewed with me.

Physicians may have the patient sign as needed for confirmation. This section helps to stimulate communication between the patient and the physician and allows for a mutual effort to write reasonable work guides. It is important for both patient and treating physician to realize that the company physician may modify the work guides further on the basis of special knowledge of the workplace.

Chapter 4

Sample Linkage Forms

Linkage, or the ability to combine the elements of the injury, the patient, and the job for the development of safe and reasonable work guides, occurs by using standard functional capacity forms. It is nearly impossible to remember each of the required elements each time functional capacity or work guides are being considered. To make the process manageable, reliable, readable, and consistent, *each physician should develop a standard return-to-work form based on his or her specific practice.* This creates familiarity and allows for linkage with science.

Tables 4-1, 4-2, 4-3, and Figure 4-1, shown earlier in this chapter, and Tables 4-4 and 4-5 shown here are the starting points. Standard forms also allow for negotiation of functional capacity with the patient. To be effective, the information must be transferred to the employee and employer with every office visit.

Table 4-4   Epidemiologic Evidence for Work-Related Musculoskeletal Disorders*

Body Part and Risk Factor	Strong Evidence (+++)	Evidence (++)	Insufficient Evidence (+/0)	Evidence of No Effect (−)
Neck and neck/shoulder				
Repetition		X		
Force	X			
Posture	X			
Vibration			X	
Shoulder				
Repetition		X		
Force			X	
Posture		X		
Vibration			X	
Elbow				
Repetition			X	
Force		X		
Posture			X	
Combination	X			

Table 4-4 *(Continued)*

Body Part and Risk Factor	Strong Evidence (+++)	Evidence (++)	Insufficient Evidence (+/0)	Evidence of No Effect (−)
Hand/wrist				
Carpal tunnel syndrome				
Repetition		X		
Force		X		
Posture			X	
Vibration		X		
Combination	X			
Tendinitis				
Repetition		X		
Force		X		
Posture		X		
Combination	X			
Hand-arm vibration syndrome				
Vibration	X			
Back				
Lifting/forceful movement	X			
Awkward posture		X		
Heavy physical work		X		
Whole body vibration	X			
Static work posture			X	

* Strong epidemiologic evidence (+++) indicates that the consistently positive findings from a large number of cross-sectional studies, strengthened by the limited number of prospective studies, provide strong evidence of increased risk of work-related musculoskeletal disorders for some body parts based on the strength of the associations, lack of ambiguity, consistency of the results, and adequate control or adjustment for likely confounders in cross-sectional studies and the temporal relationships from the prospective studies, with reasonable confidence levels in at least several of those studies. Epidemiologic evidence (++) indicates that some convincing epidemiologic evidence shows a causal relationship when the epidemiologic criteria of causality for intense or long-duration exposure to the specific risk factor(s) and musculoskeletal disorders are used. A positive relationship has been observed between exposure to the specific risk factor and musculoskeletal disorders in studies in which chance, bias, and confounding factors are not the likely explanation. Insufficient epidemiologic evidence (+/0) indicates that the available studies are of insufficient number, quality, consistency, or statistical power to permit a conclusion regarding the presence or absence of a causal association. Some studies suggest a relationship to specific risk factors, but chance, bias, or confounding may explain the association. Either there is an insufficient number of studies from which to draw conclusions or the overall conclusion from the studies is equivocal. The absence of existing epidemiologic evidence should not be interpreted to mean that there is no association between work factors and musculoskeletal disorders. No epidemiologic evidence (−) indicates that there have been no adequate studies to show that the specific workplace risk factor(s) is not related to development of musculoskeletal disorders.

Table 4-5 Workplace Risk Factors

Stressor	Attributes	Work Factors
Repetition	Exertion frequency	Production standard
	Recovery time	Pacing
	Percentage recovery	Incentives
	Cycle time	Work quantities/unit time
	Velocity and acceleration	Methods/materials
	Force	Work rotation
	Posture	Manufacturing process
		Mechanical aids
		Quality control
		Machines
Force	Amplitude probability	Friction
	Distribution	Weight of work objects
	Peak	Balance
	Average	Reaction forces/torques
	Static vs dynamic	Drag forces
	Smooth vs jerky	Mechanical aids
		Gloves/handles
		Quality control
		Machines
Posture	Range of motion	Work location
	Average	Work orientation
	Time position	Work object shape
		Methods/materials
		Machine
		Environment
Vibration	Frequency	Abrasive
	Displacement	Tool drive train
	Velocity	Bit condition
	Acceleration	Isolation/dampening
	Duration	Gloves
Temperature	Low temperature	Temperature of air
	Conductivity	Work object temperature
	Duration	Air exhaust

Chapter 4

Table 4-5   (*Continued*)

Stressor	Attributes	Work Factors
Temperature		Gloves
		Protective clothing
Contact stress	Force	Force factors
	Area	Area of contact
	Location	Location of contact
	Duration	Gloves
Unaccustomed activities	Duration	Work schedules
	Hours	Work standards
	Days	Incentives
	Percentage of time	Methods/environment

Figure 4-2 is an example of an office encounter form or charge ticket. Each office will need to modify its encounter form to accommodate its specialty. There are several important sections that all forms should have. It is very efficient and effective to have all the information for one visit on one page. This form has a carbonless copy that is given to the patient at each office visit to be taken to the employer. This makes for immediate communication between the patient and employer.

The top of the form shows the services provided during the office visit. The practice may decide to place this section on a separate form, as it is used in billing for the physician's service. The second area deals with the diagnosis. Employers may (workers' compensation) or may not (private disability) have a right to know the diagnosis without patient consent. The third area is the functional capacity guides section. The fourth contains the next appointment. The fifth is the section on patient demographics, and the last contains the patient's and/or physician's signature.

Figure 4-3 is an enlargement of the functional capacity or work guides section from Figure 4-2. There are two key points to include:

- "Please consider off work until next appointment unless alternative or transitional work is available as circled or checked below":
  — work status, hours of work and type of work, work characteristics
  — preoperative and postoperative guides
  — physician and patient signatures

Figure 4-2 Encounter Form

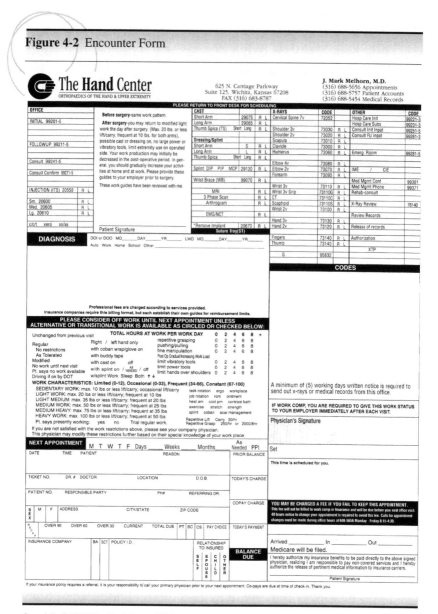

Copyright © 1991 The Hand Center, Wichita, Kansas. Reproduced with permission.

- "If you are not satisfied with the work restrictions above, you should see your company physician. This physician may modify these restrictions further based on his or her special knowledge of your workplace."

Figure 4-3   Functional Capacity or Work Guides

PLEASE CONSIDER OFF WORK UNTIL NEXT APPOINTMENT UNLESS ALTERNATIVE OR TRANSITIONAL WORK IS AVAILABLE AS CIRCLED OR CHECKED BELOW:

Unchanged from previous visit

TOTAL HOURS AT WORK PER WORK DAY   0 2 4 6 8 +

Regular
　No restrictions
　As Tolerated
Modified
No work until next visit
Pt. says no work available
Driving if ok by DOT

Right / left hand only
with coban wrap/glove on
with buddy tape
with cast on   off
with splint on / AS NEEDED / off
w/splint Work Sleep Both ↑ ↓

repetitive grasping   0 2 4 6 8
pushing/pulling   0 2 4 6 8
fine manipulation   0 2 4 6 8
Post Op Gradual Increasing Work Load
limit vibratory tools   0 2 4 6 8
limit power tools   0 2 4 6 8
limit hands over shoulders 0 2 4 6 8

WORK CHARACTERISTICS: Limited (0-12), Occasional (0-33), Frequent (34-66), Constant (67-100)

SEDENTARY WORK: max. 10 lbs or less lift/carry; occasional lift/carry
LIGHT WORK: max. 20 lbs or less lift/carry; frequent at 10 lbs
LIGHT MEDIUM: max. 35 lbs or less lift/carry; frequent at 20 lbs
MEDIUM WORK: max. 50 lbs or less lift/carry; frequent at 25 lbs
MEDIUM HEAVY: max. 75 lbs or less lift/carry; frequent at 35 lbs
HEAVY WORK: max. 100 lbs or less lift/carry; frequent at 50 lbs
Pt. says presently working: yes   no   Trial regular work.

task rotation   ergo   workplace
job rotation   rom   ointment
heat am   cool pm   contrast bath
exercise   stretch   strength
splint   coban   scar management
Repetitive Lift   Carry 30/hr
Repetitive Grasp   250/hr or 2000/8hr

If you are not satisfied with the work restrictions above, please see your company physician.
This physician may modify these restrictions further based on their special knowledge of your work place.

Additional Forms

The sample forms illustrated in the previous section are specific to the hand and upper extremity. Additional sample tables are provided to assist in the development of other practice-specific forms and include general workplace conditions (Table 4-6), lower extremity and back (Table 4-7), and specific job tasks (Table 4-8). Not all of this information is routinely required but is presented for completeness to help physicians develop their practice-specific work guide forms. In the occupational health setting, several pages of guides may be required on the initial visit, with only updates of the changed area(s) provided on follow-up visits. Although many employers will provide their own form, it is often easier for physicians to use their practice form with which they are more familiar. A copy of the functional capacity or work guides should be retained in the medical chart.

Writing Functional Capacity and Return-to-Work Guides

After reviewing the information and examples in this chapter, the physician should be ready to write the actual functional capacity or return-to-work guide. In doing so, he or she must consider the patient's symptoms, signs, risk, capacity, tolerance, job description, essential functions of the job, accommodation options, employer willingness, employee willingness, previous work guides (by the family physician, company physician, or other), response to work activity, and current work status.

Chapter 4

Table 4-6 General Workplace Conditions

	None	Infrequent	Limited	Occasional	Frequent	Continuous
Unlevel surfaces	0	1	2	4	6	8
Unprotected heights	0	1	2	4	6	8
Isolated areas	0	1	2	4	6	8
Operating cab cranes	0	1	2	4	6	8
Operating hazards, moving machinery	0	1	2	4	6	8
Dry areas only	0	1	2	4	6	8
Limit temperature <40°F or >100°F	0	1	2	4	6	8
Use of personal protective equipment	0	1	2	4	6	8
Isolated areas	0	1	2	4	6	8
Operation of company vehicles	0	1	2	4	6	8
Dry areas only	0	1	2	4	6	8
Dust >2.5 mg/cc	0	1	2	4	6	8
Respirator	0	1	2	4	6	8
Temperature <40°F or >100°F	0	1	2	4	6	8
High magnetic fields	0	1	2	4	6	8
Chemicals						
Solvents	0	1	2	4	6	8
Sealants	0	1	2	4	6	8
Skin irritants	0	1	2	4	6	8
Irritant fumes	0	1	2	4	6	8
Hearing						
Hearing ability required	0	1	2	4	6	8
Hearing aid	0	1	2	4	6	8
High noise area >85 dB	0	1	2	4	6	8
Hearing protection	0	1	2	4	6	8
Vision						
Eye goggles	0	1	2	4	6	8
Normal color vision	0	1	2	4	6	8
Peripheral vision	0	1	2	4	6	8
Depth perception	0	1	2	4	6	8
Specific visual acuity	0	1	2	4	6	8

Copyright © 1991 The Hand Center, Wichita, Kansas. Reproduced with permission.

Chapter 4

Table 4-7 Lower Extremity and Back

	None	Infrequent	Limited	Occasional	Frequent	Continuous
Bend	0	1	2	4	6	8
Twist	0	1	2	4	6	8
Stoop	0	1	2	4	6	8
Squat	0	1	2	4	6	8
Kneel	0	1	2	4	6	8
Crawl	0	1	2	4	6	8
Sit	0	1	2	4	6	8
Stand	0	1	2	4	6	8
Bench work	0	1	2	4	6	8
Walk	0	1	2	4	6	8
Climb stairs	0	1	2	4	6	8
Climb ladders	0	1	2	4	6	8

Table 4-8 Specific Job Tasks

	None	Infrequent	Limited	Occasional	Frequent	Continuous
Keyboard	0	1	2	4	6	8
Writing	0	1	2	4	6	8
Knife	0	1	2	4	6	8
Hook	0	1	2	4	6	8
Scissors	0	1	2	4	6	8
Pliers	0	1	2	4	6	8
Clamps	0	1	2	4	6	8
Pressure hoses	0	1	2	4	6	8
Telephone dialing	0	1	2	4	6	8
Drilling	0	1	2	4	6	8
Sanding	0	1	2	4	6	8
Bucking	0	1	2	4	6	8
Riveting	0	1	2	4	6	8
Deburring	0	1	2	4	6	8
Other	0	1	2	4	6	8
Above-shoulder lift in lb and time	0	1	2	4	6	8
Forward reach >18 in from body	0	1	2	4	6	8

The art of medicine requires a blending of these factors with appropriate input from the patient. The process is easier when the patient and physician work together. The first decision is whether to recommend regular work, modified work, or no work. This decision is made by considering the injury, the patient, and the job. In cases in which the physician and the patient disagree about work guides, the negotiation strategies discussed in Chapter 2 and Chapter 3 may be helpful.

A Note About Disclaimers

As America is one of the most litigious countries in the world, physicians should have standard "disclaimers" to attach to return-to-work certification forms. These may not prevent the physician from being sued, but they may make a successful suit less likely. One example of such a disclaimer, printed here, is discussed in Chapter 8:

The above statements have been made within a reasonable degree of medical probability. The opinions rendered in this case are mine alone. Recommendations regarding treatment, work, and impairment ratings are given totally independently from the requesting agents. These opinions do not constitute per se a recommendation for specific claims or administrative functions to be made or enforced.

This evaluation is based upon the history given by Mr/Ms ___, the objective medical findings noted during the examination, and information obtained from the review of the prior medical records available to me, with the assumption that this material is true and correct. If additional information is provided to me in the future, a reconsideration and an additional report may be requested. Such information may or may not change the opinions in this report.

Medicine is both an art and a science, and although Mr/Ms ___ may appear to be fit to work with the abilities and restrictions described above, there is no guarantee that he/she will not be injured or sustain a new injury if he/she chooses to return to work.

Summary

In today's environment, where outcomes are important and economics matter greatly, the treating physician is in a unique position to provide better management of work-related injuries. Improved outcomes are possible when the treating physician treats the whole patient. This whole-patient approach requires an understanding of the factors that contribute to the poorer outcomes, medical treatment plans that include options to address the biopsychosocial issues, and early return-to-work guides. These inclusive medical treatment plans aid in the patient's recovery and rehabilitation while avoiding many of the pitfalls of the workers' compensation system. This approach requires a team effort on the part of the patient, physician, employer, insurer, and government. Many physicians choose not to participate in early return to work because of concerns about liability. Therefore, appropriate legislation should be enacted in all jurisdictions to protect physicians from liability associated with appropriate return-to-work decisions.

Communication and education are key to avoiding unnecessary lost work time. The work guides must be safe and allow for speedy return to work, with the best interests of the patient being the primary responsibility. This means that at times paternalism (physician directive: "Return to work is good for you") trumps autonomy (patient choice: "I don't want to work"). Ultimately, physicians are asked for their *medical advice* as to proper work guides. Physicians are not asked to function as secretaries by recording patient preferences for work activity. To accomplish these goals, the work guides must be consistent and precise. With each visit, the treating physician should understand the current influences of the workers' compensation system, must maintain return to work as a priority in the treatment plan, and must report the diagnosis, treatment plan, disability status, and expected period of disability. These guides allow the support staff to work closely with the treating physician to provide the necessary direction and continuity to lead the worker along the complicated path of returning to work. The physician must maintain the leadership role to resolve the many barriers to early return to work. The process of developing functional capacity guides is slow, time consuming, and often frustrating for both the patient and the physician, but the benefits to the employee-patient are significant and, therefore, worth the effort.

References

1. Melhorn JM. Upper extremities: return to work issues. In: Melhorn JM, Spengler DM, eds. *Fifth Occupational Orthopaedics and Workers' Compensation: A Multidisciplinary Perspective*. Rosemont, Ill: American Academy of Orthopaedic Surgeons; 2003:256–285.

2. Mundy RR, Moore SC, Corey JB, Mundy GD. Disability syndrome: the effects of early vs delayed rehabilitation intervention. *AAOHN J.* 1994;42:379–383.

3. Christian J. Reducing disability days: healing more than the injury. *J Workers Comp.* 2000;9:30–55.

4. Atlas SJ, Chang Y, Kamman E, et al. Long-term disability and return to work among patients who have a herniated lumbar disc: the effect of disability compensation. *J Bone Joint Surg Am.* 2000;82A:4–15.

5. Burton WN, Conti DJ. Disability management: corporate medical department management of employee health and productivity. *J Occup Environ Med.* 2000;42:1006–1012.

6. Melhorn JM. *Reducing Unnecessary Workplace Disability—Treating More Than the Injury.* Sacramento, Calif: California Industrial Medicine Council; 2003.

7. Melhorn JM. Return to work: the employer's point of view. In: *2003 Safety and Health Conference.* Topeka, Kan: Kansas Department of Human Resources; 2003.

8. US Department of Labor. *The Dictionary of Occupational Titles.* Washington, DC; 1991:1012–1014. Available at: www.oalj.dol.gov/libdot.htm. Accessed October 26, 2004.

9. Millender LH, Conlon M. An approach to work-related disorders of the upper extremity. *J Am Acad Orthop Surg.* 1996;4:134–142.

10. Cocchiarella J, Andersson G, eds. *Guides to the Evaluation of Permanent Impairment.* 5th ed. Chicago, Ill: AMA Press; 2001.

11. Reed P. *The Medical Disability Advisor: Workplace Guidelines for Disability Duration.* 5th ed. Westminster, Colo: Reed Group, Ltd; 2005.

12. Denniston Jr PL. *ODG Treatment in Workers' Comp 2004.* Encinitas, Calif: Work Loss Data Institute; 2004.

13. Glass LS. *Occupational Medicine Practice Guidelines.* Beverly Farms, Mass: OEM Press; 2004.

Chapter 4

Chapter 5

Evidence-based Medicine

Elizabeth Genovese, MD, MBA

Current medical literature is replete with references to "practice guidelines" (with the assumption that they promote optimal medical practice) and to "evidence-based medicine." As a corollary, there is an implicit assumption that the former is based on "evidence" and that this evidence is sound. In reality, many practice guidelines are not based on evidence, but on consensus. When there is no consensus, common medical practices are based predominantly on opinion.

There have been attempts to formulate practice guidelines regarding return to work by organizations such as the American College of Occupational and Environmental Medicine.[1] These guidelines tend to be based on consensus rather than evidence, and while they may shape the behavior of *some* physicians who practice in this specialty, adoption by physicians in other specialties has been limited at best. This has been predominantly due to a dearth of high-quality studies clearly indicating that return-to-work benefits those who have no "tolerance" for doing so; designing studies to evaluate this is difficult, as tolerance is primarily subjective and highly individualized. An alternative is to focus, instead, on whether patients "can" work. This determination, however, assumes that we can somehow separate ability from tolerance, which is difficult to do with any degree of accuracy, as the evidence-based literature to support most assumptions regarding the extrapolation of "ability testing" to actual work environments is scant, *especially* for those who have no tolerance (or "will") to do so.

As tolerance is neither quantifiable nor verifiable, and the predictive validity of ability testing is largely unknown, we are left only with *risk*. In other words, if we wish to make credible statements regarding return to work, we need to ask whether there is literature that addresses whether returning patients with a given condition to a specific form of work places them at undue risk of injury or harm.

There is literature that addresses this topic. However, inherent in any review of the literature is the need to determine whether the conclusions are based on evidence, consensus, or anecdote. The quality of the evidence also needs to be assessed. It has been widely accepted that practice guidelines should only be classified as "evidence-based" when they reflect a scientific analysis of the available literature based on sound epidemiologic and statistical foundations. While an in-depth discussion of how one qualifies evidence is beyond the scope of this chapter and this book, it behooves all physicians to have at least a rudimentary understanding of what evidence-based medicine is, and what it is not.

Evidence-based medicine has been defined by Sackett et al[2] as the "conscientious, explicit, and judicious use of current best evidence in making decisions about the care of individual patients." As such, it means "integrating individual clinical expertise with the best available clinical evidence from systematic research."

Williams[3] notes that evidence-based medicine is "the concept of formalizing the scientific approach to the practice of medicine for identification of 'evidence' to support our clinical decisions." This in turn requires understanding critical appraisal and the basic epidemiologic principles of study design, point estimates, relative risk, odds ratios, confidence intervals, bias, and confounding.

Study Types

Studies can be experimental or observational. Experimental, blinded, randomized studies are the best way of assessing whether a treatment decision or exposure leads to a given outcome. One can standardize and randomize the choice of subjects, and control for those variables that might be etiologic for a disease or affect treatment outcomes by identifying an alternative intervention that differs only in terms of the factor being evaluated. One can also control the intensity and duration of exposure, and whether the study is *single blind* (the subject does not know whether he or she is receiving the intervention) or *double-blind* (neither the subject nor the evaluator knows who received the intervention and who did not). Table 5-1 provides a comparison of study types.

There are a number of issues that make it difficult to apply experimental study designs to the evaluation of human populations. Primary among these is difficulty in disguising the active intervention so that subjects cannot distinguish it from the control. This is clearly impossible to achieve when return to work is the intervention—hence the absence of experimental studies assessing this option. As a consequence, we utilize studies that are generally observational and epidemiologic rather than experimental in assessing the response of humans to varying exposures and treatment options.

Table 5-1 Comparison of Study Types

Study Characteristics	Experimental	Cross-Sectional	Case-Control	Historical Cohort	Nested Case-Control	Prospective Cohort
Blinded, single	Generally	No	No	No	No	No
Blinded, double	Sometimes	No	No	No	No	No
Investigator controls treatment or exposure	Yes	No	No	No	No	No
Data collected at single point in time	Sometimes	Yes	Yes (no)	Yes	Yes/no: cases are incident	No
Data collected longitudinally	Sometimes	No	Yes/no: incident	Yes	Yes	Yes
Work backward to identify exposures	No	Yes	Yes	Yes	No	No
Used to calculate disease incidence	No	Yes	No	Yes	Yes	Yes
Recall bias	No	Yes	Yes	No (?)	No	No
Nonresponse bias	Yes	No	No	No	No	Yes
Likely confounders	Sometimes	Yes	Yes	No	Sometimes	Sometimes
Suitable for rare disease processes	If designed appropriately	Yes	Yes	Yes	Yes	No
Appropriate for diseases with long latency	Not really	Yes	Yes	Yes	Yes	No
Expense	Varies	Low	Low	Low	Medium	High
Strength of evidence	No	Low	Low	Medium	Medium	Good

Epidemiologic Studies

Epidemiology is "the science concerned with the study of factors determining and influencing the frequency and distribution of disease, injury, and other health-related events in a defined human population."[4] It is primarily descriptive, and identifies the presence or absence of associations between disease and exposure in the population(s) studied. Epidemiologic studies, however, are only as good as their design and analysis. It is consequently mandatory for those involved in the assessment of causality to be able to critically evaluate these studies before automatically accepting their conclusions as valid. Furthermore, "as confident as one might be that the conclusions of an epidemiological study are scientifically sound, there is always a possibility that new discoveries or even new analyses of old data will alter those conclusions."[3]

Epidemiologic studies are, by definition, observational rather than experimental. Subjects are *not* randomly selected, and the exposure cannot be controlled. The simplest studies, case reports and case series, are descriptive rather than analytic. They simply *describe* the occurrence of a given event in a group of individuals, along with a description of the interventions or exposures they shared. While this may suggest a need for further evaluation of the relationship between the exposure or treatment and the observed outcome (which can be tested in future studies), case reports cannot be used as grounds to assert the existence of a causal relationship between the two, but are only grounds for hypotheses.

Analytic Studies

Analytic studies are, by definition, designed to evaluate hypotheses. There are three main types of analytic study: prevalence, case-control, and cohort studies.

Prevalence Studies

Prevalence (or cross-sectional) studies are the weakest form of analytic study, as conclusions are drawn from data that are collected at a single point in time. These studies allow one to conclude that there may be a potential relationship between contemporaneous exposures, symptoms, findings, or disease processes that appear at a higher rate than is ordinarily seen in populations otherwise similar to that under observation. They do *not* allow one to make conclusions regarding cause and effect, since the cases included are prevalent (have already occurred) and not incident (occurring during the study). One cannot tell, for example, whether the presence of an association indicates that a given exposure caused (or intervention helped treat) a disease, or whether those who have a given disease are simply more likely to recall the exposure or treatment under investigation (*recall bias*). It is consequently inappropriate, as a rule, to conclude anything but the possibility of a relationship between two items (without imputing cause and effect) that are found to be associated in a prevalence study.

Case-control Studies

The next level of evidence is achieved through the use of *case-control* studies. In these studies a more direct evaluation of hypotheses is possible, as those who have been exposed to a putatively harmful factor or received a potentially beneficial treatment (*cases*) are compared to those who have not (*controls*). Case-control studies differ from experiments in that they are retrospective (since this is how cases are identified), although they do often then observe both cases and controls prospectively. They also do *not* control the exposure of subjects to the factor or factors under evaluation, so careful matching of cases with controls in terms of all other potentially relevant variables is mandatory for conclusions to be valid. When this does not occur, the degree to which one can confidently assert the existence of a causal relationship between an exposure or treatment and a given outcome is diminished.

Cohort Studies

The strongest observational studies are *cohort* studies, longitudinal analyses of how disease develops (or has responded to treatment) in a well-defined source population. These studies can be prospective (beginning at a point of time with concurrent follow-up) or retrospective (historical); however, prospective studies are optimal as they minimize recall bias. In both, baseline information about the persons under evaluation is collected before a disease or treatment intervention occurs (prospective studies) or occurred (retrospective studies). The nature, quality, and degree of change in the baseline population (cohort) is then studied to assess which of the factors being evaluated (or other factors) may have played a role. Study design dictates that data from retrospective cohort studies covers only a discreet period of follow-up. When a prospective study design is used, follow-up can, if necessary, occur indefinitely—even across generations. (The Framingham study is the classic example of this.)

Compared to other observational studies, prospective cohort studies offer the best evidence regarding cause and effect, as they most closely approximate the experimental randomized controlled trial. Because observing large populations to see what develops over time is prohibitively expensive, it is generally best to use prior descriptive or prevalence studies to first generate hypotheses. Once the treatment response or condition one wishes to evaluate has been identified, it is then possible to maximize efficiency by "nesting" case-control studies inside a larger cohort study, as this reduces costs by limiting the analysis to a well-defined and, presumably, clinically relevant subset of the study population.

Chapter 5

Potential Flaws in Study Types

Study outcomes and conclusions can be influenced by study design and flaws. Understanding how these can impact the results helps the reviewer better interpret the conclusions.

Bias

As noted earlier in this chapter, observational studies demonstrate association, not cause and effect. Researchers are generally unable to control exposure and must, instead, work with existing data, which makes these studies subject to *bias*, a systematic or measurement error in the design or analysis of a study that leads to an overestimation or underestimation of the strength and significance of a given association. Bias can occur in both experimental and observational studies but is more common in the latter.

Recall bias can occur in prevalence, case-control, and retrospective studies and reflects the tendency of those who have a condition, or have undergone a particular treatment, to be more likely to recall an exposure or to focus on potential side effects of the procedure than do those who did *not* experience the condition or treatment.

Nonresponse bias is a significant potential cause of erroneous conclusions in study analysis and occurs when there are differences between those who do and do not follow up with a survey or treatment. When the response rate at follow-up is low, it is mandatory for researchers to assess the characteristics of responders as opposed to nonresponders (at least at baseline) to control for this.

Selection bias, in which one (unknowingly) compares groups that differ in ways other than their exposure to a given factor, is also a common problem affecting observational studies.

Other relevant commonly encountered forms of bias are *information bias* (when information is collected differently from the exposed and unexposed groups), *detection bias* (when a problem is detected at an earlier stage in the group that is screened than it would have been otherwise), *compliance bias* (differential rates of compliance with a treatment in the experimental and control groups), *measurement bias* (the use of testing to measure the results of an exposure or treatment that differs in predictive value when applied to cases and controls), and *procedure bias* (when matched groups of subjects do not receive identical treatment, usually due to failure to blind researchers). Procedure bias can, incidentally, be nothing more than an evaluator devoting a little more time or attention to subjects as opposed to controls. This is, however, often all that is needed to shift the balance toward finding a positive effect of treatment or negative effect of exposure in a study that would otherwise have been neutral.

Confounding

Studies can also be flawed because of *confounding*, the presence of a third, or "confounding," factor that was not accounted for in subject matching but is the "true" factor associated with both the exposure or treatment and the ultimate outcome. For example, the association between disabling back pain and decreased aerobic capacity (a measure of fitness) may well reflect an increased prevalence of "fear-avoidance" behaviors and an external rather than internal locus of control in both groups.[5–11] It would hence be inappropriate to state that fitness helps prevent back pain, as fitness is not really the relevant factor.

It is clear that assessing the significance of findings from a given study requires understanding of the strengths and weaknesses of various forms of study design. One also must understand the strengths and weaknesses of the statistical analysis used in reaching conclusions.

Statistical Analysis

Quantifiable results from a study are always characterized by a *mean*, or average value, around which most values tend to cluster, with all other values (by definition) either larger or smaller. *Standard deviation* is a measure of the dispersion, or spread, of measurements around the mean value. Standard deviation is related to variance in that greater degrees of variance in results will increase the standard deviation, which, conversely, decreases when the variance is low. In a *two-tailed test*, one in which there is no reason to expect that values will have been uniformly higher or lower than baseline, the premise is that 95% of values will fall within two standard deviations in either direction from the mean, while 99% of values will fall within three standard deviations.

Study analysis begins with the *null hypothesis*, ie, that a given intervention or exposure will *not* make a difference (will lead to results that fall within at least two standard deviations of values considered "normal" or "expected"). A test statistic is calculated on the basis of the observed data (details are beyond the scope of this chapter) and, depending on what level of significance is desired, is indicative of the cutoff values at two standard deviations from the mean. When values fall above or below this "statistic," there is a 5% probability that they are still reflective of a normal distribution (and simply represent outliers) and a 95% probability that they are *statistically significant*, ie, reflect a true effect of the treatment or exposure under investigation.

Since 99% of values should fall within three standard deviations of the mean, there is a 99% probability that values greater or less than the values at three standard deviations in either direction (for a two-tailed test) are significant, and a 1% possibility that they are still reflective of a normal distribution (ie, do *not* represent the effect of an exposure or intervention).

This information is classically communicated via *the P value*. In general, a *P* value of .05 is considered acceptable, as it indicates that the likelihood of error (or α) in classifying the observed findings as reflecting a true difference from the expected finding of no difference (the null hypothesis) is 5%. A *P* value of .01 decreases the chances that findings will be erroneously classified as significant (when they were not) to 1%. *P* values of less than .01 are optimal. Practically speaking, the best we can usually do is a *P* value of .01 to .05; *P* values of greater than .05 are generally considered to indicate an unacceptably high risk of error.

Confidence Intervals

Another way to use the same data is by calculating *confidence intervals*, which are ranges of values that represent two ($P < .05$) or three ($P < .01$) standard deviations from where one would have expected the mean to fall. Results are statistically significant in demonstrating a difference (rejecting the null hypothesis of "no difference") if the observed results after exposure or treatment do not fall into these confidence limits. The new hypothesis is then that the external event or situation was a causal factor in shifting the confidence interval away from the "original" mean. Again, this is reflective of an association between the exposure or treatment and the outcome rather than absolute proof of causality.

Odds Ratios

Alternatively, *likelihood* or *odds ratios* can be calculated, indicating the chances of observing the value seen in a given study in the normal population. If the likelihood ratio is 1.0, then the outcome was no more likely to occur (or not occur) as a result of the exposure or intervention than it was in its absence. Likelihood or odds ratio values are always listed in conjunction with a range representing, as a rule, the 95% confidence level for significance. If the value 1.0 is included within the confidence limits (at a *P* value of .05) of the calculated ratio, the observed value is most likely *not* of statistical relevance.

As noted, the *P* value conveys the degree to which a conclusion that findings represent a true deviation from the null hypothesis is erroneous, which is referred to as an α (alpha) or type I error. In other words, type I error occurs when one concludes that there is a causal relationship between an exposure and a disease, or a treatment and clinical improvement, when there really is not.

Type II error, the converse, occurs when a difference or causal relationship is *not* found, but exists. Type II error is defined as 1 minus the power; hence, if the power of a study is known, the chance of type II error can be determined. Table 5-2 can be used to better understand if there is a real difference between items such as treatment and clinical improvement.

Power is the ability of a test to appropriately reject the null hypothesis when it is false. In other words, power describes the ability of a study to detect a given difference of a given size between two outcomes if the difference really exists. The power of a statistical test is analogous to the sensitivity of a diagnostic test (ie, the ability to find a difference that is present).[4] *Power analysis* consists of determining how large a sample is required to detect an actual difference of some specified magnitude. The larger the sample, or the size of the difference one is expecting, the greater the power and the lower the risk of type II error.

There are, however, caveats to be considered in the interpretation of large studies, for if the power is large—ie, if there is a high chance of finding a difference—small differences will also be found to be statistically significant. As a *P* value of .05 *does* indicate a 5% risk of type I error (erroneously *rejecting* the null hypothesis), in situations when the ramifications of type I error are significant (for example, when the benefit of a treatment is likely to be small or short-lived and the cost, or risk, high), it would appear prudent to attempt to minimize the risk of type I error even further.

All of these factors should be kept in mind when designing a study. This process begins with assessing the level of significance or type I error one wishes to achieve (the *P* value), which in turn allows calculation of how large of a study population is required to achieve adequate power. As a corollary, a study should not be classified as contributing significantly to the evidence basis for or against a given intervention or hypothesis until the *P* value *and* the results of the power analysis are known. While most studies discuss *P* values or similar criteria (such as confidence limits or likelihood ratios), many neglect any discussion of power. It is perhaps then

Table 5-2 Type I or Type II Errors

Conclusions From Test	Reality	
	Difference Exists (H_1)	No Difference (H_0)
Difference exists (reject H_0)	Power or $1-\beta$ (correct conclusion)	Type I error, or α
No difference (do not reject H_0)	Type II error, or β	$1-\alpha$ (correct conclusion)

Chapter 5

unsurprising that type II error is quite common; this makes it difficult to determine whether "negative" studies are negative because of inadequate power or a true absence of exposure or treatment effect.[12-14]

Meta-analysis

Meta-analysis is a tool that has increasingly been applied in evidence-based medicine. In meta-analysis the results of studies with roughly equivalent subjects and interventions are pooled and analyzed as a whole. This use of the technique allows the meta-analysis to achieve greater levels of significance and power than were obtainable through analysis of the individual studies. While meta-analytic studies have flaws, as do reviews, nonetheless they are felt to represent one of the highest grades of available evidence. To the extent that they are available for a given topic, one can have a greater level of confidence in results than would otherwise be the case.

Analyzing and Applying Study Results

Even if meta-analyses and reviews are included, many available studies evaluating exposure or the effects of diagnostic or therapeutic options end with results that are inconclusive due to bias, inadequate blinding, or lack of power. When clinical practice guidelines or consensus statements are prepared, the authors must first categorize the quality of the evidence and then analyze it in conjunction with an analysis of the overall benefit vs harm to be gained from adoption or rejection of evidence in support of a given intervention.

In many cases the evidence alone is simply rated on a scale of A through D. Level A evidence represents "strong and research-based evidence provided by generally consistent findings in multiple high quality randomized control trials," while evidence is classified as level D when there are no randomized controlled trials of quality (or equivalents).[15] While this is certainly adequate to categorize the evidence itself, the scale does not include judgments regarding the risk of harm from interventions and may thus be of limited practical use.

The *Clinical Evidence* series from the BMJ Publishing Group[16] attempts to increase the practical application of categorized data by classifying interventions as "beneficial," "likely to be beneficial," "representative of trade off between benefit and harms," of "unknown effectiveness," "unlikely to be beneficial," or "likely to be ineffective or harmful." This goes beyond a simple analysis of the evidence per se.

Other schemas go even further in recognizing the contribution of consensus to the guidelines process by explicitly stating that support for or advice against a particular intervention may be based predominantly on expert opinion, or expert opinion plus fair evidence that the intervention is beneficial or carries risk in excess of benefit. As evidence-based medicine is, in its essence, the "ability to track down, critically appraise, and incorporate evidence into clinical practice,"[17] it would appear that categorization schemes that take into account research evidence, consensus opinion, and individual clinical experience optimally synthesize available information.

Even when studies are well designed, with conclusions that are statistically sound, there are other questions that still must be answered before these conclusions are used to shape clinical practice. One important question relates to the clinical relevance of the outcomes, ie, even if the treatment or exposure *does* have an impact on the outcome measured, does this change in outcome materially alter the expected overall clinical course, in the absence of the exposure or intervention, or result in a significant improvement or decrease in function? If the answer to this question is "yes," one should also ask whether the change in outcome was of such magnitude as to mandate an immediate reconsideration of current practice patterns.

Issues of cost vs benefit should be considered simultaneously, as one should be able to assess the costs (both direct and indirect) that would be associated with adoption of a new test, procedure, or means of reducing or mitigating exposure. This includes assessment of the cost of any additional testing or treatment that would not have been required otherwise. Overall, the incremental cost of adopting an intervention must be justified by the clinical benefit gained. Proponents of new tests and treatments are apt to lose sight of this very pragmatic concept, especially when they are invested financially or emotionally. When applied to the analysis of the risk of returning to work, the risk of returning patients to work when the evidence is not clear should be weighed against the cost to the patient of not doing so—and the cost to society of not suggesting return to work to patients for whom the literature suggests there is no risk.

Summary

Despite an overall trend toward the use of evidence-based practice parameters, it is difficult to achieve this goal when treatments, tests, and causes of musculoskeletal and other disorders that are defined, at least in part, subjectively are evaluated.

While there are clear guidelines for the identification of high-quality studies, there is a dearth of such studies available for review. It would appear, then, that an evidence-based approach is best described as the incorporating of results from an analysis of the literature, with consensus opinion, to

Chapter 5

formulate clinical guidelines that optimize outcome while minimizing cost and risk. Medicine has not at present reached the point where such guidelines are used routinely, especially when decisions are made regarding individual patients, yet it is reasonable to assume that the quality of available evidence will eventually increase over time so as to facilitate increased reliance on fact and decreased reliance on anecdote in assisting patients in making choices about their health care.

The area of helping patients return to work is one in which there is a particular dearth of available research for review. While only studies that discuss risk factors for work (or other activities) can be reviewed at this time, increased interest in this area should spur additional research that is critical if decisions regard an employee's ability to work are ever to become largely data driven as opposed to primarily based on anecdote and opinion.

References

1. American College of Occupational and Environmental Medicine. *ACOEM Consensus Opinion Statement: The Attending Physician's Role in Helping Patients Return to Work After an Illness or Injury.* Available at: http://acoem.org/guidelines/pdf/Return-to-Work-04-02.pdf. Accessed October 26, 2004.

2. Sackett DL, Rosenberg WM, Gray JA, Richardson WS. Evidence-based medicine: what it is and what it isn't. *BMJ.* 1996;312:71–72.

3. Williams JK. Understanding evidence-based medicine: a primer. *Am J Obstet Gynecol.* 2001;185:275–278.

4. Dawson-Saunders B, Trapp RG. *Basic and Clinical Biostatistics.* 2nd ed. Norwalk, Conn: Appleton and Lange; 1994.

5. Al-Obaidi SM, Nelson RM, Al-Awadhi S, Al-Shuwaie N. The role of anticipation and fear of pain in the persistence of avoidance behavior in patients with chronic low back pain. *Spine.* 2000;25:1126–1131.

6. Buer N, Linton SJ. Fear-avoidance beliefs and catastrophizing: occurrence and risk factor in back pain and ADL in the general population. *Pain.* 2002;99:485–491.

7. Fritz JM, George SZ, Delitto A. The role of fear-avoidance beliefs in acute low back pain: relationships with current and future disability and work status. *Pain.* 2001;94:7–15.

8. Fritz JM, George SZ. Identifying psychosocial variables in patients with acute work-related low back pain: the importance of fear-avoidance beliefs. *Phys Ther.* 2002;82:973–983.

9. Klenerman L, Slade PD, Stanley IM, et al. The prediction of chronicity in patients with an acute attack of low back pain in a general practice setting. *Spine.* 1995;20:478–484.

10. Mannion AF, Junge A, Taimela S, Muntener M, Lorenzo K, Dvorak J. Active therapy for chronic low back pain, part 3: factors influencing self-rated disability and its change following therapy. *Spine.* 2001;26:920–929.

11. Waddell G, Newton M, Henderson I, Somerville D, Main CJ. A Fear-Avoidance Beliefs Questionnaire (FABQ) and the role of fear-avoidance beliefs in chronic low back pain and disability. *Pain.* 1993;52:157–168.

12. Moher D, Dulberg CS, Wells GA. Statistical power, sample size, and their reporting in randomized controlled trials. *JAMA.* 1994;272:122–124.

13. Freiman JA, Chalmers TC, Smith H Jr, Kuebler RR. The importance of beta, the type II error and sample size in the design and interpretation of the randomized control trial: survey of 71 "negative" trials. *N Engl J Med.* 1978;299:690–694.

14. Pocock SJ, Hughes MD, Lee RJ. Statistical problems in the reporting of clinical trials: a survey of three medical journals. *N Engl J Med.* 1987;317:426–432.

15. Agency for Health Care Research and Quality. *Clinical Practice Guidelines Online.* Available at: www.ahrq.gov/clinic/cpgonline.htm. Accessed October 27, 2004.

16. British Medical Journal. *Clinical Evidence.* Available at: http://www.clinicalevidence.com/ceweb/conditions/index.jsp. Accessed October 27, 2004.

17. Rosenberg WM, Sackett DL. On the need for evidence-based medicine. *Therapie.* 1996;51:212–217.

Chapter 5

Chapter 6

Causation Analysis

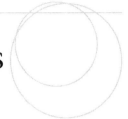

Elizabeth Genovese, MD, MBA

Physicians usually only think about causation when seeking explanations for symptoms or physical findings or attempting to assess what risk factors patients may have for future disease. The topic of causation is relevant only by virtue of its impact, or potential impact, on testing and treatment options.

Once physicians become involved in caring for patients with workers' compensation claims, the relevance of causation changes dramatically. Workers who have decided that they cannot tolerate their jobs often develop symptoms that are not based on physiologic alterations in bodily function (symptoms occur in the absence of impairment), and often do so while performing activities or sustaining exposures that would not ordinarily be expected to result in the symptoms or disorder being claimed. Causation analysis is consequently necessary at the initiation of care (to assess whether the claim is compensable), during care (to ascertain whether new symptoms or findings alter compensability or the ability to return to work), and at the termination of care (to determine whether symptoms or physical findings that may limit work are due to the compensable injury or unrelated medical problems, or are, alternatively, unaccompanied by objective evidence of pathology). Causation analysis is also relevant to the management of patients who have been out of work for reasons other than workers' compensation claims, as it is useful to know the degree to which the presence of specific physical findings, impairment, or disease processes would be expected to limit work options.

Hill Criteria for Causation Analysis

The Hill Criteria are widely cited as the basis for causation analysis. The criteria, listed in Table 6-1, include temporality, biological plausibility, predictive performance, gradient, reversibility, strength of the association, consistency of the association/coherence, experimental evidence/analogy, and specificity.[1]

Table 6-1 The Hill Criteria

Temporality	Related in time—factor occurs *before* disease process
Biological Plausibility	Mechanism, duration of exposure consistent with what one would expect given the nature of the disease process
Predictive Performance	Ability of the association to "predict" future disease in those exposed (especially relevant with long latencies)
Gradient	Dose-response relationship between exposure and result
Reversibility	Disappearance (or partial disappearance) with cessation of exposure
Strength of Association	Degree to which association is demonstrated in the literature—refers to strength, not frequency, of association
Consistency of Association/ Coherence	Consistency of association across studies, subjects, and time—in keeping with other knowledge
Experimental Evidence/ Analogy	Experimental models corroboratory—if done with animals, can extrapolate to humans
Specificity	Degree to which effect is unique to exposure

Temporality refers to the logical need for a cause to precede an effect; however, this should not be interpreted to mean that succession always implies causation. Nonetheless, the temporal relationship between the exposure or injury and the medical condition (or symptoms suggestive of the condition) is the first factor that must be assessed. The illness or disease should occur after the exposure (referred to as "temporal ordering") and within a time period that is reasonable given the nature of the exposure ("temporal contiguity"). In certain situations (such as asbestos, lead, and benzene exposure) there is a long latency between the time of exposure and the appearance of disease. Hence, regardless of whether a temporal relationship appears to be present, determining causality also requires one to assess whether a causal relationship is biologically plausible.

The presence of a *biologically plausible* explanation for a causal relationship between an exposure or injury and a subsequent disease process or event is mandatory. A causal relationship is biologically plausible when the following criteria are met:

1. The relationship between the medical condition and the exposure or injury can be explained anatomically and/or physiologically.
2. The duration, intensity, and/or mechanism of exposure or injury was or is sufficient to cause the illness or injury in question.

Predictive performance is related to biologic plausibility and refers to the ability of an association between an exposure and initial physical finding or disease process to predict future health problems related to that exposure.

Gradient (or dose-response) refers to the expectation that the relationship between the disease process and the risk factor will result in demonstrable increased estimates of risk associated with increased levels of exposure. This is also referred to as *contiguity*. Likewise, the effect would also be expected to be reversible (at least in the early phases of many disease processes) with cessation of exposure. Some exposures lead to an "all or nothing" response, so while evidence of a gradient helps prove causation, absence of a demonstrable dose-response relationship does not necessarily imply that a causal relationship is absent.

Strength of association implies that the stronger the relationship between an independent variable (the risk) and a dependent variable (the disease or injury), the less the likelihood that it is due to an extraneous variable. Strength of association can be assessed by searching the literature for high-quality studies that support the existence of a relationship between the exposure and the disease process or symptoms under evaluation. One must have a thorough understanding of study design and statistical significance to determine whether studies that describe a significant relationship between two events are indeed accurate in doing so.

Consistency of the association is related to strength of association but, rather than relating to an individual study, refers to the degree to which multiple observations or prior studies indicate a continuing association between an exposure and a disease process across different subjects, under different circumstances, and with different measurement instruments. Consistency can be modified by the degree to which certain individualized circumstances and subject characteristics affect the results of a given exposure. This is similar to *coherence*, the degree to which a cause-and-effect explanation for an association is consistent with other knowledge.

Experimental evidence corroborating the results of observational studies and hypotheses will increase the plausibility of inferences that the association between exposure and disease is indicative of a causal relationship. Related to this is the concept of *analogy*, ie, the ability to generalize the results from studies performed with animal models to humans, as often the only experimental studies will have been done with the former.

Specificity is present when an exposure leads to one effect rather than a series of effects—especially if the effect is rarely seen in the absence of the exposure in question. Conversely, in the presence of several different potential causes for a given disease process, specificity also refers to the ability to clearly identify one factor as causal.

Chapter 6

Addressing Causation

In some situations causation is *presumptive*, ie, automatically accepted on the basis of case law or legislation, or has been established through litigation. Under these circumstances causation does not need to be formally addressed, even when there is reason to suspect that the legal construct of presumptive causation may not necessarily be accurate (an example is the policy of municipalities to accept that all coronary artery disease in firefighters is related to their employment).

On the other hand, causality always must be addressed when the referral source has significant doubts regarding the legitimacy of a patient's complaints as related to the initial injury (or alleged injury). Furthermore, even when a clear causal relationship *is* present between an accident and subsequent physical pathology, one may need to state whether an exacerbation, recurrence, or aggravation of a prior condition occurred and to apportion liability accordingly.

The need for apportionment reflects our knowledge that most medical conditions are *multifactorial* in etiology, ie, reflective of more than one physiologic or environmental process. Thus, while in some situations a discrete exposure appears to bring out ("unmask," "light up," or "precipitate") a given condition, the same exposure might not lead to the condition in those who are not predisposed to it by virtue of genetics or anthropomorphic factors. Likewise, an individual who does a great deal of overhead lifting at work may, while painting his or her house, do even more overhead work at home. If the shoulder starts hurting at work it is work related; if it occurs at home it is not. In reality, *both* exposures play a role regardless of where the patient is when his or her shoulder begins to ache.

In some jurisdictions there is no apportionment, as it is held that the patient should be taken "as is." If it is a work injury that causes the patient to become symptomatic or require treatment significantly in excess of what was required previously, this is the employer's sole responsibility. Other states have some degree of apportionment, or apportion for one type of injury (motor vehicle accidents) and not others. Regardless of the need to apportion, physicians should understand the terminology involved and be able to apply it when necessary.

Apportionment

Apportionment involves determining to what extent a condition is related to an event, injury, preexisting condition(s), or unrelated disease process(es). To apportion, the examiner must know the temporal factors and exposures that support the alleged association between the exposure or injury and the disease.

Table 6-2 Terminology Used in Apportionment Analysis

Presumption	Disease process is legislatively determined to result from an exposure or in association with a particular occupation
Precipitation	Injury or exposure causes a "latent" or potential disease process to become manifest
Aggravation	A particular event or exposure permanently worsens a prior condition
Exacerbation	An exposure or injury temporarily worsens a prior condition
Recurrence	Signs or symptoms attributable to a prior illness or injury occur in the absence of a new provocative event

This should be analyzed in conjunction with data from the physical examination and any tests that were performed, along with information regarding the medical history (especially prior injuries) and activities outside the workplace. Table 6-2 outlines the terminology used in apportionment analysis.

As noted earlier in this chapter, an injury or exposure can "precipitate" a disease process for which the claimant was at risk but that had not yet become manifest. A classic example is when a patient has a myocardial infarction while at work (since we can be almost certain that this would have occurred eventually, possibly in a nonwork setting). This differs from *aggravation*, the permanent worsening of a prior condition by a particular event or exposure, in that the latter implies that the condition was already symptomatic or, at the very least, active at the time of the exposure.

Exacerbation is the transient worsening of a prior condition by an injury or illness, with the expectation that the situation will eventually return to baseline. It is often difficult to distinguish exacerbation from aggravation if the patient's condition was already slowly worsening, as one would need to quantify how the condition would have worsened in the absence of the exposure. In situations such as this, one needs to reassess biological plausibility in the context of the prior condition, as in many cases it can be determined that a true injury actually did not occur, ie, the increase in symptoms reflected an inability to tolerate an activity that would not have led to symptoms in the absence of prior disease. Even if symptoms do ultimately diminish, return-to-work decisions are complicated by the expectation that symptoms will again occur once the patient resumes the inciting activity.

A *recurrence* is similar to an exacerbation, but it generally involves the reappearance of signs or symptoms attributable to a prior injury with minimal or no provocation and does not necessarily occur at work. An example of this is the reappearance of radicular symptoms in a patient with a work-related disk herniation while performing an activity that would not ordinarily have been expected to lead to symptoms.

Given the frequency with which terms such as *precipitation* and *aggravation* may be inappropriately applied to link symptoms to work activities in the absence of true injury, it is clear that physicians must evaluate the validity and strength of all postulated causal mechanisms both at the time of "injury" and when a patient returns to work. Biological implausibility should be identified at the patient's initial examination by asking whether the mechanism and duration of exposure could realistically account for the clinical presentation. One must ask "can it occur" (is it possible that the mechanism of injury could account for the symptoms or physical findings?), "does it occur" (has this association been demonstrated in the literature?), and "did it occur" (is the history as provided by the patient accurate—is a causal link operative in *this* situation?).

This is especially important when one considers that the legal definition of a causal relationship often is based on determining whether an association was "probable" or "possible." It is *probable* if the chance of an exposure (or alleged exposure) and the symptoms or findings being related is greater than 50%. It is *possible* if the chance of a relationship is deemed to be less than 50%. This ultimately can be reduced to determining whether the probability of association was 49% (possible) or 51% (probable); there is little in the field of medicine that can allow one to make this inherently subjective determination with any degree of accuracy. While the United States Supreme Court, in the *Daubert* case, held that federal court testimony must be grounded in the methods and procedures of science and must be based on more than simply subjective belief or unsupported speculation to be held as relevant and reliable,[2] this standard is not routinely used in many jurisdictions. Thus, regardless of what would be dictated by science, decisions regarding causation often are founded on the use of legal terminology that is anything *but* scientific.

Causality Determination

There is a logical process that should be used to assess causation both when a patient initially presents with claims of having sustained an injury and when determinations are made regarding return to work.

At the time of initial presentation, the patient should be asked to describe *precisely* (in his or her own words) what happened, and a comprehensive medical history should be obtained. Possible questions are as follows:

- What were you doing at the time your symptoms occurred? (This would include a complete description of the activity being performed, body positioning [including a description of how any weights or other relevant materials were being held and managed], relevant environmental factors, the duration of the activity, what symptoms developed initially, and how they then progressed.)

- Have symptoms worsened or improved since the time of injury? (If they have worsened, it may be appropriate to ask the patient to provide an opinion regarding *why* this occurred, especially if he or she has not continued to do the provocative activity. Alternatively, if symptoms did not occur until some time after the alleged injury, the patient must be asked why he or she nonetheless believes that they are linked to the putatively causal event.)
- Do any of your coworkers have similar symptoms? (This question would be applied to scenarios in which a patient claims that symptoms are reflective of overuse or a repetitive stress disorder.)
- Have you ever had symptoms like this before? If so, did they occur as a result of a clearly identifiable exposure or injury, or did they occur spontaneously?
- Do you have any other symptoms or medical problems? (Particular attention should be paid to eliciting a history of prior conditions that might be relevant to the current situation.)
- What are your hobbies or other activities outside of work? Have these ever led to symptoms similar to those with which you are presenting today?
- Do you like your job? Why or why not? How well do you get along with your supervisor and coworkers? (It might be necessary to be somewhat indirect in getting this information.)
- What are you doing with your time now that you are not working? (This is asked if the patient is out of work.)
- Have you had any prior problems with depression or drug or alcohol dependence?

During the physical examination, the physician should do the following:

- Thoroughly evaluate the body part(s) or organ system(s) that would be responsible for symptoms or could have potentially sustained injury.
- Assess whether the patient's movement patterns are consistent with the symptoms and injury being claimed.
- Perform other maneuvers to assess the possibility of symptom magnification (if appropriate).
- Review all relevant diagnostic testing, if any.
- Determine whether any of the physical findings limit performance of some, or all, work activities.

Chapter 6

If there are any doubts regarding causation, the physician should:

- Attempt to obtain any relevant medical records that are known to exist.
- Contact the patient's supervisor or employer to see whether there are any current or potential conflicts that may be relevant.
- Review the medical literature to determine the extent, nature, and quality of any studies that would support or refute the existence of a causal relationship.

Should the presence of a causal relationship be accepted, it is important to continue to assess causation on an ongoing basis. Possible questions to ask include the following:

- Is the patient progressing as expected? If not, is there a physiologic explanation for his or her lack of progress? In particular, if symptoms have worsened, one must ask whether this is consistent with the natural course of the disorder or whether the patient is doing other activities that might account for it.
- Are there symptoms or are body parts involved that were not involved initially? If so, is there a biologically plausible explanation?

Finally, when it becomes time to return the patient to work, the following questions should be asked:

- Have symptoms resolved? If so, does the nature of the underlying disorder suggest that it will again become manifest if the patient returns to his or her prior activities? If symptoms have not resolved, is there a physiologic explanation for their continuation?
- If there *is* a physiologic explanation for the continuation of symptoms, is there any reason to believe that return-to-work activities will result in physiologic alterations that cause them to worsen? If not, are there any other *objective* data that suggest the patient is no longer capable of doing his or her former job?
- If there is *not* a physiologic explanation for the continuation of symptoms, is there any other medically defensible rationale for work restrictions?

Summary

Causation assessment is an important component of return to work, as the determination of whether there is a relationship between work activities and symptoms, physical findings, or disease processes affects whether patients have a compensable injury and, regardless of compensability, whether they should be restricted from some forms of work. Temporal relationship and biological plausibility are the most critical criteria that must be met to state that a causal relationship exists, and these criteria are optimally accompanied by at least several other criteria such as gradient, reversibility, strength and consistency of association, coherence, corroboratory physical evidence, and analogy in the medical literature.

If criteria for causation have been met, and patient symptoms are consistent with a physiologically definable process, it would appear reasonable to apply available data in assessing whether there should be any work restrictions. After the patient has had adequate time to recover (and during the treatment course), causation analysis should be applied toward assessing the physiologic basis of continued complaints and determining to what degree continued or further work restrictions are warranted. When objective evidence of a causal link between patient symptoms and work activities is not apparent, it should be recognized that symptoms most likely reflect an intolerance of work and not an inability to work. The focus then should be on identifying whether there are any risk factors that preclude work. In the absence of these, it should be stated that there are no medical contraindications to the patient working.

Chapter 6

References

1. Hill AB. The environment and disease association or causation? *Proc R Soc Med.* 1965;58:295–300.

2. Annas GJ. Burden of proof: judging science and protecting public health in (and out of) the courtroom. *Am J Public Health.* 1999;89:490–493.

The Functional Capacity Evaluation: Is It Helpful?

David C. Randolph, MD, MPH, Trang H. Nguyen, MD, and Phillip Osborne, MD

The *functional capacity evaluation* (FCE) is a test designed to evaluate an individual's physical ability to perform certain tasks or activities generally associated with work. The *Dictionary of Occupational Titles*,[1] published by the United States Department of Labor, provides 20 separate functions on which work capabilities are based:

- Lifting
- Climbing
- Balancing
- Stooping
- Kneeling
- Crouching
- Crawling
- Reaching
- Pushing/pulling
- Standing

- Carrying
- Talking
- Hearing
- Tasting/smelling
- Near/far acuity
- Sitting
- Walking
- Handling
- Fingering
- Feeling

When properly performed, the FCE can systematically evaluate these functions. The performance of the functional test should be predicated on information objectively obtained by an appropriately trained medical professional. Information and interpretation gained through the functional test should take into account the historical, medical, and physical examination findings, and the psychological and motivational status of the individual.

Individuals may be removed from the work force for a variety of reasons. The physician attempting to evaluate an individual's capability of returning to work activity needs to understand the nature of the absence from work to ensure that the condition that has resulted in the absence has stabilized so that returning to work activities will not pose a threat to the health and well-being of the patient or the coworkers. Clearly, the physical and medical status of the individual must then be a part of this evaluation process before any such formal evaluation of an individual's capabilities is undertaken.

Psychological issues can occur in association with absence as either a primary or a secondary phenomenon. Such psychological issues, like medical issues, can impact the return-to-work status. These issues must be at the forefront of consideration with respect to work abilities.

Assuming the stability of the medical and psychological issues, the practicing physician may legitimately search for answers to questions with respect to an individual's ability to perform work. This is the purpose behind the FCE: to provide objective, verifiable information with respect to the patient's ability and safety in terms of returning to tasks and activities associated with work.

The FCE and statements of return to work should consider the patient's medical history and procedures, his or her overall medical and psychological status, the results of a well-performed physical examination, physiologic measurements (ie, heart rate, blood pressure, and respiratory rate), height and weight, pertinent psychosocial issues, pain issues, and unrelated health issues. In other words, the family physician will have the advantage of evaluating multiple aspects of the individual's clinical presentation to ensure that return-to-work recommendations are appropriate and well founded.

It should be remembered that the FCE can provide input and direction in the process of determining work and activity ability. The FCE should not be considered alone without considering related medical factors and issues.

The Purpose of the Functional Capacity Evaluation

A variety of questions can be addressed through the performance of an FCE. Most commonly the test is used to provide direct input with respect to an individual's "safe" ability to return to the workforce. Specific questions addressing lifting ability and/or unique activity tolerances (ie, manual dexterity, overhead lifting) can also be assessed. The primary care physician may wish to specifically address these issues when requesting the FCE.

Simply put, the FCE addresses whether the individual can return to work and whether there are work limitations (things the individual is not able to do). *FCEs do not assess risk,* but rather tolerance, and/or occasionally capacity.

The FCE can also be used to monitor progress through rehabilitation, guide further treatment recommendations, assist in disability rating, or set rehabilitative goals.[2] From a more global standpoint, the FCE can be used to match an individual to a particular occupation or job task or to determine his or her overall work capabilities. Each type of FCE can become progressively more involved and is therefore more time consuming.

The Elements of a Functional Capacity Evaluation

The process of determining functional ability has several parts, all with factors and issues about which the primary care physician should be familiar. The physician needs to understand the evaluator, the evaluation process, the results, and the report interpretation. These factors will be individually addressed and discussed in this section.

The Evaluator

Currently, no standards exist with respect to who can actually perform the FCE.[3] Individuals from a variety of backgrounds are performing these tests. Evaluators include athletic trainers, chiropractors, vocational evaluators, registered nurses, physical therapists, occupational therapists, trained assistants in those fields, and exercise physiologists.

Commonly, FCEs are offered through freestanding physical therapy centers, occupational medical clinics, "evaluation centers," or hospital-based physical therapy centers. It is not uncommon for such centers to use certain commercial systems for the functional test. These systems became popular in the 1980s and 1990s, and some of them are no longer commercially available. While validity and reliability will be discussed later in this chapter, it should be noted that most of these systems and/or testing protocols have very little published scientific credibility.[4]

The evaluator and the evaluation facility should be carefully chosen, as the results often reflect the evaluator's training and medical knowledge. The quality of the return-to-work decision should be based on a cautiously

Chapter 7

performed and well-explained process. If FCEs are to be used regularly, the primary care physician should become familiar with the evaluator, the process, and the facility. If FCEs are not to be used regularly, physicians should consider referring the return-to-work decision to a physician who handles such decisions routinely. All parties involved should be comfortable with the facility and the evaluator so that the decision provided is readily believable.

The Evaluation Process

A standard FCE can be expected to take 2 to 3 hours; however, the duration of the examination is highly variable. Some tests last only 1 hour, and some last up to several days. There are no standards with respect to testing duration.[3]

The process itself should begin with consent forms, various historical and patient information forms, and an understanding between the evaluator and the evaluee regarding the safety issues of the functional test. Specifically, the examination process can be terminated at will by either the evaluator or the evaluee, and this understanding should be a part of the formalized process at the very beginning. The totality of the test process should be explained and a clear understanding of that process by the evaluee should be documented before testing begins. The introductory process should include an opportunity for questions and answers. A signed consent form should be obtained before the FCE begins, with clear written parameters outlined.

The process of evaluating an individual's work ability should address certain physically definable activities. These physical activities are listed at the beginning of this chapter. Information obtained from the FCE can be applied to work-related demands and capability recommendations can be provided.

Some of these physical demands (eg, sitting) can be evaluated during an interview or by observation of the individuals while completing the test forms. Others (eg, lifting) should be independently tested by means of an objective, written protocol.

Endurance

Aerobic capacity becomes an extremely important issue with respect to functional capabilities, as the individual must be capable of performing work activities at a set pace for a period of approximately 8 hours. While a large variety of tests exists for determination of aerobic ability (ranging from cardiac treadmill testing to the simpler submaximal step testing), some form of acceptable cardiac endurance testing should accompany the functional testing process. A list of treadmill protocols and their conversion into metabolic equivalents (or energy units) (METs) can be found in the American Medical Association's (AMA's) *Guides to the Evaluation of Permanent Impairment,*

Fourth Edition[5] and *Fifth Edition.*[6] A thorough documentation of aerobic capability should be included in the report. MET levels should be calculated and provided with this portion of the evaluation. The MET levels can be readily converted into work capabilities (ie, light, moderate, and heavy work) by means of Table 5.8 in Chapter 5 of the AMA's *Guides, Fifth Edition.*[6]

If the FCE needs to be terminated before completion for any reason, the rationale behind the test discontinuation should be properly recorded in the report. For example, if the individual indicates that after walking on a treadmill at a particular pace he or she became short of breath, this should be documented and vital signs and observations of the presence or absence of dyspnea recorded. This process can aid the physician in determining the presence of a physiologic basis for incapacity.

Strength/Lifting

Lifting is one of the more popular components of the functional test. It remains an important portion of the questions posed to the primary care physician with respect to return-to-work issues. Some of the common approaches to strength testing will be discussed. Usually the term *strength* refers to lifting ability. Lifting can be tested in a number of different ways.[7,8] Isometric lifting correlates poorly to real-world function. Isometric testing (pulling on an immovable object) is a technique for approximating infrequent maximum lifting capacity. It is a reasonably safe technique in terms of testing lifting capacity.[9,10] Isometric testing should not be interpreted alone but rather should be correlated with the results of dynamic strength testing obtained through isoinertial techniques (eg, lifting weights in a crate).[11-14] In these protocols, the maximum safe lifting capacity is predetermined on the basis of gender- and age-specific maximum heart rate. Isoinertial testing is accomplished through a "progressive dynamic lift" procedure where an individual is provided gradually increasing weights with continuous observation of body mechanics. The use of accessory muscles, pulse, blood pressure, and respiratory rate are monitored during testing to determine a maximum safe lifting ability. Lifting activities are often performed from floor to knuckle height (lumbar), elbow height, and shoulder height (cervical).[15] Again, there are no standard protocols with respect to lifting.

Grip strength is often referred to as a test of upper-extremity strength. It should be noted that grip strength does not necessarily correlate with the functional level of performance of activities of daily living. The AMA's *Guides, Fifth Edition* provides a description of this test in Chapter 16.[6] In general, it can be used to obtain information on hand strength and the level of participation and consistency during the evaluation process.[16,17] One grip strength protocol involves five-position testing using a Jamar dynamometer (testing grip strength at each of five different spacings or separation

Chapter 7

distances for the handles of the instrument). The results should reveal a bell-shaped curve with a peak force between position number two and number three. "Flat" curves or linear lines may reflect incomplete participation in the examination process due to symptom magnification, or due to pain during testing. The findings should correlate with the physical examination. Normative data for grip strength based on age and gender can be found in Table 16-32 in Chapter 16 of the AMA's *Guides, Fifth Edition.*[6,18]

Pain
Monitoring levels of pain in response to a physical challenge is an important adjunct to determining work capacity. If an individual reports heightened levels of pain during the testing process, vital signs should be documented at that time to determine and verify physiologic correspondence to the pain levels. Again, this helps provide a physiologic basis to work and activity capacity.

Coordination and Balance
Suspicions regarding difficulties with coordination and balance should be detected during the pretest history and physical examination. Should symptoms or examination findings raise significant concerns, further diagnostic studies are mandated. During the FCE, balance and coordination can be verified through simple observation (eg, during the performance of endurance testing with either the treadmill or the step test). Coordination and balance can be further verified during observation of lifting and strength testing activities. Verification of observations made during the FCE should be correlated with the physical examination findings before any judgment with respect to altered function or work incapacity is considered.

Results and Report Interpretation
The FCE report is often lengthy and filled with a number of graphs, tables, and charts. Information and data provided may be of limited value or meaning. A good FCE will have a summary making recommendations for return-to-work abilities under safe circumstances. These should be confirmed by a quick review of the raw data provided by the evaluator. For example, if an individual is deemed unable to lift more than 20 lb, then raw data provided by the evaluator should confirm not only that inability but also some physiologic parameter change (ie, alterations in pulse, blood pressure, and/or respirations) indicating that the evaluee provided adequate effort during the performance of that phase of the test. The report should fully explain less-than-predicted results or the early termination of testing, eg, whether the observed findings and recommendations were due to pain, marked elevation of vital signs, or unsafe lifting practices. The conclusions presented should be well documented and provide the primary care physician with medical substantiation to make sound clinical judgments with respect to work activity. Conclusions provided by the FCE report should be accompanied by

objective physiologic measures and should provide some statement with respect to effort during the testing process. The report should provide summary recommendations in a clear, concise fashion with reference to portions of the test demonstrating the source of the conclusions. It is unacceptable to provide no summary and recommendations, or to provide recommendations without substantiation. Raw data should always be provided with the test summary and conclusions.

Validity and Reliability of the Functional Capacity Evaluation

Validity refers to whether a particular test or procedure measures what it is supposed to measure. The results of a test should be used to make inferences and, more specifically, to make recommendations for return to work. *Reliability* refers to the reproducibility of the result of a given test, in other words, whether it can reasonably be expected that a similar result will be obtained if the same test is performed on different days or by a different examiner. Reliability must be established for a test to have validity. Unfortunately, most commercially available functional systems do not have published reliability or validity data.

In 1994, Lechner et al[19] briefly summarized the reliability and validity of 10 existing FCE systems. Four systems (Smith, Isernhagen, Matheson-Work Tolerance Screening, and Sweat) had some types of validity studied. Only the Smith FCE evaluated predictive validity that was published in a peer-reviewed journal.[20] Because of the small sample size, the high rate of loss to follow-up, and inadequate subject description, the predictive validity of this system remains questionable. During this period examined by Lechner et al, only two systems had studied reliability (Matheson and Baltimore Therapeutic Equipment [BTE]). The BTE reliability study was not published, and the authors did not provide details for the study by Matheson et al.

In 1998 King et al[4] reported that only the Physical Work Performance Evaluation had peer-reviewed published validity. However, the evidence to evaluate the validity of this study was not provided. It was unclear from the King et al article whether the original studies were evaluated. A review of the original study by Lechner et al[19] indicated inadequate evidence of validity and reliability secondary to questionable randomization of subjects (subjects were volunteers), possible confounders (ie, educational level, age, gender, and social economic status), which were not considered in the statistical analysis, and lack of information on the work level recommended and the actual work level correctly and incorrectly determined. In 1999, Innes and Straker[21] reviewed the validity of 28 FCE systems or protocols. Validity

Chapter 7

was graded on a scale of zero to five and "good, moderate, poor, or un-known" according to how the data were presented. A level of zero meant no validity, and a level of four referred to studies published in non-peer-reviewed journals. A level of five meant results were reported in a peer-reviewed journal. Although some FCE studies are published in peer-reviewed journals, the methodologies for most of these studies have been question-able. The author cautioned that systems or protocols with a validity level of four to five are not necessarily equated with sound scientific methodology.[21]

Recently published articles have studied sensitivity, specificity, and predic-tive validity of FCE. Lemstra et al[22] concluded that when the FCE was used to differentiate submaximal and maximal effort, sensitivity was 65% and specificity was 84%. The FCE was not considered helpful in determining the accuracy of submaximal effort. In other words, if an individual perform-ing the functional test produces less than a maximal effort, the evaluator's ability to detect this is questionable.

Gross et al[23,24] examined the validity of the Isernhagen FCE protocol in pre-dicting timely return to work. The FCE results showed that few participants could pass all protocol components, yet most had benefits terminated and returned to work. The follow-up study showed a 20% reinjury rate. The conclusions were that the FCE had little predictive validity in safe return to work. The outcome measure in the study (reinjury) was based on historic administrative data. The conclusion is limited by the small sample size. These recent studies have limitations such as lack of blinding of subjects, possible randomization bias, small sample size, and questionable definitions used to analyze the study's outcomes. Conclusions provided by the study should be interpreted in light of these limitations. Further research in this area is warranted.

Despite these issues, the properly performed FCE can be a helpful adjunct, along with historic information, physical examination, and diagnostic stud-ies, to assist the primary care physician in the return-to-work process.

Using a Functional Capacity Evaluation to Make Return-to-Work Recommendations

The primary care physician will often find cooperation in a return to work if the patient or injured worker is an active participant in the process. To be most successful, the process of returning an individual to work starts from the day that absence begins. Returning the individual to meaningful activity should be an ongoing conversation and discussion. This approach will often avoid hostility or confrontations when the time to return to work draws near.

Open communications and repeated discussions about returning to work will further open conversations and address issues of potential conflict with respect to this process. If there are such issues present (eg, personality conflicts with the supervisor), these can be addressed and discussed early on rather than only at the final office visit.

Ultimately, the decision to return someone to work, and under what, if any, restrictions, is one that should be based on the total clinical picture, including a good physical examination. The FCE remains only a portion of that decision. Hall et al[25] found that the group of workers with back injuries who returned to work without restrictions (ignoring those recommended by an FCE) had a higher rate of successful outcome than the group provided with restrictions based on an FCE. Clearly, there is a need for future studies regarding the utility of FCE in the return-to-work process.

Again, even with the aforementioned limitations of the FCE, meaningful conclusions can be made with respect to an individual's ability to work. With information gathered from lifting observations and endurance testing, real-world conclusions can be reached with respect to an individual's ability to work an 8-hour day and lift objects of a given weight on a full-time basis.

The information gleaned from the functional test should be openly discussed with the patient-injured worker. An open discussion with respect to the mechanics of the actual job should accompany a review of the FCE.

Summary

It is apparent that solid scientific information with respect to functional testing is still lacking. Therefore, physicians should exercise caution when interpreting these data in drawing conclusions or making recommendations regarding activity capability.

The information from the FCE should be coupled with a thorough understanding of the individual's medical problem and correlated with his or her medical history, an understanding of the injury, and the job tasks to make an educated decision with respect to the individual's capability of performing any particular task or activity.

References

1. US Department of Labor. *The Dictionary of Occupational Titles.* 4th ed. Washington, DC: US Department of Labor; 1991. Available at: www.oalj.dol.gov/libdot.htm. Accessed October 27, 2004.

2. Isernhagen SJ. *Functional Capacity Assessment.* London, England: Churchill-Livingstone; 1990.

3. Rothstein JM, Campbell SK, Echternach JL. Standards for tests and measurements in physical therapy practice. *Phys Ther.* 1991;71:589–622.

4. King PM, Tuckwell N, Barrett TE. A critical review of functional capacity evaluations. *Phys Ther.* 1998;78:852–866.

5. Doege TC, Houston TP. *Guides to the Evaluation of Permanent Impairment.* 4th ed. Chicago, Ill: AMA Press; 1993.

6. Cocchiarella L, Andersson GB. *Guides to the Evaluation of Permanent Impairment.* 5th ed. Chicago, Ill: AMA Press; 2001.

7. Aghazadeh F, Ayoub MM. A comparison of dynamic- and static-strength models for prediction of lifting capacity. *Ergonomics.* 1985;28:1409–1417.

8. Garg A, Mital A, Asfour SS. A comparison of isometric strength and dynamic lifting capability. *Ergonomics.* 1980;23:13–27.

9. Chaffin DB. Human strength capability and low-back pain. *J Occup Med.* 1974;16:248–254.

10. Chaffin DB. Ergonomics guide for the assessment of human static strength. *Am Ind Hyg Assoc J.* 1975;36:505–511.

11. Jay MA, Lamb JM, Watson RL, et al. Sensitivity and specificity of the indicators of sincere effort of the EPIC lift capacity test on a previously injured population. *Spine.* 2000;25:1405–1412.

12. Mayer TG, Barnes D, Kishino ND, et al. Progressive isoinertial lifting evaluation, I: a standardized protocol and normative database. *Spine.* 1988; 13:993–997.

13. Matheson LN. Relationships among age, body weight, resting heart rate, and performance in a new test of lift capacity. *J Occup Rehabil.* 1996; 6:225–237.

14. Matheson LN, Mooney V, Jarvis G. Progressive lifting capacity with masked weights: reliability study. Presented at the meeting of the International Society for the Study of Lumbar Spine; Boston, Mass; 1990.

15. Karwowski W, Marras WS. *Occupational Ergonomics Handbook.* Boca Raton, Fla: CRC Press LLC; 1999.

16. Bohannon RW. Test-retest reliability of hand-held dynamometry during a single session of strength assessment. *Phys Ther.* 1986;66:206–209.

17. Bohannon RW, Andrews AW. Interrater reliability of hand-held dynamometry. *Phys Ther.* 1987;67:931–933.

18. Mathiowetz V, Kashman N, Volland G, Weber K, Dowe M, Rogers S. Grip and pinch strength: normative data for adults. *Arch Phys Med Rehabil.* 1985; 66:69–74.

19. Lechner DE, Jackson JR, Roth DL, Straaton KV. Reliability and validity of a newly developed test of physical work performance. *J Occup Med.* 1994;36:997–1004.

20. Smith SL, Cunningham S, Weinberg R. The predictive validity of the functional capacities evaluation. *Am J Occup Ther.* 1986;40:564–567.

21. Innes E, Straker L. Validity of work-related assessments. *Work.* 1999;13:125–152.

22. Lemstra M, Olszynski WP, Enright W. The sensitivity and specificity of functional capacity evaluations in determining maximal effort: a randomized trial. *Spine.* 2004;29:953–959.

23. Gross DP, Battie MC, Cassidy JD. The prognostic value of functional capacity evaluation in patients with chronic low back pain, part 1: timely return to work. *Spine.* 2004;29:914–919.

24. Gross DP, Battie MC. The prognostic value of functional capacity evaluation in patients with chronic low back pain, part 2: sustained recovery. *Spine.* 2004;29:920–924.

25. Hall H, McIntosh G, Melles T, Holowachuk B, Wai E. Effect of discharge recommendations on outcome. *Spine.* 1994;19:2033–2037.

Chapter 7

Chapter 8

The Medical and Legal Aspects of Return-to-Work Decision Making

Paul F. Waldner, JD, and Lezzlie E. Hornsby, JD

*T*he jury was riveted on the scene being played out in front of them. On the witness stand was an orthopedic surgeon, a middle-aged guy with a hairline headed toward the occiput, crow's feet that stretched from the corners of his eyes almost to his ears, and a paunch you could set your coffee cup on. His suit looked as if it had been made for a smaller, shorter man—tight at the shoulders and arms, too much wrist showing, cuffs riding about three inches above the top of sagging, faded black socks, exposing bleached, hairless legs. He was sweating like an NBA player in the fourth quarter, with face flushed, eyes darting around the courtroom, fidgeting like he was sitting on top of a bed of fire ants. By contrast, the lawyer standing in front of him was tall and trim, tanned, confident, dressed in a custom-made, navy blue gabardine suit. He looked like he had just stepped from the pages of Esquire. Sporting a look of barely perceptible amusement, he was speaking to the physician much like a concerned parent scolding a petulant child.

"Now doctor," he asked, "Certainly you're familiar with the state's workers' compensation act, aren't you?"

"Well . . . I guess I know parts of it," the surgeon replied with considerable hesitation.

"Would one of those parts be that section which has to do with the circumstances under which a gravely injured worker," and then he paused, gesturing toward his client, the apparent Gravely Injured Worker, "will be allowed to return to his job?"

"I . . . I . . . guess so," the surgeon acknowledged, in a low, shaky voice, laced with trepidation and uncertainty.

"The fate of my client's family is at stake in this proceeding and you're going to sit there and guess about your testimony?" the lawyer growled at him, simultaneously sporting a look of disdain and incredulity.

It had never occurred to the physician when he had dictated his narrative to the compensation carrier early one evening, as he tried to rush through the mountain of paperwork on his desk to get home to his family and have dinner with them for the first time in weeks, that the fate of the gravely injured man's family hinged on the adjectives dribbling out of his mouth. He had thought that he was just dictating a report. No one had told him during his orthopedic residency and fellowship that the practice of orthopedic surgery is really a mix of law and medicine—a whole bunch of law and medicine. He loved the medicine, but the law part of his practice had about as much appeal to him as colon cancer.

Many physicians have had some of the same feelings as the orthopedic surgeon in the preceding tragedy. Are law and medicine really like oil and water, or can they peacefully coexist? Can physicians *ever* master the seemingly hundreds of statutes, regulations, and legal principles that seem to pop up all the time in those miserable depositions?

One of the issues that many physicians—family practitioners, orthopedic surgeons, neurologists, etc—frequently are faced with is when and under what circumstances a patient can be told that he or she is free to return to work. Can he go back to the same job? Can she perform her usual tasks without restrictions? What are their usual tasks? Is a finding of permanent impairment or disability inconsistent with releasing a patient to return to work? Is there a legal test floating around somewhere that has to be considered before the phrase "return to work" is even uttered? Does any law apply to the decision to return a patient to work and, if so, what law is it? What portion of the law applies? Are there any exceptions? Does this patient come under any of them?

This chapter discusses the hows and whys of returning a patient to work and attempts to enlighten, guide, and reassure physicians that most (though, admittedly, not all) of the anxiety can be eliminated. The chapter explores the various statutes that most commonly come into play, focuses on the relevant portions of them, and advises physicians on how to comply with them and stay out of trouble.

Promoting the Return to Work: The Physician's Responsibility

Is work good for people? Are human beings better off as productive individuals than as nonproductive, dependent souls? If an injury, disease, or condition has caused a temporary hiatus in an individual's employment, should he or she be encouraged to resume usual activities as soon as possible?

Obviously, each of these questions has the same answer. As discussed in Chapter 1, work *is* good for people. Being productive and independent *is* preferable to the alternative. Return to work *should* be encouraged. However, there are certain disincentives that have to be addressed and overcome. Some citizens are injured under circumstances that actually promote staying off work. What are the responsibilities of the physician when faced with this type of situation? Do any or all of the answers to the questions in the previous paragraph turn from yes to no?

It is rumored that occasionally an injured worker will hire an attorney, and that the attorney will actually suggest to the treating physician that his or her client should be kept off work. There are also rumors that the same suggestion will be made to the injured worker. What is a physician to do when caught between the goal of returning a patient to work as soon as possible and the pressures that may be applied to keep that person off work?

The solution is obvious. If morals and ethics were eliminated from the discussion, and only what is best *medically* were considered, the patient would be better off returning to work than staying at home. Without question, the patient would be better off *psychologically* at work as opposed to staying at home. In that case, one might ask, why in the world would an injured person want to stay off work? There would have to be some perceived economic benefit in doing so. Would there be a larger workers' compensation settlement or car wreck claim? Does the injured person feel that the additional dollars the lawyer may be able to obtain will be far in excess of what the person would have earned had he or she gone back to work earlier? Is there a point where a legitimate claim for injuries, disability, or impairment converts to a scam? Certainly there can be, and the treating physician is in the best position to head that nonsense off "at the pass."

Early in the physician–patient relationship, it is important that the physician establish goals with the patient. The physician should ask the following questions of the patient: "Do you agree that our goal is to restore you as closely as we can to your preaccident condition? Do you feel that your job is more important to you and your family than your claim is? Do you expect

Chapter 8

me to be truthful and honest with you about your condition? Do you realize that the longer you're off work, the greater the chance that your job will be given to someone else?" The partnership that must develop between the physician and the injured worker must be based on a mutual agreement of just what the goal is.

Any suggestion or hint—from the patient or the patient's lawyer—that the period a patient stays off work be extended should be met quickly with considerable resistance. The same is obviously true if pressure is applied from an insurance company or claims personnel to encourage a premature return to work. The treating physician has the last, loudest, and most important word on this issue. Attempts to usurp that authority or to abuse that responsibility should never be tolerated.

Knowing the Job Requirements and Knowing the Law

An insurance agent breaks his ankle in a company softball game and he can go back to work in a few days. An ironworker suffers an identical injury on the job and he might be off work for months. A statute might allow an injured employee to return to work only when he or she can perform the complete requirements of the job. Another statute might require that an employee return to work when recovery has progressed to the point that *any* work can be performed.

And where does all of this leave the treating physician? The answer to most return-to-work questions is not in *Campbell's Operative Orthopedics.*[1] It may or may not be in the revised fourth edition of *The Dictionary of Occupational Titles*[2] or *The Transitional Classification of Jobs.*[3]

It would certainly be advisable for any physician who is going to be faced with making return-to-work decisions to have *some* idea about the physical requirements of the work itself, even if not hands-on knowledge. The two best sources for this information are the employer and the employee. A questionnaire could be developed to be used at the time of the first office visit and, possibly, a similar questionnaire could be sent to the employer. The return-to-work decision made by a physician is a lot easier to defend if the physician has documented information about the job itself. Of equal importance is having some knowledge of the applicable rule, statute, or regulation regarding the issue of returning to work after an injury. What law applies? What *section* of the law applies? Would it be covered by state or federal law—or both? Can the patient be returned to light duty with some restrictions or only full duty with no restrictions?

One certain way to determine the circumstances under which a patient may return to work is to simply write the party paying the bill and ask. Whether it is the employer, the workers' compensation insurance company, or the state or federal agency, they should be able to address medical–legal questions about the circumstances that control the return to work. Additionally, the reply letter to the physician's inquiry is valuable documentation in the patient's chart.

Some Statutes That Apply to Return-to-Work Determinations

A variety of statutes may apply to the rights, obligations, and benefits of an injured worker. Determining which statute has application in a specific case is usually done by considering who the employer is and what kind of work was being performed. The overwhelming majority of on-the-job injuries will be covered by workers' compensation—a state statute. There are specialized federal statutes, however, that exist to protect workers in certain industries (eg, maritime, railroad, mining) that Congress has deemed to be essential to commerce. Some of the statutes are administered by state or federal agencies, some by commissions, and some by the courts. While many of the statutes are discussed in this chapter, the following practice tips should apply, irrespective of the applicable statute:

1. Determine at the first office visit which statute applies.
2. Notify the administering entity that the claimant is being treated.
3. Ask for printed rules or guideline for return-to-work determinations.

State Statutes: Workers' Compensation

All 50 states have their own workers' compensation statute. Essentially, workers' compensation is a compromise between an employer and its employees. The employee receives all of the reasonable and necessary medical care for his or her injuries and a predetermined percentage of wages, together with a lump-sum settlement based on disability and/or impairment. In return, the employer is given a limitation of liability regardless of the extent of the injury. Neither the employee nor the employer is required to prove negligence to activate the statute—only that an accidental injury (or occupational disease) was incurred in the course and scope of employment.

Workers' compensation requires reasonable and necessary medical treatment and temporary and permanent disability benefits for an employee sustaining a work-related injury.[4] It also provides benefits for partial and total disability. In many states, an employer with one employee is a covered

Chapter 8

employer. An employee who incurs an injury that arises out of and in the course of the employment relationship is protected.[4] An employee who has a preexisting condition that is aggravated or accelerated by the workplace is also protected.[4] It is unlawful to terminate an employee's employment for exercising rights under the workers' compensation statute.

An employee must report a work-related injury within a specific number of days of the occurrence of the illness or injury. However, failure to report within the specified time period may not foreclose financial recovery. State variations apply.[4]

One of the purposes of the various workers' compensation statutes is to avoid litigation. Employers who carry workers' compensation insurance make themselves immune to suit by their employees for injuries, with very few exceptions (eg, gross negligence resulting in death, intentional acts). While most workers' compensation claims are handled within the specific agency that administers the statute, some states provide for jury trials as a method of appeal.

Physicians need to be aware that some workers' compensation statutes treat *disability* and *impairment* as virtually the same determination. Some statutes actually assign disability awards out of impairment guides. Irrespective of the state in which the injury occurs, the principal determinations will be the nature and extent of the disability, including whether it is temporary or permanent, partial or total.

Federal Statutes
As stated earlier, Congress has identified certain industries as those that are critical to commerce. Accordingly, workers within those industries are given the protection of federal statutes.

Maritime and Railroad Workers
Working on a ship and working around railroads are two of the most hazardous areas of employment in the country. Many ships are just floating petrochemical plants—except that they are wet, rolling, and pitching. Injuries on ships are often unavoidable. Working on, around, or between railroad cars is just as dangerous because of the weight of the cars and the fact that, once in motion, it takes considerable time and distance to stop them. However, the maritime and railroad industries are both vital to commerce. To attract and retain qualified, skilled workers, Congress deemed them to be worthy of special protection.

In 1920, Congress enacted the Jones Act (41 Stat 988, c 250, Merchant Marine Act 1920, §33, 46 App USCA §688) to remove the maritime law's bar to a seaman's (or woman's) suit for negligence. Under the Jones Act, which makes the provisions of the Federal Employers' Liability Act (FELA) (45 USCA §§51-60) applicable to seamen injured in the course of their employment, employees have a right of recovery for injuries resulting from the negligence of their employer and its agents or employees.[5] As a result, an injured seaman can recover damages from the employer when the employer's or a coworker's negligence causes an injury—just like their counterparts in the railroad industry. The Jones Act applies only to seamen, who are persons with an employment-related connection to a vessel in navigation and who contribute to the vessel's function or mission, ie, persons who do the ship's work. A person whose work is covered under the Longshore and Harbor Workers' Compensation Act may be treated as a Jones Act seaman in some cases.[6] Additionally, the Jones Act ensures that the United States keeps and maintains a fleet of ships staffed by US crews and owned by US companies.[7]

Before the passing of the Jones Act in 1920, there were no laws (statues) written by Congress to ensure that US seamen would be provided for if they were injured. For many years, injured seamen relied on maritime law for their recovery. Maritime law or admiralty law is a mixture of common law, traditions, and practices adopted by ancient seafaring nations, and incorporated into the American legal system over time.[7] The Jones Act provision authorizing such suits enlarges the rule of liability under the maritime law by conferring on seamen or their representatives the right afforded by the FELA to recover damages resulting from an employer's negligence.

The Jones Act covers not only the members of a crew, but the masters of that crew as well, ie, anyone who has a connection that is substantial in both nature and duration to a specific vessel, or to a fleet of vessels, and whose duties contribute to the function or mission of that vessel or fleet. Generally, anyone who spends more than 30% of his or her time on a vessel that is in navigation will qualify as a Jones Act seaman. It is important to understand that the terms *duration* and *nature*, when talking about someone's connection to a ship, are traditionally construed by the courts to be exceptionally broad when determining whether an employee qualifies for Jones Act coverage.[7]

The FELA governs the liability of every common carrier by rail engaging in interstate or foreign commerce for the work-related injury of an employee. It imposes liability on the railroad for injuries or death resulting from negligence in the use of its cars, engines, appliances, machinery, track, roadbed, works, boats, or other equipment.

Chapter 8

Both the Jones Act and the FELA shift to the respective industries the "human overhead" of doing business.

In treating a Jones Act seaman or a FELA railroad worker, the physician must be very careful in making the return-to-work decisions. These are extremely hazardous occupations. Rarely are there minor injuries on ships or in railroad yards. Workers with significant disabilities may very easily constitute a significant threat not only to themselves but to their coworkers as well.

Longshore and Harbor Workers

The Longshore and Harbor Workers' Compensation Act (LHWCA) (33 USC § 901, et seq, 20 CFR 701-704) is a federal act that provides compensation benefits and medical care for maritime workers who are not seamen.[8] The law fills a gap that exists between the Jones Act, which protects seamen, and state workers' compensation, which covers injuries occurring within a particular state, but not usually on navigable water.[8] The act was initially passed by the US Congress in 1927 and provided coverage to longshore workers working on navigable waters of the US in instances in which no state workers' compensation law applied.[9] In 1984, however, Congress substantially amended the LHWCA in an attempt to give all longshore and harbor workers the same type of protection.[9]

Coverage is determined under the LHWCA dependent on the location where the employee was working and whether the type of work performed had a traditional relationship to maritime employment.[9] The LHWCA covers injuries that occur during maritime employment on navigable waters of the US.[8] Navigable water can include places on land that adjoin water. For example, a worker who is injured on a pier, wharf, dry dock, or terminal can be compensated under the Act. Areas near a pier or wharf can also be included in navigable waters, such as areas for loading, unloading, repairing, or building vessels. Maritime employment includes the loading and unloading of vessels, repairing vessels, and building vessels.[8]

Return-to-work decisions for longshore and harbor workers should be made with the same considerations as those for merchant seamen and railroad workers. These men and women also work in a very high-risk environment and, if released to return to work prematurely, might pose a significant risk to themselves and others.

The Americans With Disabilities Act of 1990

There probably has not been a federal statute or regulation in the last generation that has impacted return-to-work issues as much as the Americans With Disabilities Act of 1990 (ADA)[10]—not the Occupational Safety and

Health Administration (OSHA), not the Employee Retirement Income Security Act (ERISA), and not OSHA and ERISA *combined*. In almost a decade and a half, the ADA has caused considerable head-scratching in board rooms, in human resources departments, in union halls, and in physicians' offices.

It all began with the congressional acknowledgment that disabled people were not being treated fairly in the workplace. It was difficult to inspire disabled individuals to attempt to overcome their disabilities when they were never really given the opportunity to do so.

The ADA was passed to combat discrimination—discrimination against disabled citizens in the workplace who may or may not need special accommodations to assist them in doing their jobs. Like most federal statutes, it contains its own vernacular: *reasonable accommodation; major life activity; physical or mental impairment; essential functions; qualified individual;* and on and on. All of these phrases together add up to the requirement that employers make reasonable accommodations for present or prospective qualified individuals who have a physical or mental impairment that limits a major life activity if that individual can perform the essential functions of the job.[11]

Unquestionably, the onus of ADA compliance sits squarely atop the shoulders of the employer. It is the employer's responsibility to determine whether a person with a disability is able to perform the essential functions of a job.[11] Even if an employee has sustained a work-related injury and has made his or her way through the state's workers' compensation system, the disability determination made as a result of the employee's workers' compensation claim (eg, permanent partial disability) does not relieve the employer of the "reasonable accommodation" requirement, and does not even classify the employee as "disabled" under the ADA.[11] Before the enactment of the ADA, employers were free to deny employment to disabled individuals if they felt that the disability created a risk of future injury. It would seem that legitimate areas of concern for an employer would be the safety of the disabled employee and his or her coworkers, the cost of workers' compensation insurance, etc. The ADA changed all of that. The employer now has to establish that the employee currently would pose a direct threat in the position to justify the decision not to allow him or her to return to work.[11]

Under the ADA, it is the *employer*—not the physician—who has the ultimate responsibility for deciding whether an employee with a disability-related occupational injury is ready to return to work. Therefore, the employer, rather than a rehabilitation counselor, physician, or other specialist, must determine whether the employee can perform the essential functions of the job, with or without reasonable accommodation, or can work without posing a direct threat.[11] Without question, however, the employer may and usually does rely on healthcare providers of varied disciplines to provide information essential to making return-to-work decisions. Considering the weight of the responsibility the ADA places on employers regarding these issues, physicians who treat injured workers should appreciate that they will frequently be a very important part of this process. Physicians not only will be called on to provide information regarding disability and impairment, but also will be consulted about proposed accommodations, risk of future injury, etc.

When called on to assist the employer in making the return-to-work decision, the physician should make sure that sufficient information regarding the job has been provided. That information should include a detailed description of the physical requirements for the job, possible risks and hazards, some information about the work environment and the employer's operations, and any possible reasonable accommodations the employer might propose.[11]

There are circumstances under the ADA in which an employer may require that an employee undergo a medical examination, but the examination has to be job related and has to be consistent with business necessity. The purpose of the examination would usually be to determine whether the employee is physically capable of performing the essential functions of the job, or whether there is sufficient residual functioning to perform the job if reasonable accommodations are made.[11]

The most important thing for physicians to remember about the ADA is that Congress has placed great emphasis on the importance of assisting disabled persons in obtaining and retaining employment. While the final decision is the responsibility of the employer, that decision by necessity will have to be made in conjunction with medical evidence about disability, restrictions, etc.

Family and Medical Leave Act of 1993

Catastrophic events within a family can seriously impact employee availability and productivity. The birth of a child, the death of a spouse, or the serious health condition of an aging parent can all disrupt if not destroy the relationship between an employee and employer. The most dedicated, loyal, and trustworthy employee would probably admit that critical needs of the family come before critical needs of the company.

In late 1992 and early 1993, Congress debated the details of the Family and Medical Leave Act (FMLA). On February 5, 1993, it was signed into law by President Clinton.[12]

The Act applies to employers with 50 or more employees. It establishes that those employees are entitled to 12 work weeks of *unpaid* leave during any 12-month period. The circumstances that give rise to this entitlement are as follows:

- The birth of a son or daughter of the employee and the care of such son or daughter
- The placement of a son or daughter with the employee for adoption or foster care
- The care of a spouse, son, daughter, or parent of the employee who has a serious health condition
- A serious health condition of the employee that makes the employee unable to perform the essential functions of his or her position.[13]

The Act also provides that when an employee returns from FMLA leave, he or she must be returned to the same position or an equivalent position. They are also to receive the same pay, benefits, and other terms and conditions of employment.[13]

Like any federal statute, the FMLA has its own definitions and vernacular. From a physician's standpoint, the most important phrase in the statute probably is *serious health condition*. Typically, an employee with a serious health condition will exhaust all of his or her sick leave and vacation before opting for FMLA leave. Following is the definition of *serious health condition* exactly as it is set out in the Act[12]:

Serious Health Condition: (1) Serious health condition means an illness, injury, impairment, or physical or mental condition that involves-(i) Inpatient care (i.e., an overnight stay) in a hospital, hospice, or residential medical care facility, including any period of incapacity or any subsequent treatment in connection with such inpatient care; or (ii) Continuing treatment by a healthcare provider that includes (but is not limited to) examinations to determine if there is a serious health condition and evaluations of such conditions if the examinations or valuations determine that a serious health condition exists. Continuing treatment by a healthcare provider may include one or more of the following—(A) A period of incapacity of more than 3 consecutive calendar days, including any subsequent treatment or period of incapacity relating to the same condition, that also involves—(1) Treatment two or more times by a healthcare provider, by a healthcare provider under the direct supervision of the affected individual's healthcare provider, or by a provider of healthcare services under orders of, or on referral by, a healthcare provider; or (2) Treatment by a healthcare provider on at least one occasion which results in a regimen of continuing treatment under the supervision of the healthcare provider (e.g., a course of prescription medication or therapy requiring special equipment to resolve or alleviate the health condition). (B) Any period of incapacity due to pregnancy or childbirth, or for prenatal care, even if the affected individual does not receive active treatment from a healthcare provider during the period of incapacity or the period of incapacity does not last more than 3 consecutive calendar days. (C) Any period of incapacity or treatment for such incapacity due to a chronic serious health condition that—(1) Requires periodic visits for treatment by a healthcare provider or by a healthcare provider under the direct supervision of the affected individual's healthcare provider, (2) Continues over an extended period of time (including recurring episodes of a single underlying condition); and (3) May cause episodic rather than a continuing period of incapacity (e.g., asthma, diabetes, epilepsy, etc.). The condition is covered even if the affected individual does not receive active treatment from a healthcare provider during the period of incapacity or the period of incapacity does not last more than 3 consecutive calendar days. (D) A period of incapacity, which is permanent or long-term due to a condition for which treatment may not be effective. The affected individual must be under the continuing supervision of, but need not be receiving active treatment by, a healthcare provider (e.g., Alzheimer's, severe stroke, or terminal stages of a disease). (E) Any period of absence to receive multiple treatments (including any period of recovery) by a healthcare provider or by a provider of healthcare services under orders of, or on referral by, a healthcare provider, either for restorative surgery after an accident or other injury or for a condition that would likely result in a period of incapacity of more than 3 consecutive calendar days in the absence of medical intervention or treatment (e.g., chemotherapy/radiation for cancer, physical therapy for severe arthritis, dialysis for kidney disease). (2) (Serious health condition does not include routine physical, eye, or dental examinations; a regimen of continuing treatment that includes the taking of over-the-counter medications, bed-rest, exercise, and other similar activities that can be initiated without a visit to the healthcare provider; a condition for which cosmetic treatments are administered, unless inpatient hospital care is required or unless complications develop; or an absence because of an employee's use of an illegal substance, unless the employee is receiving treatment for substance abuse by a healthcare provider or by a provider of healthcare services on referral by a healthcare provider. Ordinarily, unless complications arise, the common cold, the flu, earaches, upset stomach, minor ulcers, headaches (other than migraines), routine dental or orthodontia problems, and periodontal disease are not serious health conditions. Allergies, restorative dental or plastic surgery after an injury, removal of cancerous growth, or mental illness resulting from stress may be serious health conditions only if such conditions require.

Boiled down to the essentials, all of this means that if an employee is absent for more than three consecutive calendar days and also has been treated two or more times by a healthcare provider, or maybe even *once* if that treatment resulted in a regimen of continuing treatment (like therapy), then the employee is eligible.

The employer may require that employees who have been off work under the FMLA because of their own serious health condition provide a *fitness for duty certification* on return to work.[14] The Act sets out the guideline for the certifications, with the expected prohibitions against discriminatory application, etc, and limiting the certification requirement to only the condition that caused the FMLA leave.

There are two circumstances in which a physician may become involved in the fitness-for-duty certification. The first would be as a physician for the employee. A certification may have to be submitted on the employee's behalf, but it need only be a simple statement verifying the employee's ability or inability to return to work. The second would be if the physician were retained by the employer to clarify or confirm the employee's fitness or lack of fitness for returning to work. Under those circumstances, the physician must first obtain the employee's permission to speak with his or her physician, and the only information that may be acquired is that relating to the serious health condition for which the FMLA leave was taken.

Physician Liability in Making Return-to-Work Decisions

Any discussion of medical–legal issues would not be complete without some mention of physician liability. To what extent may a physician be held liable in making return-to-work decisions? To whom would such liability extend? What can be done in advance to either negate or greatly reduce exposure?

The extent to which a physician may be liable for these decisions is greatly determined by state law. Since there are 50 of them out there, a very wide range of possibilities exists. However, the rules are generally very similar and there are very few variants.

Most states, for example, have established that physicians are not responsible for injuries to third parties. For example, an ironworker patient has recovered very well from his knee surgery, and the physician sends him back to work. While walking a girder 40 floors above the street, his knee buckles, he drops his load, and an electrician on the fifth floor is hit on the head. Is the physician liable to the electrician? In most states, the answer would be a resounding "no." There are two reasons for this: the injury itself was not foreseeable, and the physician owes no duty to the electrician. The physician–patient relationship exists between the physician and the iron-worker, and that relationship establishes a legal *duty*. The physician has the duty to use ordinary care, ie, to do that which the ordinary, prudent physi-cian would do under like or similar circumstances. Since the physician has no such relationship with the electrician, there is no duty. If there is no duty, there is no liability.

Under the ironworker and electrician example, are there circumstances in which the physician may be held liable? There are. For example, perhaps re-habilitation has not gone well. The knee is swollen and unstable. The physi-cian forgets what this patient does for a living and thinks he is an insurance agent or a tollbooth operator. The ironworker is walking the same girder and the same knee buckles. This time, however, the ironworker falls 40 floors, miraculously surviving the fall but sustaining a number of fractures. The physician could well have a liability problem under those circumstances, if it can be shown that the ordinary prudent physician would not have returned the patient to ironwork.

Following are some practice pointers that the ordinary, prudent physician should consider.

Form a Friendly Relationship With a Lawyer
Having a friendly relationship between a lawyer and a physician can yield great benefits to both. Over the years, they may trade thousands of dollars worth of medical and legal information and advice at no cost to either party. If the lawyer is wading through medical records or operative reports and gets confused, he or she can simply call the physician. If the physician is faced with a patient confidentiality issue or is having a problem with a lawyer, he or she can call the lawyer friend.

The ideal lawyer friend is not a tax lawyer, estate planner, or traffic ticket fixer. He or she should be a trial lawyer, someone who toils daily in a per-sonal injury practice and is familiar with the issues, which overlap with those of a busy medical practice. There are plenty of trial lawyers who would jump at the opportunity to enter into such a relationship with a physician. This mutually beneficial relationship would be enlightening to both participants and would go a long way in fostering goodwill between the two professions.

Patient Confidentiality
The passage of the Health Insurance Portability and Accountability Act of 1996 (HIPAA) is testimony to the importance of protecting the health infor-mation of patients. HIPAA took effect on April 14, 2003. Developed by the Department of Health and Human Services, it provides patients with

access to their medical records and more control over how their personal health information is used and disclosed. It represents uniform, minimal privacy protections for patients across the country.

Any time a physician is called to testify about the treatment or condition of a patient, he or she should make sure that the patient has given consent for such testimony. The physician–patient privilege belongs to the patient; however, the physician has a duty to invoke that privilege on behalf of the patient. The privilege protects information whether it is written, unwritten, electronic, or in some other form.

The physician should never discuss a patient's health information with anyone—not even the patient's attorney—until he or she has obtained a written authorization, signed by the patient, to do so. Moreover, a written authorization, once obtained, does not give the physician carte blanche to discuss the patient's health information with anyone he or she pleases. The authorization should state specifically what information is to be released and to whom.* If the authorization does not specify what information is to be released, the physician should not discuss any aspect of the patient's health with anyone. Instead, he or she should insist that the patient sign an authorization that clearly specifies the exact information that can be given out.

A physician may obtain the patient's permission to discuss his or her health with third parties; however, such permission should be documented, preferably in the patient's chart. Sometimes a court may order a physician to release information about a patient in spite of the patient's objection. In this case, the judge would make a determination as to the relevancy of such information. If the judge decides that the patient's health information is relevant, the physician should insist on having the judge make a ruling on the record or sign an order requiring him or her to testify.

Disclaimers

Many—if not *most*—disability evaluations, fitness certifications, return-to-work decisions, etc, are made in the form of a report or letter. The words the physician chooses to use in the report will be where all of the scrutiny is

---

* Often, insurance companies (and sometimes attorneys) will request that opposing attorneys have their clients sign medical authorizations addressed to: "To whom it may concern." Such an authorization is overly broad because is allows the insurance company to obtain information that is not necessarily related to the litigation. For example, with that authorization, the insurance company could request medical records from the claimant's gynecologist even though the claim pertains to a back injury incurred in an auto accident. Allowing an insurance company to use its discretion in obtaining medical records is ill-advised. A patient should *never* rely on others to protect his or her health information. To avoid this situation, the patient's attorney should always ensure that any authorization his or her client signs is made out to a particular doctor, hospital, clinic, etc.

given if something goes wrong. At the conclusion of the report, just above the signature line, should be a disclaimer that sets out what the report is and what it is not. Below are two sample disclaimers. The first is used if the physician making the report is the treating physician:

The above statements have been made within a reasonable degree of medical probability. The opinions rendered in this case are mine alone. Recommendations regarding treatment, work, and impairment ratings are given totally independently from the requesting agents. These opinions do not constitute per se a recommendation for specific claims or administrative functions to be made or enforced.

This evaluation is based upon the history given by Mr/Ms___, the objective medical findings noted during the examination, and information obtained from the review of the prior medical records available to me, with the assumption that this material is true and correct. If additional information is provided to me in the future, a reconsideration and an additional report may be requested. Such information may or may not change the opinions in this report.

Medicine is both an art and a science, and although Mr/Ms ___ may appear to be fit to work with the abilities and restrictions described above, there is no guarantee that he/she will not be injured or sustain a new injury if he/she chooses to return to work.

The following is a version of the disclaimer to be used by a physician who reviewed a file but did not see the person.

The opinions rendered in this case are the opinions of the reviewer. The review has been conducted without a medical examination of the individual reviewed. The review is based on documents provided with the assumption that the material is true and correct. If more information becomes available at a later date, an additional service/report/consideration may be requested. Such information may or may not change the opinions rendered in this report. This report is a clinical assessment of documentation and the opinions are based on the information available. This opinion does not constitute per se a recommendation for specific claims or administrative functions to be made or enforced.

These disclaimers say, in effect, "I have given my opinions on the basis of the information I had at hand at the time I stated them. If more information becomes available, give it to me and my opinions *may* change."

Summary

There is some risk in everything people do in life, and that includes work, regardless of whether they are healthy. Understanding the legal considerations can help the healthcare provider when assigning work guides. Communication is key to improving return to work. Realizing that tolerance, not capacity or risk, is often the limiting factor can reduce the physician's legal risk in return-to-work decision making.

References

1. Canale SL, ed. *Campbell's Operative Orthopedics*. 10th ed. Philadelphia, Pa: Mosby; 2003.

2. US Department of Labor. *The Dictionary of Occupational Titles*. 4th ed. Washington, DC: US Department of Labor; 1991. Available at: www.oalj.dol.gov/libdot.htm. Accessed October 27, 2004.

3. *The Transitional Classification of Jobs*. 6th ed. Athens, Ga: Elliott & Fitzpatrick Inc; 2004.

4. Bevan TW. State workers' compensation programs. In: Demeter SL, Andersson GB, eds. *Disability Evaluation*. 2nd ed. St Louis, Mo: Mosby; 2003.

5. ALR Federal Alert, West Group, Volume 169, Admiralty, Jones Act—Supreme Court, p 3.

6. Maritime Injury Lawyers. Jones Act: protecting injured seaman. Available at: www.maritimeinjurylawyers.com/pages/jonesact.html. Accessed October 27, 2004.

7. *The Jones Act*. Available at: www.shipguide.com/the-jones-act.html. Accessed October 27, 2004.

8. Maritime Injury Lawyers. *Longshore & Harbor Workers' Compensation Act*. Available at: www.maritimeinjurylawyers.com/pages/longshoreandharboract. html. Accessed October 27, 2004.

9. *What is the Longshore and Harbor Workers' Compensation Act?* Available at: http://law.freeadvice.com/admiralty_maritime/maritime_worker_injury/ longshore_workers_comp.htm. Accessed October 27, 2004.

10. 42 USCA §12101, et seq, July 26, 1990.

11. *Equal Employment Opportunity Commission Enforcement Guidance: Workers' Compensation and the Americans With Disabilities Act*. Washington, DC: US Department of Labor, Equal Employment Opportunity Commission, ADA Division, Office of Legal Counsel; September 3, 1996.

12. 29 USCA §2601, et seq, 29 CFR 825, February 5, 1993.

13. Office of Personnel Management. Family and medical leave. Available at: www.opm.gov/oca/leave/HTML/fmlafac2.asp. Accessed October 27, 2004.

14. US Department of Labor, Office of the Assistant Secretary for Policy. Employment law guide: family and medical leave. Available at: www.dol.gov/asp/ programs/guide/fmla.htm. Accessed October 27, 2004.

Chapter 8

Chapter 9

Can This Patient Work?
A Disability Perspective

John LoCascio, MD*

> *Capacity is a construct that indicates, as a qualifier, the highest probable level of functioning that a person may reach in a domain in the Activities and Participation list at a given moment.*
>
> — INTERNATIONAL CLASSIFICATION OF FUNCTIONING, DISABILITY, AND HEALTH[1]

> *What is this parroting of numbers? Give me one look into the mind of Flaminius.*
>
> —HANNIBAL BARCA

It all starts with the sample attending physician's statement (Figure 9-1). The sample attending physician's statement was synthesized from disability applications gathered from five commercial disability insurers representing approximately 50% of the United States market in terms of covered lives.

A patient hands the physician a disability application. The physician hesitates. He has not been trained in disability assessment. He provides care. Maybe he is not sure whether the patient is disabled. Maybe he has not given disability a thought in this case. Perhaps the physician did not know the patient was out of work. Maybe he has only the vaguest idea of what the patient does for a living.

* The opinions in this chapter reflect the views of the author alone and should not be attributed to the UNUMProvident Corporation or its subsidiaries and affiliates.

Figure 9-1 A Sample Attending Physician's Statement

InsureCo

Sample Attending Physician's Statement

Patient's Name:	Date of Birth:	Social Security Number:

Primary Diagnosis:

Objective Findings:

Subjective Symptoms:

Are there any Secondary Conditions impairing your patient's work capacity? If so, what are they?

Please list relevant tests and procedures:

Please list current treatments, medications and dosages:

Please list any other relevant caregivers:

Limitations (*what the patient cannot do*) :

Restrictions (*what the patient should not do*) :

Date restrictions and limitations began:	Date you expect restrictions and limitations to end:

Name:	Degree:	Medical Specialty:
Address:		Phone:

Signature   Date

Please attach any applicable office treatment notes, test results, discharge summaries, etc.

But the physician would like to help, and the patient clearly expects his support. That evening the application is in his paperwork. His staff has completed the Patient Information and Diagnosis section. The physician begins.

The Disability Decision Maker

When faced with a disability application, clinical caregivers naturally assume that they are being asked whether the patient is disabled. However, the application does not ask this question. In addition to the familiar demographics and diagnosis, it asks what the person can and cannot do (sometimes using the terms *limitations* and *restrictions*).

This is because, in commercial programs, neither the attending physician nor any physician consulted by the insurer is the *disability decision maker*. The decision maker is the claim administrator, usually a lay business person. This arrangement is the natural result of the structure of the disability decision.

Defining Disability

In 1980, disability was defined by the World Health Organization (WHO) as ". . . any restriction or lack . . . of ability to perform an activity in the manner or within the range considered normal for a human being."[2]

The WHO required a broad definition of disability because it is concerned with the effect of medical conditions on all populations, at all ages, in all countries and cultures of the world. In the US and other Western countries, however, we think of disability in a narrower sense, as the inability to earn a living as a result of illness or injury.

Even within this narrower concept, confusion arises because we are confronted with a variety of governmental and commercial programs with differing contracts, regulations, and procedures, such as Social Security, workers' compensation, and commercial disability products.

The Core Idea

All of these programs, however, contain the same core element. They all balance functional capacity against occupational demand. Thus, a disability decision is a supply and demand decision, where "supply" is functional capacity as modified by a medical condition; "demand" is the

Chapter 9

sum of the required tasks of the occupation; and the balancing procedure is defined in the contract, which functions as the "scales." (In governmental programs such as US Social Security Disability, the "contract" takes the form of the act or law that creates the program, together with the regulations that are issued to administer it.) Figure 9-2 illustrates this concept.

If a particular functional capacity is equal to or greater than the corresponding, required occupational demand, the patient is not "disabled." If one or more demands outweighs one or more required capacities, then the patient is "disabled." While practice is rarely as simple as principle, this basic concept is vital to understanding the physician's role in the disability process.

Whether a particular task is "required" by an occupation is often a point for vocational experts. While many tasks reported by the patient are "required," others may not be because they are idiosyncratic to the employee (ie, not performed in that way by fellow employees), they can be "reasonably accommodated," etc. Such determinations are not the responsibility of the physician but of vocational experts.

The Decision Maker in Context

Disability determination requires three types of knowledge: medical, occupational, and contractual. Figure 9-3 illustrates the interaction between these three types of knowledge.

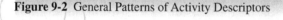

Figure 9-2 General Patterns of Activity Descriptors

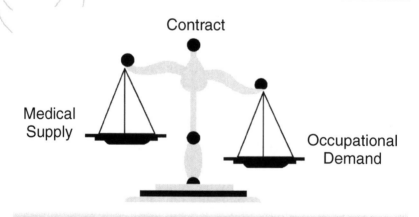

Figure 9-3 The Relationships of Medical, Contractual, and Occupational
Elements With Disability

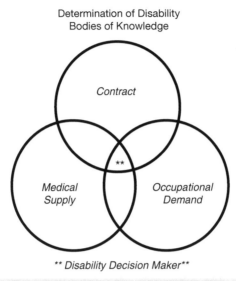

Determination of Disability
Bodies of Knowledge

Contract

**

Medical
Supply

Occupational
Demand

** Disability Decision Maker**

While most issues are straightforward, each body of knowledge has its own
experts and potential complications. For example, the contract may define
the occupation as any of the following:

- The patient's actual occupation at the time he or she applies for benefits
- Any occupation for which the patient is qualified on the basis of "training,
  education, and experience"
- Any occupation existing in the general economy.

The contract may cover one of the following:

- Short-term disability (where coverage usually begins after a waiting
  period of one to two weeks and lasts from three to six months)
- Long-term disability (where coverage usually begins after a waiting
  period of three to six months and often lasts to age 65 years).

Finally, is coverage in force at all? Depending on dates of employment or
payment of premium, a patient who is clearly unable to continue employment from the medical perspective may not be eligible for benefits.

Figure 9-3 also illustrates why the physician is not the disability decision
maker. The physician cannot be expected to be an expert in all three required
bodies of knowledge, only in the medical facts of the case. The claims

administrator is the disability decision maker because he or she is trained in the interaction of all three bodies of knowledge and is expected to obtain in-depth advice from physicians, attorneys, or vocational resources as required.

The Physician's Role

If the application does not ask whether the patient is disabled, then what does it ask? The answer is simpler than it appears: The physician must com-municate and support a reasonable clinical estimate of what the patient can do and can no longer do.

Although many physicians are sometimes uncomfortable formulating such an estimate, it is clinically familiar as an "activity prescription" for rehabilitation. Such a prescription aims to define baseline function and maximize functional outcomes within the limits of reason and safety. As in the rehabilitation set-ting, such an estimate is based first on medical facts and expectations. While it must also recognize reasonable patient concerns (including tolerance for symptoms), it cannot be based solely on or be dominated by such concerns.

This is not an issue confined to rehabilitation specialists. Behavioral health professionals also turn to medical colleagues for assistance in such judg-ments. Additional guidance may be found in the *Diagnostic and Statistical Manual of Mental Disorders, Fourth Edition, Text Revision (DSM-IV-TR)*, which states (in part): "Objective findings should be evaluated without undue reliance on subjective complaints."[3]

Basic Concepts and Terminology

The concepts of *diagnosis, impairment, functional capacity, limitation,* and *restriction* are critical to understanding and easily completing a dis-ability application.

Diagnosis

Diagnosis is subtly different when viewed from a disability perspective. In disability analysis, a solid *pathophysiologic* diagnosis is important because it allows easier demonstration of underlying pathology. Thus, it is easier to estimate whether pathology is proportional to reported impairment. On the other hand, *syndromic* diagnoses are characterized by symptoms that are dis-proportionate to objective findings. These include chronic fatigue syndrome and chronic pain syndrome, but also include by extension all conditions and diagnoses in which symptoms in excess of findings are the primary basis for reported impairment.

This is not to say that syndromic diagnoses cannot be offered or must be invalid. However, it is important to recognize the objective limits of clinical data in this setting. In 1950, some patients with thyroid disease would have qualified for the 1988 Centers for Disease Control and Prevention criteria for chronic fatigue syndrome.[4] Patients who now have Parkinson disease then had Parkinson syndrome. How well medical data support a reported functional impairment is the critical issue in any disability application. However, it is easier to gather and assess functional data for pathophysiologic conditions than for syndromic conditions.

"Diagnosis does not equal disability" is an axiom that lies at the heart of the Americans With Disabilities Act. From the perspective of a disability application, a solid diagnosis helps support the contention that a patient is incapable of one or more tasks. However, the vast majority of patients with a solid pathophysiologic diagnosis are probably not disabled. If, on the basis of diagnosis alone, it is not possible to tell which patients are "disabled," then disability cannot be "proved" on this basis alone to an insurer. However, a diagnosis may result in "disability" if it produces one or more impairments.

Impairment

Impairment is related to the clinical concept of "end-organ damage." It is defined as "a loss, loss of use, or derangement of any body part, organ system, or organ function"[5] (another definition would be functional capacity below "certain generally accepted population standards,"[1] but the application of this absolute standard is cumbersome and impractical). In other words, regardless of baseline, if a patient has diminished organ or system function as a result of injury or disease, he or she is impaired.

By this definition, a nonprofessional athlete who runs a 4-minute mile, develops subclinical asthma, and then runs an 8-minute mile is technically impaired. However, such an individual is hardly "disabled" in the common sense of the word. The athlete may become disabled, however, if the asthma worsens and prevents an essential occupational function.

Thus, *impairment also does not equal disability* but may result in disability depending on its nature, its severity, and how it reduces a specific functional capacity or capacities.

Functional Capacity

From the disability perspective, the idea of a "task" is the central concept of functional capacity.

A task is a complex physical or mental action with a defined result (eg, climbing stairs, writing, reading, calculating, multiple simultaneous attention). After reduction by impairment, what is left is a residual functional capacity, which is usually expressed as a limit:

- Lift up to 20 lb, occasionally.
- Type up to 30 minutes at a time, up to four hours a day.

Impairment can reduce functional capacity by two mechanisms: limitation and restriction. Understanding these concepts is important to properly express and support the physician's estimates of residual functional capacity.

Limitation

Limitation is what a person cannot do as a result of illness or injury. For example, a person is limited from (physically incapable of) driving an automobile while having a generalized seizure, as he or she is unconscious during the seizure. By virtue of this definition, limitation is usually measurable or objectifiable. In practice, an estimate of reduction in functional capacity by limitation is usually supported because it is judged clinically proportionate to a demonstrated impairment. (See also "Estimating Functional Capacity" later in this chapter.) Less commonly, a functional capacity may be indirectly measured.

Certain functional capacities can be directly measured on formal functional capacity evaluations (for more information about functional capacity evaluation, refer to Chapter 7 of this book and *Disability Evaluation*[6]). Less specific functional measurements can be obtained from procedures such as pulmonary function testing or cardiac or pulmonary exercise tests. The results of these tests can be used in two ways: by extrapolating exercise levels to standard patterns of activity, such as those defined in the US Department of Labor *Dictionary of Occupational Titles* (see the section on "Physical Demand Levels from the Dictionary of Occupational Titles" at the end of this chapter), or by observing whether the activity performed in the course of the test is consistent with the reported impairment.

Restriction

Restriction is what a person should not do because of illness- or injury-related risk to self or others. The patient *must be capable* of performing an action from which he or she is restricted. For example, a patient who has fully recovered from a seizure is now physically capable of driving an automobile but is told not to do so until certain criteria are met (that is, until the risk of a recurrent seizure is deemed "acceptable").

Because restrictions are based on risk, they are rarely well quantified or objectified. A person may resume driving after meeting certain regulatory criteria that include a defined seizure-free interval. However, all of these criteria vary from state to state because, while there is reasonable agreement on the risk in general, there are too many variables to measure the risk precisely.

A person who has had a seizure is not *limited* from driving an automobile, but is *restricted* from driving. By extension, he or she may also be restricted from activities such as climbing to heights and using power machinery.

Restriction from driving after a seizure is seldom controversial because it is codified by jurisdiction. However, the vast majority of medical restrictions (lifting restrictions in back pain, carrying restrictions after total knee replacement, prohibitions from performing surgery because of potential spread of infection, prohibitions from reentering certain environments because of psychological conditions) are based more on each physician's anecdotal experience and common sense than on data. Supporting and administering such restrictions is sometimes difficult because their justification depends on a medicolegal concept of the "immediacy" of the risk. In the absence of data, estimating the degree of risk is difficult.

Restrictions and limitations (often abbreviated as R/Ls) can be combined. For example, after a laminectomy, a 150-lb (70-kg) man may know from experience that he is no longer physically capable of lifting 75 lb (35 kg) (deconditioned from inactivity), but that he can still lift 50 lb (25 kg). He is *limited* to 50 lb. However, the physician advises him not to lift more than 35 lb (15 kg) to reduce the risk of reinjury. He is *restricted* to 35 lb. Assuming the restriction is justified, his residual functional capacity is 35 lb.

Finally, impairments can result in multiple R/Ls, and a particular restriction or limitation can affect multiple functional capacities. They must do so, however, in a manner that is physiologically consistent across functional capacities.

Patient Interview: Defining Pertinent Functional Capacities

Occupations consist of hundreds of tasks or capacities. How can the physician determine which are the most affected in any particular case? The simplest way is to ask the patient:

In your job, what can you no longer do? And why can't you do it?

It is reasonable to assume that the patient will identify the most important problem or problems first, the symptoms that reduce that capacity, and the point at which they stop. For reasons of clarity, the physician should limit his or her attention to the first one or two tasks identified by the patient. More can be added later if questions arise.

This type of questioning may seem clinically unfamiliar, but patients usually present to physicians with reference to a functional capacity:

"It hurts when I do this."
"I'm getting too weak to do that."
"I can't hear any more."
"Dad can't balance his checkbook any more."

In fact, a history that lacks spontaneous reference to specific functional capacities or has physiologically inconsistent references across related functional capacities is a potential concern. The longer the history and list of observers, the greater the concern.

Estimating Functional Capacity

In most cases, functional capacity is not measured but must be estimated from clinical data. Unfortunately, there is no formula that allows physicians to derive specific functional capacities from clinical findings.

The starting point is objective data. Are there soft physical findings that require a great deal of physician judgment and patient cooperation (like tenderness, spasm, manual muscle testing, or range of motion), or hard physical findings, like gross muscle atrophy, that can be measured? Are there laboratory or imaging findings?

From the extent and character of these findings, and based on his or her experience, the physician will naturally form a mental picture of a population of similar patients with similar findings: a "reference population."

Independent of the patient's history and using the functional capacities identified by questioning, the physician next thinks about what a normal distribution of functional capacities in the "reference population" would look like. Would a clear majority of such patients be reasonably capable of lifting 10, 20, or 50 lb, climbing a flight of stairs, or concentrating well enough to drive a car?

This estimate is meant to be as "proportionate to findings" (ie, objectifiable) as possible.

This estimate is compared with the symptoms and capacities reported by the patient. If they roughly correspond, the R/Ls (or residual functional capacities) the physician reports on the application are less likely to result in questions from the insurance company. However, if the reported symptoms and impairments are greatly in excess of the physician's expectations, the application for benefit is likely highly subjective.

Symptoms in excess of findings are the hallmark of subjectively based R/Ls. Whenever the physician is required to address such issues (on a disability application or elsewhere), it is far better to simply acknowledge what is objectively supported and what symptoms are reported in excess of findings. As discussed above, such estimates are not necessarily invalid, but they are more difficult to support.

Supporting Symptoms in Excess of Findings

There are certain assumptions that all clinicians use:

> . . . clinicians use certain, understandable and appropriate assumptions in their daily work: for example, until proved otherwise, clinicians assume that patients' histories are accurate and that the patient has strong conscious and unconscious drives to recover. These assumptions are appropriate to the overwhelming majority of patients seen in practice. They are also necessary; without them medical practice would be impossibly cumbersome and inefficient.[7]

Clinical assumptions, like all assumptions, are unspoken. However, they influence what is or is not asked of patients and, therefore, what is or is not noted in the record. In applications for short-term disability, such assumptions are rarely a problem, as, with time, recovery demonstrates support for the diagnosis and treatment. However, if the patient fails to recover after a reasonable period for workup and therapy, three clinical scenarios are possible:

1. Severe impairment is objectively supported as a basis for R/Ls.
2. The patient is reasonably referred for consultation in a timely manner.
3. Time and consultation have demonstrated that the symptoms are likely to remain unexplained, or poorly explained, and in excess of findings.

When asked about R/Ls for patients in group 3, clinicians commonly reply that they believe what the patient tells them because they have no reason to disbelieve. This is simply an expression of the *reasonable clinical assumptions* discussed at the beginning of this section. However, assumptions are correctly applied to the majority of cases. The patients in group 3 are an exceedingly small minority of the patients seen by clinicians. For that reason, the usual assumptions no longer apply.

However, in the "Diagnosis" subsection it was stated that syndromic diagnoses are conditions in which symptoms in excess of findings are the primary basis for reported impairment, which does not mean that syndromic diagnoses cannot be offered or must be invalid. If assumptions cannot be used to validate symptoms in excess of findings, what can the physician offer?

Objective and Subjective: Different Issues, Different Tests

A critical insight in supporting disability applications is to understand that different tests apply to objectively based impairment and subjectively based symptoms in excess of findings.

• The test and support of impairment are data: hard signs, laboratory data, imaging, or measurement of functional capacity.
• The test of symptoms in excess of findings is consistency.

Dimensions of Consistency

As discussed earlier in this chapter, limitations, restrictions, and residual functional capacity (ie, patient behaviors) must be consistent across time, observers, and related functional capacities. In terms of minimal breadth and depth, the clinical data must be adequate under "usual and customary" standards with respect to diagnosis, therapy, and consultation.

For example, if a patient always describes a pain in the same way to the same observer, the report is consistent in one dimension (time). If the patient describes the same pain to two observers who question in two different ways, the report is consistent in two dimensions. If the patient describes the same pain across time and observers and the pain is physiologically consistent across functional capacities, then the report is consistent in three dimensions. If the reported pain is also physiologically consistent with distraction or other tests of validity (eg, Waddell's signs of pain behavior in patients with back pain), it is consistent in four dimensions, and so on.

It is also important to think about activities outside the work setting. Patients who cannot sit for extended periods usually cannot drive or take extended air flights. Patients with constant neck pain usually have difficulty participating in Dix-Hallpike maneuvers. Patients with severe low back pain are not expected to achieve high metabolic equivalent levels on cardiac exercise testing.

Disability Applications and Supporting Medical Data

The sample attending physician's statement asks the physician to append "applicable data." This is rarely a problem in the majority of applications, which are reasonably supported by objective data.

In applications in which the physician decides to support significant R/Ls on the basis of symptoms in excess of findings, the consistency and adequacy standards should be kept in mind. The physician should either forward observational data that supports the contention, or inform the carrier of other physicians or institutions where relevant data can be obtained. (The sample attending physician's statement in Figure 9-1 asks for this information.)

Chapter 9

Psychiatric Claims for Disability

Psychiatric diagnoses are syndromic in character. This is not to deny the biological substrate of all mental processes and their behavioral expressions. It is, however, the practical result of current medical knowledge and understanding. *DSM-IV-TR* diagnostic criteria do not refer to laboratory testing. Laboratory testing can assist in monitoring therapy, and psychometric or neuropsychiatric testing can partially objectify impairment as well as provide an objective framework to assess response bias (another dimension of consistency). However, the bulk of psychiatric diagnosis and care still rests on patient report and professional observation and interpretation.

The analytic approach to syndromic conditions described previously also works well in psychiatric applications for disability benefit with one important proviso. Psychiatry is the one area of medical specialty that has:

- Uniform and comprehensive standards for syndromic diagnoses (the *DSM-IV-TR*)

- A large group of behavioral health professionals trained in the application of these standards
- A uniform reporting system (the five-axis diagnosis) that includes a standard descriptor of function (axis 5, the global assessment of functioning).

These advantages do not eliminate the syndromic character of psychiatric impairment. They do, however, make it easier for mental health professionals to evaluate and report observed behaviors and functional levels, and for disability evaluators to assess the consistency of reports against known standards.

Examples of Attending Physician Statements

Figures 9-4 and 9-5 illustrate two sample attending physician statements (APSs) for patient "Jane Doe." Keeping in mind the principles discussed in this chapter. What thoughts and questions do these sample statements raise?

From the disability perspective, the short-term APS is straightforward and internally consistent. It reports conditions that are easily objectified and the required data are probably already attached. The R/Ls are proportionate to the findings, and the estimated recovery time is proportionate to the reported procedure.

The long-term APS is obviously very different. The long list of diagnoses suggests that an extensive search for the cause of persistent back pain has occurred. The search was probably unsuccessful because the patient is still reporting pain and the APS does not focus on a specific pain generator. Pain is now reported in multiple systems (migraine, irritable bowel syndrome [IBS]) and is nonfocal (fibromyalgia) as well as chronic. A new diagnosis (hypothyroidism) may explain fatigue and perhaps "depression" if it is uncompensated, but there is no way to know from the data available. Psychiatric diagnoses and therapy have appeared, but there is no mention of a behavioral health professional. If the psychiatric diagnoses are supported, this may or may not be an area of concern, depending on the duration and response to therapy. The patient apparently is now seeing a new primary care provider (Dr Wilson instead of Dr Smith). Why? Finally, the R/Ls are both extreme ("no lifting, sitting, standing," if taken literally, describes a bed-bound status) and vague ("totally disabled" adds nothing to our knowledge and is technically a disability decision).

Figure 9-4 Sample Attending Physician Statement (Short-term Disability)

InsureCo

Short-Term Disability
Sample Attending Physician's Statement

Patient's Name: Jane Doe	Date of Birth:	Social Security Number:

Primary Diagnosis:
   Left L5 Radiculopathy

Objective Findings:
   Diminished sensation in left L5 dermatome, foot drop.

Subjective Symptoms:
   Low back pain with left L5 radicular pain.

Are there any Secondary Conditions impairing your patient's work capacity? If so, what are they?

   No.

Please list relevant tests and procedures:

   Extruded disc fragment on MRI. (See attached.)

Please list current treatments, medications and dosages:

   2 weeks s/p L4-L5 laminectomy (04/14/2002, see attached operative note)

Please list any other relevant caregivers:

   P Smith MD (Family Practice), 212 Main Street, Fargo   (123) 456-7890

Limitations (what the patient cannot do):
               Current abilities, limited by tolerance: Lift > 10 lbs, walk > 20 feet,
               sit/ stand more than 20 minutes without a break.

Restrictions (what the patient should not do):
   Same.

Date restrictions and limitations began:	Date you expect restrictions and limitations to end:
04/14/2002	4 to 6 weeks depending on recovery.

Name: E Brandt	Degree: MD	Medical Specialty Orthopedic Surgery
Address: 4567 Western Avenue, Suite J, Fargo		Phone: (098) 765-4321

04/28/2003

_____   _____
Signature   Date

Please attach any applicable office treatment notes, test results,
discharge summaries, etc.

Chapter 9

Figure 9-5 Sample Attending Physician Statement (Long-term Disability)

InsureCo

Long-Term Disability
Sample Attending Physician's Statement

Patient's Name:	Date of Birth:	Social Security Number:
Jane Doe		

Primary Diagnosis: Low back pain, radiculopathy, facet syndrome, degenerative disc disease, fibromyalgia, migraines, fatigue, anxiety, depression

Objective Findings:

Decreased back motion, abnormal EMG, tender points, abnormal LFTs

Subjective Symptoms:

Constant pain and severe fatigue

Are there any Secondary Conditions impairing your patient's work capacity? If so, what are they?

Hypothyroidism, depression and anxiety, headaches, IBS.

Please list relevant tests and procedures:

L5-S1   Laminectomy, 11/18 tender points,

Please list current treatments, medications and dosages:

Celebrex, Ativan prn, Duragesic, Synthroid, Celexa, Ultram prn

Please list any other relevant caregivers:

The patient had surgery with Dr. Brandt in April. Sees Dr. Campos for Rheumatology, Dr. Erikson for Neurosurgery.

Limitations (what the patient cannot do):

No lifting, sitting, standing. Avoid stress.

Restrictions (what the patient should not do):

Totally disabled.

Date restrictions and limitations began:	Date you expect restrictions and limitations to end:
September 21, 2001	Indefinite

Name:	Degree:	Medical Specialty:
J. Wilson	MD	Internal Medicine

Address:	Phone:
4567 Kings Highway	(333) 444-5555

_____   09/11/2003
Signature   Date

Please attach any applicable office treatment notes, test results, discharge summaries, etc.

The point is not that anyone can answer these questions from the APS alone. The point is that the more these questions can be anticipated, the less likely they are to arise in an APS and the more likely the physician is to proactively address them with attached data.

Physical Demand Levels from the *Dictionary of Occupational Titles*

Table 9-1 is a summary of familiar categories of work. They are formally known as physical demand levels (PDLs) and were developed by the US Department of Labor for the *Dictionary of Occupational Titles* (DOT).[8]

The DOT was last updated in 1991, although it is still available from the US Government Printing Office in Washington, DC. It was to be replaced by the O*Net,[9] which contains no similar classifications of work. In fact, a fifth edition[10] of the DOT was published in 2003. It combines the fourth edition of the DOT with O*Net definitions. In part, this is because the system of PDLs has proven to be so useful and so well known that it is in constant use to this day. Even though they may not be recognized, PDL definitions are frequently seen in insurance applications, functional capacity evaluations, and various other reports. For that reason, a general understanding of their structure is useful to almost all medical practitioners.

The PDL table contains five descriptors, each with three categories or patterns:

- Lifting
- Frequency
- Characteristic tasks

Table 9-1 Physical Demand Characteristics of Work

Work Pattern	Occasional (0%–33% of the Work Day)	Frequent (34%–66% of the Work Day)	Constant (67%–100% of the Work Day)
Sedentary	10 lb		
Light	20 lb	10 lb and/or walk/ stand, push/pull, or arm/leg controls	Pull/pull or arm/leg controls while seated
Medium	50 lb	20 lb	10 lb
Heavy	100 lb	50 lb	20 lb
Very Heavy	Over 100 lb	Over 50 lb	Over 20 lb

By identifying a lifting limit and a frequency, the physician can estimate a general pattern of activity that matches the descriptors sedentary, light, medium, heavy, and very heavy. Table 9-2 identifies each descriptor.

Lifting in pounds is a fairly straightforward concept. (The lift is assumed to be from floor to counter height.) Frequency is more difficult to estimate, even for trained resources. However, if a person is engaged in an activity for one third of the time it is described as occasional, for two thirds, frequent, and for three thirds, constant. The point, however, is common sense. The descriptor that best fits the general occupational pattern should be chosen.

Table 9-2 General Patterns of Activity Descriptors*

(S) Sedentary Work

Exerting up to 10 lb of force *occasionally* and/or a negligible amount of force *frequently* to lift, carry, push, pull, or otherwise move objects, including the human body. Sedentary work involves sitting most of the time, but may involve walking or standing for brief periods of time. Jobs are sedentary if walking and standing are required only *occasionally* and all other sedentary criteria are met.

(L) Light Work

Exerting up to 20 lb of force *occasionally*, and/or up to 10 lb of force *frequently*, and/or a negligible amount of force *constantly* to move objects. Physical demand requirements are in excess of those for sedentary work. Even though the weight lifted may be only negligible, a job should be rated light work: (1) when it requires walking or standing to a significant degree; or (2) when it requires sitting most of the time but entails pushing and/or pulling of arm or leg controls; and/or (3) when the job requires working at a production rate pace entailing the constant pushing and/or pulling of materials even though the weight of those materials is negligible. NOTE: The constant stress and strain of maintaining a production rate pace, especially in an industrial setting, is physically exhausting.

(M) Medium Work

Exerting 20 to 50 lb of force *occasionally*, and/or 10 to 25 lb of force *frequently*, and/or greater than negligible up to 10 lb of force *constantly* to move objects. Physical demand requirements are in excess of those for light work.

(H) Heavy Work

Exerting 50 to 100 lb of force *occasionally*, and/or 25 to 50 lb of force *frequently*, and/or 10 to 20 lb of force *constantly* to move objects. Physical demand requirements are in excess of those for medium work.

(V) Very Heavy Work

Exerting in excess of 100 lb of force *occasionally*, and/or in excess of 50 lb of force *frequently*, and/or in excess of 20 lb of force *constantly* to move objects. Physical demands are in excess of those for heavy work.

* "Occasionally" indicates that an activity or condition exists up to one third of the time; "frequently" indicates that an activity or condition exists from one third to two thirds of the time; "constantly" indicates that an activity or condition exists two thirds or more of the time.

Chapter 9

This general pattern of lifting and frequency is a *lifting proxy*, a pattern of lifting that stands for and helps to define a general pattern of all activities in the occupational categories sedentary, light, etc.

These categories make intuitive sense. Administrative assistants, attorneys, consultants, and executives tend to share general patterns of lifting, walking, stair climbing, etc. The same can be said for large groups of technicians, sales people, and field representatives; for tradesmen and stock clerks; and so on.

Characteristic tasks are self-explanatory. Within wide limits, sedentary occupations have a prominent sitting component, light occupations have a prominent standing component, etc.

Can a system that has not been revised in more than 10 years still be useful? The answer is "yes," because:

- It is in widespread and ongoing use by vocational and rehabilitation professionals
- The general patterns have not changed, even as specific occupations come and go and evolve
- The descriptor is being applied to a patient's reported pattern of activity, which is medically reasonable. How this corresponds to actual occupational requirements is a vocational question.

What if a patient has a special or unusual physical demand that does not seem to fit the standard patterns?

- The physician simply notes any special circumstances of which he or she is aware. If, after investigation, these circumstances are found to be relevant, they can be added to the basic pattern.

Summary

The following points should be kept in mind when a disability attending physician statement is completed:

- Pathophysiologic diagnosis is helpful but does not "prove" disability.
- Syndromic diagnosis will require support for symptoms in excess of findings.
- "Limitations" are described by physicians. Impairment and limitation should be proportional to objective findings.
- "Restrictions" are imposed by physicians. Restriction is based on risk. The estimate of risk should be explained.

• Symptoms in excess of findings, as a basis for R/Ls, require a multidimensional demonstration of consistency across an adequate database:
  — Consistency in time (different visits with the same physician)
  — Consistency in different examinations (do other physicians describe the same symptoms and limitations?)
  — Consistency in activities (do limitations in potential work activities make physiologic sense in view of nonwork activity abilities?)
  — Consistency despite distraction (are limitations consistent when the patient is not aware of observation of an ability?)

References

1. World Health Organization. *International Classification of Functioning, Disability, and Health.* Geneva, Switzerland: World Health Organization; 2001.

2. World Health Organization. *International Classification of Impairments, Disabilities and Handicaps.* Geneva, Switzerland: World Health Organization; 1980.

3. American Psychiatric Association. *Diagnostic and Statistical Manual of Mental Disorders, Fourth Edition, Text Revision.* Washington, DC: American Psychiatric Association; 2002.

4. Holmes GP, Kaplan JE, Guntz NM, et al. Chronic fatigue syndrome: a working case definition. *Ann Intern Med.* 1988;108:387–389.

5. Cocchiarella L, Andersson G, eds. *Guides to the Evaluation of Permanent Impairment.* 5th ed. Chicago, Ill: AMA Press; 2001.

6. Demeter SL, Andersson BJ, eds. *Disability Evaluation.* 2nd ed. Chicago, Ill: AMA Press; 2003.

7. Halligan P, Bass C, Oakley D, eds. *Malingering and Illness Deception.* Oxford, England: Oxford University Press; 2003. (Material used with permission from Oxford University Press.)

8. US Department of Labor. *Dictionary of Occupational Titles.* Rev 4th ed. Washington, DC: US Department of Labor; 1991.

9. O*Net OnLine. Available at: http://online.onetcenter.org. Accessed October 28, 2004.

10. US Department of Labor. *Dictionary of Occupational Titles.* 5th ed. Washington, DC: US Department of Labor; 2003.

Chapter 10

Medications, Driving, and Work

Gerald M. Aronoff, MD, Michael Erdil, MD, and Natalie P. Hartenbaum, MD, MPH

Healthcare provider (HCP) recommendations regarding driving abilities and work activities for patients who use prescription and over-the-counter (OTC) medications must consider a number of factors. These include the medical condition(s) for which drugs are used, the effects of drugs on cognitive and motor skills, the synergistic effects when multiple drugs are used, and how a drug might further impair abilities already compromised by the medical condition itself. Healthcare providers must also consider the risks associated with driving and work activities, legal and ethical issues, the limitations of existing literature regarding this issue, and the challenge of making appropriate work fitness and risk decisions.

Driving requires complex psychomotor abilities, as do many work activities with heavy machinery such as forklifts, power presses, and power tools. Working at heights where falls are a risk may also be a hazard for those taking certain medications. There is literature that demonstrates that medications can impair psychomotor performance and can increase the risk of traffic accidents. Because of space limitations, this chapter is not meant to be a comprehensive resource detailing the effects of specific medications used in clinical practice. Rather, the intent is to describe issues regarding medication use, the potential cognitive and motor problems affecting driving and work, and the potential liabilities to provide a framework for decision making.

Healthcare providers must acknowledge that, despite our society's dependence on the automobile, the ability to travel to and from work does not necessarily mean that one must drive to get to work. Many workers do not have a driver's license or a vehicle. An HCP should not state "unable to work" just because an individual who is used to driving to work may be currently unable to drive (for example, with initiation of potentially sedating medication treatment). Also, employers cannot require driving ability as a prerequisite for work *unless* the job itself involves driving.

Chapter 10

Magnitude of the Issue

Use of prescription and OTC medication is ubiquitous. Many medications can affect alertness, judgment, vasomotor responses, motor skills, and other abilities required for safe driving and/or potentially hazardous work. The *Physician's Desk Reference* contains more than 700 medications with warnings to use caution when driving a motor vehicle or operating machinery.[1] Among the many studies evaluating medication use and traffic accidents, there are a few population-based epidemiologic studies using linked databases (eg, health care, hospital, pharmacy, and motor vehicle). Four studies evaluated older drivers and two studies evaluated drivers of all ages.[2] These studies[3-8] suggest that benzodiazepine use increases accident risk up to 50%, with highest risk for increasing dose, daytime use, initial therapy, and/or combined benzodiazepine use. Cyclic antidepressants were associated with a twofold increased accident risk in two studies. Further research is necessary to characterize the impact of other types of medications on motor vehicle safety.

Many other medications, such as the sedating antihistamines and various OTC medications (including those containing alcohol), have similar potential effects on traffic safety. Healthcare providers need to inquire and counsel patients about the combined effects of these agents. In some occupations, employees are specifically warned about the risks of using potentially impairing medications, and in some (eg, motor vehicle operators) drug testing is performed, primarily to identify those who are using illicit drugs. The 2000 National Household Survey on Drug Abuse[9] estimated that 14 million Americans used illegal drugs in the month prior to the survey, with 7 million reporting driving under the influence of drugs. Seventy-seven percent of these individuals also reported driving under the influence of alcohol. In one voluntary study from Washington State's Operation Trucker Check,[10] a significant number of truck drivers were found to be using potentially impairing substances. Of drivers who volunteered for testing, 21% were positive for illicit substances or for potentially impairing prescription or OTC medications.

Potential Risks

Prescribing a medication to an individual encompasses more than just determining which medication can best treat the symptoms or disease, choosing the proper dose, and issuing the prescription. The HCP prescribing potentially sedating medications must be aware of the activities the patient participates in, both vocationally and recreationally. While individuals may choose not to engage in recreational activities when affected by impairing medications, financial pressures may influence them to not miss work given the same degree of impairment. In many cases, similar to observations with alcohol, an individual may not be able to accurately assess his or her degree of impairment. Cognitive impairment not only may affect the ability to drive or operate machinery safely, but also may affect judgment, decision-making abilities, and alertness. Any of these could place the individual, his or her coworkers, or the public in danger.

Safety-Sensitive Workers

Workers in safety-sensitive positions, such as commercial motor vehicle drivers, nuclear plant operators, or railroad engineers, may be prohibited by federal law and regulations from taking medications that might impair their ability to work safely. In many settings, this prohibition is not medication specific or absolute, but requires review and determination by the treating provider as to whether the individual can safely perform duties while taking the specific medication. For example, the federal medical standards for commercial drivers states that a person is physically qualified to drive a commercial motor vehicle if that person:

(i) Does not use a controlled substance identified in 21 CFR 1308.11 Schedule I, an amphetamine, a narcotic, or any other habit-forming drug.

(ii) Exception. A driver may use such a substance or drug, if the substance or drug is prescribed by a licensed medical practitioner who:

(A) Is familiar with the driver's medical history and assigned duties; and

(B) Has advised the driver that the prescribed substance or drug will not adversely affect the driver's ability to safely operate a commercial motor vehicle.

In addition, the medical examiner is required not only to review which medications the individual is taking but also to discuss with the driver the "potential hazards of medications, including OTC medications, while driving." The National Transportation Safety Board has investigated many accidents where it was determined that medications played a causal role. The Department of Transportation has repeatedly advised transportation industries "of potential threat to public safety caused by the on-duty use of some OTC and prescription medications by persons performing some safety sensitive duties."[11] In most cases, there is little official guidance from the federal agencies, and employers defer the decision as to whether an individual is safe to drive to the treating provider. However, several guidance documents are available from the Department of Transportation to assist with HCP decisions.[12–14] The HCPs must be familiar with specific statutes and regulations pertinent to safety-sensitive workers.

Chapter 10

State Department of Motor Vehicles

Healthcare providers must provide clear advice to patients to avoid driving when there is impairment from a medical condition or medication. This will occur most commonly when medications are initiated or doses are increased. Many states have regulations that prohibit motor vehicle operation when under the influence of medication, legal or illicit, which may interfere with safe motor vehicle operation.[15] Healthcare providers may be *required* to report drivers with medical conditions that impair safe driving. Providers should be familiar with state Department of Motor Vehicles reporting requirements to minimize medical–legal risks. Up-to-date information is available through most Department of Motor Vehicles Web sites. Considerations regarding whether to report include assessment of the degree of risk posed by the patient, safety of the patient and the public, and legal requirements including confidentiality. Healthcare providers should carefully document the specific reasons for concerns regarding driving safety, the methods used to assess driving safety, and the recommendations made to the patient about driving and medication use.

Other Legal Considerations

Healthcare providers may be liable for prescribing impairing medications and not adequately warning their patients of the potential hazards. Courts in Hawaii,[16] Michigan,[17] and Washington[18] have found HCPs responsible to third parties for injuries sustained when an HCP did not adequately warn the individual of the risk of driving. This may include failure to provide information regarding medication side effects and medical conditions that affect ability to drive.[15] Decisions and actions regarding return to hazardous work should consider these issues and mitigation strategies as well, since potential liability can occur if a worker on medication(s) sustains an injury attributed to the medication(s).

State-specific "drug-free workplace" statutes may pose an additional legal hazard for physicians. Several states have laws that require drug testing after workplace accidents. These laws state that if a postaccident drug test is positive for illegal drug use, the drug use is presumed to have caused the accident, and the worker loses workers' compensation coverage for the injury. Thus, if a worker borrowed an opioid from a family member or bought an opioid illegally, the presence of opioids on the postaccident drug screen provides the (rebuttable) legal presumption that the drug use caused the injury. If instead opioids are prescribed for a worker by a physician, and the worker has an accident at work with a postaccident drug screen detecting the presence of the opioids, the injured worker's lawyer can argue by analogy that the physician's prescription of opioids caused the worker's accident.

Decision Making

Driving and work task performance can be affected by several types of medication side effects. These include decreased alertness, impaired insight and judgment, euphoria, delayed reaction time, dizziness, blurred vision, blood pressure or pulse abnormalities, and extrapyramidal reactions. Patients may *not* recognize the degree of impairment associated with medication use.[19–23] The medical history should document impairing symptoms from illness and/or injury, as well as impairment from prescription and OTC medications, alcohol, and illicit substances. The history should inquire about new medications, recent dose adjustments, side effects, and potential synergistic effects of combined medication use with alcohol.

The occupational history should include the essential job tasks and psychomotor requirements. Job tasks that may involve increased risk to self or others (including public safety) include work-related driving, public safety, working at heights where falls are a risk, use of hazardous equipment and tools, work with hazardous chemicals, and the like. Healthcare providers must understand regulatory issues that may preclude work if certain medications are used or side effects are experienced, such as federal motor safety regulations (49 CFR 391.41) for commercial motor vehicle operators.[24] It is unknown whether shift workers have increased risk of injury or increased psychomotor risks with certain medications. However, the potential for synergistic effects of fatigue and sleep deprivation from shift work and sedating medications should be considered. The history of work accidents, near misses, and driving record may add additional insight, as may information from employers or family members raising safety concerns.

Physical examination to assess safety to drive and perform potentially hazardous work tasks requires evaluation of the underlying physical condition for which the patient is taking medications, including vital signs, vision, hearing, and cognitive and motor skills. The Mini-Mental State Examination, including psychomotor task performance using calculators or computers, can enhance traditional HCP examination findings and impressions.

Chapter 3 of the *HCP's Guide to Assessing and Counseling Older Drivers*[15] describes a battery of tools to assess driving-related skills in the elderly population. This includes visual acuity and visual fields, the timed Trail-Making Test (alternately connecting randomly arranged numbers and letters), clock drawing, timed rapid-pace walking (10 feet and turning around), manual test of range of motion, and motor strength. Specific scoring, interpretation, and intervention strategies are provided. While not targeted to the working population, the publication offers good suggestions on assessment of psychomotor skills and driving abilities.

Chapter 10

Questions regarding driving safety after evaluation should prompt evaluation by a driving rehabilitation specialist. These professionals may be located from inquiries to hospitals or rehabilitation centers, driving schools, or Departments of Motor Vehicles, or by searching the Association for Driver Rehabilitation Specialists online directory at www.driver-ed.org or www.aded.net. Driving evaluations may employ actual or computer-simulated driving skill assessment, depending on availability. Supervised work trials or work site evaluations can be used to assess performance of work-required tasks. Vocational rehabilitation specialists, physical therapists, or occupational therapists can work with employers and HCPs to design and assess work trials in difficult situations.

Driving and the performance of potentially hazardous work tasks should be supported by physicians in settings where patients have been carefully evaluated regarding mental acuity and cognitive functioning and have been found to be alert with appropriate concentration and attention span. These patients must have no evidence of drug effects that would interfere with safe job performance or endanger themselves or coworkers. For work activities covered by specific regulations (eg, commercial motor vehicle drivers), HCPs must be familiar with those regulations and consider any available guidance documents (eg, Psychiatric, Neurologic, and/or Cardiac Federal Motor Carrier Conference Reports[12–14]). These are available online at http://www.fmcsa.dot.gov/rulesregs/medreports.htm. Patients who have restrictions limiting driving or hazardous work may still be able to work in a temporary modified work capacity. Again, because someone should not drive to work does *not* mean that individual cannot be at work and do appropriate work tasks. Healthcare providers should support continued work while seeking appropriate treatments that promote return to regular duty.

Healthcare providers should, whenever possible, prescribe treatments and medications with the lowest possible risk of impairment. For example, patients with musculoskeletal disorders may have options of treatment with acetaminophen or nonsteroidal anti-inflammatory agents for pain control rather than potentially sedating muscle relaxants or opioids. Topical agents and self-applied thermal treatments may be useful pain control interventions. Transcutaneous electrical nerve stimulation units, acupuncture, physical therapy, and chiropractic care may provide nonmedication treatment options for others. These options are described elsewhere.[25,26] When prescribing new medications, HCPs should consider medical problems that may make patients more sensitive to medication side effects and the impact of other prescription and OTC medication use that may pose synergistic or additive effects. Use of the lowest effective dose can limit risks. Patients must be educated about the use medications as prescribed, the potential medication risks and side effects, the risks of combined medication use, the increase in side effects when there is a change or increase in the dose of medications, the potential for the patient not to recognize impairment, the need to avoid hazardous activities if sedated, and the need to report symptoms. When using medications with higher risks of sedation or side effects, or when increasing dosing, patients should be advised to take the first few doses in settings where they have lower risks of injury (at home, after work). Patients may need to be instructed to cease driving or operating hazardous machinery temporarily while they adjust to medication changes. Temporary restriction from hazardous work tasks and alternative transportation arrangements can help avoid lost work time. Finally, patients using OTC medications should be advised to carefully read labels regarding potential side effects causing sedation or decreased psychomotor fitness.

Specific Medications

Literature reviews[27] have shown that many medications can impair psychomotor performance. Certain classes of medications, including benzodiazepines,[3,4,27] muscle relaxants,[28] sedating antihistamines,[16,27,29,30] neuroleptics,[31,32] anxiolytics,[15] narcotic analgesics,[33] and some nonnarcotic analgesics and sedatives, have been shown to impair performance of driving tasks, at times to a similar degree as alcohol. Much like the individual impaired by alcohol, the driver impaired by medications may be unable to accurately assess his or her degree of impairment. Alcohol can also potentiate the central nervous system effects of prescribed medications, and patients should be counseled appropriately. An extensive review of the effect of medications on psychomotor performance is beyond the scope of this chapter. This information is available elsewhere;[15,27,34,35] a brief review follows.

Antidepressants and Psychoactive Agents

Patients with active suicidal, psychotic, manic, anxiety, or other significant psychiatric symptoms will require temporary activity limitations consistent with their condition, regardless of what medication is being used or started. Psychoactive medications have the potential to alter psychomotor and driving performance. Initiation of sedating medications or alteration of dosing may prompt physician-imposed temporary activity restrictions (based on risk). Tricyclic antidepressants are prescribed, at times, to treat musculoskeletal disorders. Potential side effects with these drugs include sedation, orthostasis, blurred vision, and cardiac effects.[36] The Federal Highway Administration Conference on Psychiatric Disorders and the Commercial Driver[12] recommended that for commercial motor vehicle drivers:

- Some antidepressants do produce impairment that can be mitigated over time but not completely removed with chronic use. Individuals on antidepressants that may interfere with performance should not be allowed to drive commercial vehicles. Amitriptyline was specifically mentioned as an antidepressant to be avoided because of its sedating effects. (By analogy, all cyclic antidepressants are considered problematic for commercial drivers.)

- Given strong evidence of impaired psychomotor performance associated with the use of all antipsychotic drugs, drivers should be qualified only after the effects of the illness and the neuroleptic have been reviewed by a psychiatrist familiar with the regulations and safety risks associated with medications and commercial driving.
- Lithium, in a stable, long-term dose and plasma level, is permissible for regularly monitored asymptomatic drivers.

Antihistamines
Older antihistamines (eg, diphenhydramine and chlorpheniramine) may have significant potential for psychomotor and driving impairment, and these effects may not be recognized by patients.[15,16,22,27,29,30] Newer nonsedating antihistamines used in recommended doses offer alternative treatment with lower risks.[36]

Antihypertensives
Potential side effects of antihypertensive treatment include dizziness, fatigue, and hypotension. Temporary caution may be required during initiation of treatment and during dose changes. Some agents, such as clonidine, methydopa, guanabenz, reserpine, and prazosin, may have more significant central nervous system or other side effects.[14] Electrolyte problems and dehydration can also affect driving abilities.

Anxiolytics and Hypnotics
Psychoactive medications such as the benzodiazepines[37-39] have been demonstrated to impair psychomotor performance, including driving, and increase the risk of motor vehicle accidents. Longer-acting agents have greater effects than short-acting agents on function, including daytime function after nocturnal administration. The Federal Highway Administration Conference on Psychiatric Disorders and the Commercial Driver recommended[12]:

- "Individuals requiring anxiolytic medications should be precluded from commercial driving. This recommendation would not apply to patients treated effectively with non-sedating anxiolytics such as buspirone."
- "Individuals requiring hypnotics should only use drugs with half lives of less than 5 hours for less than 2 weeks under medical supervision and only at the lowest effective dose."

- Some shorter-acting hypnotics such as zaleplon may permit driving as soon as five hours after use. Considerations with medication use include selection of shorter-acting agents, patient counseling about impairment and lack of recognition, possible avoidance of driving, and hazardous work during initiation or dose changes.

Muscle Relaxants

Drowsiness and dizziness have been reported to occur in up to 30% of patients taking muscle relaxants compared with placebos.[40] Some agents (eg, cyclobenzaprine or carisoprodol) may have greater effects on psychomotor performance than less sedating medications.[15] Lower-dose cyclobenzaprine may have less sedative effects than historical doses.

Opioids

In the context of a rehabilitation focus for patients with chronic pain, it is important to address concerns about the use of opioids while patients are driving or performing potentially hazardous work tasks. Some literature on new-onset, uncomplicated, acute work-related low back pain suggests an association between prolonged opioid use and longer duration of work disability.[41] It is unclear whether prolonged disability could reflect more significant pathology, improper opioid use, provider or employer decision making against return to work, or other causes. Guidelines from the Agency for Health Care Policy and Research regarding acute low back pain state, "opioids appear to be no more effective in relieving low back symptoms than safer analgesics, such as acetaminophen or aspirin or other NSAIDs [nonsteroidal anti-inflammatory drugs]."[40] However, opioids are commonly used for control of pain unresponsive to other interventions. Some authors believe that the effects of opioids on performance have been exaggerated.[42] There is some evidence that patients habituate to the sedative and psychomotor effects of long-term opioids,[43] permitting safe return to work. While many HCPs restrict their patients from driving while on opioids, emerging research and opinion[44–54] suggest that patients with a normal mental status who are on stable doses of long-acting or sustained-action opioids may have acceptable risks for driving and work, and that uncontrolled pain itself is a greater risk factor for injury than is pain controlled by a long-term, stable opioid dose. New (acute) opioid use and intermittent opioid use are more likely to produce mental and/or psychomotor impairment than is long-term use of an opioid on a fixed dosing schedule. Thus, acute use of an opioid or intermittent opioid use may require temporary modification of activities (work restriction based on risk) until stability occurs and task safety is documented.

Fishbain et al[55,56] performed two evidence-based literature reviews regarding opioids and driving. The 2002 review[55] concluded that "opioids are not

Chapter 10

associated with intoxicated driving, MVA [motor vehicle accidents] and MVA fatalities. . . . As in all clinical decisions, this determination should be individualized according to clinical factors." The 2003 review[56] suggested that stable opioid use had no significant impairment of psychomotor abilities, cognitive function, psychomotor abilities, or impairment when measured in driving simulators. Fishbain concluded that "the majority of the reviewed articles appeared to indicate that opioids do not impair driving-related skills in opioid-dependent/tolerant patients. . . ."[56] Fishbain did suggest the need for additional controlled studies.

Galski et al,[57] in a pilot study to determine the effects of medically pre-scribed, stable opioid use on the driving abilities of patients with persistent, nonmalignant chronic pain, assessed patients with a comprehensive off-road driving evaluation using measures shown to be sensitive in predicting on-road driving performance. Patients on long-term opioid therapy did not have significantly impaired perception, cognition, coordination, or behavior that would affect on-road driving. However, the authors noted that "methodolog-ical problems may limit the generalizability of results and recommendations are made for research beyond a pilot study."

Careful medical supervision is required while managing patients on chronic opioid analgesic therapy. Opioid contracts have been used by many HCPs to document patient responsibilities and informed consent. Assessment of mental status and physical ability for driving in the elderly was previously discussed.[15] In addition, one of us (G.A.) monitors reaction time by using the "Aronoff test of reaction time." This test is not validated but can be a useful tool for observing reaction time. With the patient not anticipating the event, the physician throws a soft rubber or foam ball at the patient. The patient's reaction is observed. A normal response is for the patient to react appropriately and catch the ball (or reach for the ball to avoid being struck). The author (G.A.) believes that a sedated patient with decreased mental acu-ity or impaired reflexes will generally not be able to catch or deflect the ball, and thus will be struck by the ball. This has not been tested for scientific validity, nor is it being endorsed for widespread use at this time. However, the author (G.A.) believes that this test combined with a detailed mental status examination gives a good estimate of whether a patient has adequate reaction time to function in a number of situations, including driving, and therefore is a clinically useful tool.

Follow-up examinations should include assessment of mental acuity, cogni-tive function, evidence of a thought disorder, attention span and concentra-tion, and mood/affect. If the mood appears to be depressed, it is essential to inquire about suicidal ideation or intent. Each time the dosage of opioid is increased, HCPs must caution patients not to drive, not to operate potentially dangerous equipment, and not to put themselves (or others) in at-risk situations if somnolent or if mentally "slow" until they acclimate to the new dose. As with other medications, patients may not recognize impairment, and periodic objective HCP assessment is beneficial. For medical–legal purposes, HCPs may wish to restrict comments in patient records as to whether or not there is a medical or psychiatric basis to recommend restricting the patient from driving, since HCPs generally do not have knowledge about actual driving skills of patients. A useful entry in the patient's record is "based on today's evaluation, I find no basis to restrict this patient from driving or working, if he/she so chooses. Mr/Ms _____ knows that if at any time he/she is not fully alert or if he/she experiences any decrease in mental acuity, he/she is not to drive or engage in potentially hazardous activities."

Patients whose work involves safety-sensitive operations, such as public safety workers and those operating a train, bus, or truck, where impairment may endanger others, are a special category. Primary care physicians should not clear these patients for safety-sensitive work while the patients are using opioids (or other potentially impairing medications) without full knowledge of the applicable state and federal (Department of Transportation, etc) regulations, and without specialist consultation.

In practice, whether patients taking opioids are "allowed" by their HCPs and employers to return to work may be independent of actual patient functioning or the presence (or absence) of medication side effects, since return to work also involves medical, legal, and regulatory issues, attitudes, etc. However, an injured worker with chronic pain who is appropriately evaluated, treated, and monitored and who is using stable doses of opioids might be able to be medically cleared to return to work according to the framework discussed in this chapter. Again, as with all potentially impairing medications, new (acute) opioid use and intermittent opioid use are more likely to produce mental and/or psychomotor impairment than is long-term use of an opioid on a fixed dosing schedule. Thus, acute use of an opioid or intermittent opioid use may require temporary modification of activities (work restriction based on risk) until stability and task safety are documented.

Stimulants

Stimulants may be prescribed for conditions such as attention deficit disorder. Increased accident rates have been observed in adolescent drivers, and HCPs should screen for learning disabilities and other conditions that could affect driving safety.[15] The Conference on Psychiatric Disorders and the Commercial Driver recommended the following[12]:

> CNS [central nervous system] stimulants, in therapeutic doses, impair driving by a variety of mechanisms. A person using these drugs should not

be medically qualified to drive commercially. Legitimate medical use (ADHD [attention deficit–hyperactivity disorder], for example) with no demonstrable impairment or dosage escalation tendency, may receive an exemption after expert review.

While the increased alertness during peak stimulant effect may intuitively seem to be beneficial, the decreased alertness that frequently occurs when the stimulant blood levels are decreasing may lead to mistakes and accidents.

Summary

Information is available regarding the side effects of prescription and non-prescription medications. There is a need for additional literature to clarify the impact of many drugs on driving, and especially on work performance. Guidance documents for regulated positions (eg, Department of Transportation) need to be updated to reflect current patterns of medication use and current understanding of side effects. Cost-effective and validated tools to objectively assess patient-employee abilities and enhance decision making are needed. Furthermore, strategies need to be developed to enhance HCP and patient awareness about this topic.

The appropriate use of most prescription and OTC medications is not usually a major issue in return-to-work decision making, as there is usually little impairment of psychomotor faculties. There are medications and there are safety-sensitive jobs for which these issues require considerable information gathering and discussion between the physician and the patient, and perhaps with the employer.

References

1. Hartenbaum NP. *The DOT Medical Examination: A Guide to Commercial Drivers' Medical Certification.* 3rd ed. Beverly Farms, Mass: OEM Health Information Inc; 2003.

2. Stevens J. Testimony on epidemiology of transportation safety and potentially sedating or impairing medications. FDA/NTSB Joint Public Meeting, Washington, DC, November 14, 2001.

3. Barbone F, McMahon AD, Davey PG, et al. Association of road-traffic accidents with benzodiazepine use. *Lancet.* 1998;5:239–244.

4. Hemmelgarn B, Suissa S, Huang A, Boivin J-F, Pinard G. Benzodiazepine use and the risk of motor vehicle crash in the elderly. *JAMA.* 1997;278:27–31.

5. Leveille SG, Buchner DM, Koepsell TD, McCloskey LW, Wolf ME, Wagner EH. Psychoactive medications and injurious motor vehicle collisions involving older drivers. *Epidemiology.* 1994;5:591–598.

6. Neutel CI. Risk of traffic accident injury after a prescription for a benzodiazepine. *Ann Epidemiol.* 1995;5:239–244.

7. Oster G, Huse DM, Adams SF, Imbimbo J, Russell MW. Benzodiazepine tranquilizers and the risk of accidental injury. *Am J Public Health.* 1990;80: 1467–1470.

8. Ray WA, Fought RL, Decker MD. Psychoactive drugs and the risk of injurious motor vehicle crashes in elderly drivers. *Am J Epidemiol.* 1992;136:873–883.

9. *Summary of Findings from the 2000 National Household Survey on Drug Abuse.* Washington, DC: Department of Health and Hunan Services, SAMHSA, Office of Applied Studies; September 2001.

10. Couper FJ, Pemberton M, Jarvis A, Hughes M, Logan BK. Prevalence of drug use in commercial tractor trailer drivers. *J Forensic Sci.* 2002;47:562–567.

11. National Transportation Safety Board. *Safety Recommendation, I-00-1 through I-00-4.* Available at: www.ntsb.gov/Recs/letters/2000/I00_1_4.pdf. Accessed May 21, 2004.

12. US Department of Transportation, Federal Highway Administration. *Conference on Psychiatric Disorders and Commercial Drivers.* Washington, DC: Office of Motor Carriers; 1991. Publication FHWA-MC-91-006. Available at: www.fmcsa.dot.gov/Pdfs/psych1.pdf; www.fmcsa.dot.gov/Pdfs/psych2.pdf; www.fmcsa.dot.gov/Pdfs/psych3.pdf; www.fmcsa.dot.gov/Pdfs/psych4.pdf. Accessed July 2, 2004.

13. US Department of Transportation, Federal Highway Administration. *Conference on Neurological Disorders and Commercial Drivers.* Washington, DC: Office of Motor Carriers; 1988. Publication FHWA-MC-88-042. Available at: www.fmcsa.dot.gov/Pdfs/neuro.pdf; www.fmcsa.dot.gov/Pdfs/neuro2.pdf. Accessed July 2, 2004.

14. US Department of Transportation, Federal Highway Administration. *Cardiovascular Advisory Panel Guidelines for the Medical Examination of Commercial Motor Vehicle Drivers.* Washington, DC: Office of Motor Carriers; October 2002. Publication FMCSA-MCP-02-002. Available at: www.fmcsa.dot.gov/pdfs/cardio.pdf. Accessed July 2, 2004.

15. Wang CC, Kosinski CJ, Schwartzberg JG, Shanklin AV. *Physicians' Guide to Assessing and Counseling Older Drivers.* Washington, DC: National Highway Traffic Safety Administration; 2003. Available at: www.ama-assn.org/ama/pub/category/10791.html. Accessed October 27, 2004.

16. McKenzie et al *v* Hawaii Permanante Medical Group Inc et al. Hawaii Supreme Court, June 10, 2002.

17. Duvall *v* Goldin, 362 NW 2d 275 (Mich App 1984).

18. Kaiser *v* Suburban Transportation System, 65 Wash 2d 461, 398 P.2d 14 (Wash 1965).

19. Mattila M. Acute and subacute effects of diazepam on human performance: comparison of plain tablet and controlled release capsule. *Pharmacol Toxicol.* 1988;63:369–374.

20. Roache JD, Griffiths RR. Comparison of triazolam and pentobarbital: performance impairment, subjective effects and abuse liability. *J Pharmacol Exp Ther.* 1985;234:120–133.

Chapter 10

21. Aranko K, Mattila MJ, Bordignon D. Psychomotor effects of alprazolam and diazepam during acute and subacute treatment, and during the follow-up phase. *Acta Pharmacol Toxicol.* 1985;56:364–372.

22. Weiler JM, Bloomfield JR, Woodworth GG, et al. Effects of fexofenadine, diphenhydramine, and alcohol on driving performance: a randomized placebo-controlled trial in the Iowa driving simulator. *Ann Intern Med.* 2000;132:354–363.

23. Kay GG, Quig ME. Impact of sedating antihistamines on safety and productivity. *Allergy Asthma Proc.* 2001;22:281–283.

24. FMCSR Physical Qualification of Drivers; Medical Examination; Final rule; *Fed Reg* 2000;65(October 5):59363–59380.

25. Erdil M, Dickerson OB, eds. *Cumulative Trauma Disorders: Prevention, Evaluation and Treatment.* New York, NY: Van Nostrand Reinhold; 1997.

26. American College of Occupational and Environmental Medicine. *Occupational Medicine Practice Guidelines.* Arlington Heights, Ill: American College of Occupational and Environmental Medicine; 2004.

27. Basselt RC. *Drug Effects on Psychomotor Performance.* Foster City, Calif: Biomedical Publications; 2001.

28. Logan BK, Case GA, Gordon AM. Carisprodol, meprobamate, and driving impairment. *J Forensic Sci.* 2000;45:619–623.

29. Kay GG. The effects of antihistamines on cognition and performance. *J Allergy Clin Immunol.* 2000;105(6 suppl, pt 2):S622–S627.

30. O'Hanlon JF, Ramaekers JG. Antihistamine effects on actual driving performance in a standard test: a summary of Dutch experience, 1989–94. *Allergy.* 1995;50:234–242.

31. Grabe HJ, Wolf T, Gratz S, Laux G. The influence of clozapine and typical neuroleptics on information processing of the central nervous system under clinical conditions in schizophrenic disorders: implications for fitness to drive. *Neuropsychobiology.* 1999;40:196–201.

32. Wylie KJ, Thompson DJ, Wildgust HJ. Effects of depot neuroleptics on driving performance in chronic schizophrenic patients. *J Neurol Neurosurg Psychiatry.* 1993;56:910–913.

33. Linnioila L, Hakkinen S. Effects of diazepam and codeine, alone and in combination with alcohol on simulated driving. *Clin Pharmacol Ther.* 1974;15:368–373.

34. DeHart RL. Medication and the work environment. *J Occup Med.* 1990;32:310–312.

35. Aronoff GM. *Handbook on Pharmacological Management of Chronic Pain.* Indianapolis, Ind: ML Wavecrest Publishing. In press.

36. Ray WA, Purushottam BT, Shorr RI. Medications and the older driver. *Clin Geriatr Med.* 1993;9:413–438.

37. Vermeeren A, Danlou PE, O'Hanlon JF. Residual effects of zaleplon 10 and 20 mg on memory and actual driving performance following administration 5 and 2 hours before awakening. *Br J Clin Pharmacol.* 1999;48:367–374.

Chapter 10

38. Vermeeren A, Muntjewerff ND, van Boxtel M, et al. Residual effects of zaleplon and zopiclone versus the effects of alcohol on actual car driving performance [abstract]. *Eur Neuropsychopharmacol.* 2000;10(suppl 3):S394.

39. Volkerts ER, Verster JC, Heuckelem JHG, et al. The impact on car-driving performance of zaleplon and zolpiden administration during the night [abstract]. *Eur Neuropsychopharmacol.* 2000;10(suppl 3):S395.

40. Bigos SJ, Bowyer O, Braen G, et al. *Acute Low Back Problems in Adults. Clinical Practice Guideline No. 14.* Rockville, Md: Agency for Health Care Policy and Research, Public Health Service, US Department of Health and Human Services; 1994. AHCPR Publication 95-0642.

41. Mahmud MA, Webster BS, Courtney TK, Matz S, Tacci JA, Christiani DC. Clinical management and the duration of disability for work-related low back pain. *J Occup Environ Med.* 2000;42:1178–1187.

42. Aronoff GM. Opioids in chronic pain management: is there a significant risk of addiction? *Curr Rev Pain.* 2000;4:112–121.

43. Sjogren P, Thompsen AB, Olsen AK. Impaired neuropsychological performance in chronic nonmalignant pain patients receiving long-term oral opioid therapy. *J Pain Symptom Manage.* 2000;19:100–108.

44. Zacny JP. A review of the effects of opioids on psychomotor and cognitive functioning in humans. *Exp Clin Psychopharmacol.* 1995;3:432–466.

45. Chesher GB. Understanding the opioid analgesics and their effects on skills performance. *Alcohol Drugs Driving.* 1989;5:111–138.

46. Hanks GW, O'Neill WM, Simpson P, et al. The cognitive and psychomotor effects of opioid analgesics, II: a randomized controlled trial of single doses of morphine, lorazepam, and placebo in healthy subjects. *Eur J Clin Pharmacol.* 1995;48:455–460.

47. Hanks GW. Morphine sans morpheus. *Lancet.* 1995;346:652–653.

48. Kappes S, Laux G. Driving performance of opiate addicts under methadone supported rehabilitation. *Pharmacopsychiatry.* 1995;28:191.

49. Lodeman E, Leifer K, Kluwig J, et al. An investigation of the cognitive effects of repeated doses of opioid analgesics in volunteers. *Pharmacopsychiatry.* 1995;28:1999.

50. O'Neill WM, Hanks GW, McIntyre E, et al. An investigation of the cognitive effects of repeated doses of opioid analgesics in volunteers. *Eur J Clin Invest.* 1995;25:379.

51. Smith AM. Patients taking stable doses of morphine may drive. *BMJ.* 1996;312:56–57.

52. Starmer GA. A review of the effects of opioids on driving performance. In: O'Hanlon JF, de Fier JJ, eds. *Drugs and Driving.* London, England: Taylor Francis; 1986:251–269.

53. Vainio A, Ollila J, Matikainen E, et al. Driving ability in cancer patients receiving long-term morphine analgesia. *Lancet.* 1995;346:667–670.

54. Zacny JP. Opioids and chronic pain. *Clin J Pain.* 1998;14:89–91.

Chapter 10

55. Fishbain DA, Cutler RB, Rosomoff HL, Rosomoff RS. Can patients taking opioids drive safely? A structured evidence-based review. *J Pain Palliat Care Pharmacother.* 2002;16:9–28.

56. Fishbain DA. Are opioid-dependent/tolerant patients impaired in driving-related skills? A structured evidence-based review. *J Pain Symptom Manage.* 2003;25:559–577.

57. Galski T, Williams JB, Ehle HT. Effects of opioids on driving ability. *J Pain Symptom Manage.* 2000;19:200–208.

Chapter 10

Chapter 11

How the Primary Care Physician Can Help Patients Negotiate the Return-to-Work/ Disability Dilemma

Mark D. Pilley, MD

Completion of a family medicine residency enables new primary care physicians to feel confident that the scope of recent clinical training will provide the level of skills necessary to cope with disease and chronic illness, and the challenges accompanying long-term disability. Clinical residency experiences are like all life experiences in that true experience occurs when coping with a life event requires the application of knowledge for crisis resolution. Healthcare concepts presented remain concepts until applied in dealing with the impact of impairment and the challenge of recovery.

Understanding the Role of the Primary Care Physician

The role of the primary care physician seems perfectly obvious to the objective observer until external forces take charge. Understanding the impact of impairment in reference to presumed disability, and understanding the terms *risk assessment*, *capacity*, and *tolerance,* are needed to be effective in the prevention of long-term disability. Patient advocacy is best served by providing advice and directives that support recovery to maximum activity and return to work. Physicians should avoid enabling inappropriate work absence, thus preventing avoidable long-term disability. Understanding the patient's social obligations, personal resources, family needs, and demands is central in providing insightful and appropriate patient education and advice.[1]

Physicians are frequently asked for notes confirming that work absence was medically necessary and/or that return to work is now appropriate. When a physician–patient encounter involves documenting loss of time from work because of illness or injury, the issues surrounding why the absence occurred need to be clearly understood. Knowing the patient's history and the secondary gains driving illness behavior helps in determining barriers that cause delayed recovery. There are no "poor historians," just poor history takers. Establishing reliability in the historical information obtained is essential and necessary. Some patients attempt either consciously or unconsciously to deceive their physicians, either by exaggerating or by minimizing the severity of their medical condition.

The current economics of US medicine are part of the problem. With currently declining reimbursement rates for office visits, it is harder for primary care physicians to incorporate health promotion and disease prevention into routine single-problem office visits. Similarly, taking the time to inquire about the various job tasks a patient must perform and to inquire about the psychosocial factors that impact disability is difficult, especially because that time is generally not "codable" or "reimbursable." It takes much less time to sign a form certifying disability than to both explore whether the patient can work and educate the patient that return to work is both medically appropriate and in his or her best interest. However, history is obviously the driver directing the next steps in diagnosis, treatment, recovery, and return to work.

An additional pressure on the primary care physician is living up to the, at times, unreasonable expectations of a patient's extended family. Many times a physician will recognize that a request from a patient for disability certification is not medically appropriate, but the physician will be threatened with the loss of the entire extended family as patients in the practice if he or she refuses to certify the inappropriate disability.

Sometimes primary care physicians certify inappropriate medical disability because they fail to realize that being out of work may be detrimental to a patient's physical, mental, and social well-being, as discussed in Chapter 1.

Avoiding the Impact of Delay

One of the objectives for the physician, employer, and insurer is to avoid the impact of delay. Delayed understanding of the issues in "medical leave" leads to delayed intervention and delayed recovery that places the patient at risk for permanent work absence (permanent disability). Approximately 50% of people off work for 8 weeks will not return to work. More than 85% of persons off work for 6 months will not return to long-term employment and are at risk of long-term disability. Their lives seldom recover fully, physically, mentally, spiritually, and/or financially.

Billions of dollars are lost annually because of work absence. In 1994 it was estimated that $36.2 billion was unrecoverable from wage protection programs.[2] Today this figure may have doubled. This is equivalent to an annual stock market crash resulting in unrecoverable dollars. Recurrent cyclic trends are well documented by the insurance industry. When companies reorganize, when the economy adjusts to major crisis such as the terrorist attacks on September 11, 2001, and when jobs are eliminated and transferred to another country, the incidence of persons claiming disability increases in a parallel manner. At the same time that disability claims increase, the demands for healthcare services increase.

Understanding the factors contributing to long-term disability is very important. Age, education, external vs internal locus of control, motivation, and job or career satisfaction are known predictors or indicators of the risk of long-term disability.[3] Family dynamics such as the number of children under the age of 20 years, proximity to a viable labor market (rural vs city), and single vs multiple diagnoses or illnesses are additional contributors to the risk of long-term disability and failure to return to work.[4] Secondary forces such as active or pending litigation, progressive vs nonprogressive medical conditions, and compensation factors such as disability benefit coverage play major roles in delayed return to work.

Improving Chances for Successful Return to Work: Sample Cases

Early physician intervention and communication of the physician's anticipation of recovery during the initial period of illness and/or injury (the temporary phase of disability) improves the chances for successful return to work and the avoidance of unnecessary long-term disability. The temporary limitations and/or restrictions that are appropriate just after an injury or just after disease onset do not necessarily become permanent. Recovery, at least to some degree, is usually expected. As recovery occurs, it is usually appropriate to encourage increased activity, both at home and at work (decreased work limitations and restrictions). Subjective components such as job dissatisfaction, burnout, personal feelings, and limitations in coping with change have a major impact on prolonged absence behavior.[1] Despite the contribution of subjective and social determinants, there is evidence that "early activation" or early intervention through appropriate resumption of activity decreases the risk of prolonged absence behavior and promotes improved return-to-work outcomes.[5]

Returning the ill or injured person to work is a process that begins with the physician's understanding of not only the health status and impact of functional status, but also the patient's absence behavior and the social environment that provides support for such behavior. Unlike specialists, who tend to see patients as deranged organ systems, primary care physicians are able to see the whole person as a person and so are uniquely qualified to determine the factors that hinder return to work and to intervene. Understanding and insight are only part of the equation. A plan of action will assist in overcoming barriers that prevent "early activation" and return to work.
The following two cases are examples of true experiences in which patients overcame significant medical and psychosocial challenges and successfully returned to work.

Case 1: Myocardial Infarction
Becoming 40 years old began an important transition period for this man. His children were nearing the age for college, his career in information technology was very successful, the house was almost paid for, and he and his wife were experiencing a wonderful relationship. His personal and family medical history were unremarkable. His only known cardiac risk factor was cigarette smoking.

The man unexpectedly suffered an acute myocardial infarction. Revascularization with a percutaneous coronary intervention was performed, but when anticoagulation treatment was stopped, the stented artery reclotted and the posterolateral infarct extended, resulting in cardiogenic shock. Two weeks later the patient was stable enough to be weaned off of the aortic balloon assist pump. With an initial ejection fraction of 19%, he was considered a potential candidate for cardiac transplantation. By the time he was assessed for transplantation, his ejection fraction was 26% to 29%, and he was no longer a candidate.

While the patient had lost a considerable portion of his myocardium and pumping ability, he had no residual ischemic myocardium at risk for infarction from other coronary lesions. After recovery, he did not have angina, but rather fatigue as his dominant problem. He had no ventricular arrhythmias. His cardiologist prescribed the expected angiotensin-converting enzyme inhibitor, β-blocker, diuretic, aspirin, and hydroxymethyl glutaryl coenzyme A reductase inhibitor (statin). His primary care physician's recovery plan for the patient was focused on smoking cessation, improvement of function, increased activity, and resumption of as normal a life as possible, with return to work being considered part of the recovery process.

Presumed Disability

The Social Security Administration's criterion for total disability (no job the patient can be expected to do) is as follows[6]:

> The inability to engage in any substantial, gainful activity by reason of any medically determinable physical or mental impairment(s), which can be expected to result in death or which has lasted or can be expected to last for a continuous period of not less than 12 months.

Risk Assessment

Cardiogenic shock occurring after acute myocardial infarction has a mortality rate varying between 50% and 80%.[7-11] The first 48 hours are critical, with most deaths occurring during this time.[11,12] Patients who survive until discharge have a 1-year survival rate of 88%.[11,13]

With no residual ischemia (and thus no angina) and with no documented arrhythmia, risk is not a significant issue for this man, whose work is primarily sedentary and whose job demands are primarily cognitive. Thus, he does not require physician-imposed work restrictions.

Some individuals will have a level of cardiac pump function after cardiogenic shock that will never allow them to resume gainful employment, resulting in permanent disability.[14] This is based in capacity and not in risk. Risk assessment involves issues like the risk of reinfarction and the risk of sudden arrhythmic death.

Capacity

Compensated congestive heart failure is this man's clinical diagnosis. Limitation of functional capacity for an individual recovering from myocardial injury severe enough to cause cardiogenic shock is related to the degree of pump function reserve available to support the physical and metabolic demands of activity. Capacity is reflected by clinical symptoms experienced with increasing levels of activity, including the ability to respond to emotional stress, infection, and work demands, and is measurable with exercise testing.[14] If the person's work requires performing strenuous tasks, then restrictions may need to be imposed, limitations may need to be described, and potential accommodations may need to be described. Reassignment and/or transfer to a less demanding job may be indicated. (See Chapter 15 for further details.)

After discharge from the hospital, this man had a marked limitation of physical activity capacity. Even though he was comfortable at rest, light physical activity caused fatigue and dyspnea. Exercise testing demonstrated that he was able to achieve 3 to 3.5 metabolic equivalents, placing him in functional class III.

Tolerance

Postinfarction congestive heart failure may result in permanent or long-term disability. This man had no previous medical problems and there were no comorbid conditions contributing to a delayed recovery or prolonged work absence other than his history of cigarette smoking. Cardiogenic shock itself was the major complication of his acute myocardial infarction. Other organ systems did not demonstrate significant injury caused by the hypoperfusion of cardiogenic shock.

Phase II cardiac rehabilitation was started approximately 6 weeks after myocardial infarction and was continued until the patient returned to working partial days, at which time phase III or maintenance cardiac rehabilitation therapy began. Cardiac rehabilitation provided an opportunity to regain not only physical strength and endurance (capacity) but confidence (tolerance) and hope. The man was able to acquire additional skills in coping through behavioral modification. By participating in the recovery process with other persons who also had had a severe myocardial infarction, he was able to realize through a shared experience that he could still have an active life. After 12 weeks of cardiac rehabilitation he was able to exercise up to 5 metabolic equivalents, placing him at class II functional status.

The Primary Care Physician's Role

One of the most important challenges and focuses for the family physician is in assisting with and supporting a patient in the recovery of emotional and social well-being. Approximately 65% of people experience symptoms of depression after a myocardial infarction. Major depression may affect 15% to 22% of such patients.[15] Depression by itself is considered an independent risk factor in the development and mortality associated with cardiovascular disease.[16] Persons who have preexisting cardiovascular disease and are depressed have a 3.5 times greater risk of death than those who have cardiovascular disease and are not depressed.[17,18] Cognitive-behavioral therapy is considered the preferred form of psychological treatment. This, combined with use of a selective serotonin reuptake inhibitor, is considered to be the most effective approach.[19]

Pharmacotherapy for depression was offered but declined. The man did not want to "take drugs to feel better." Counseling was also declined. A series of 20-minute office visits was the option selected. Frequent office visits gave the family physician the needed opportunity to conduct cognitive-behavioral therapy. By being an astute observer and letting the patient communicate what he felt the physician needed to know about his life, the physician learned about the impact of the man's disability on the rest of the family: wife, son, daughter, mother, father-in-law, and cousins. His wife was protective and at times reluctant to consider allowing her husband to return to work. His children were anxious and fearful of the unknown future without their father. His parents and extended family were hopeful and reverent, as they felt "it was in the hands of a higher power." He was the son to be proud of. He provided the largest portion of the family income. If he didn't work, how would his children go to college? He was the "responsible" and loved son, father, and spouse. Paradoxically, he was seen as too young to be disabled, but yet not too young to have almost died. He had declined seeing a psychologist, but he needed to express these thoughts and feelings. He needed help accepting his feelings and how life changed. The primary care physician was there to listen and advise (cognitive therapy) and to prescribe and supervise his cardiac rehabilitation (behavioral therapy).

All of the patient's extended family felt the impact of his disease, impairment, illness, and disability. What was at risk here was the health and well-being of an entire family. The primary care physician, who also cared for other members of this family, saw the fear and insecurity felt by the wife and children. Uncertainty and concern were expressed by the parents and cousins. Those who smoked began to smoke more. Hostility and argumentativeness increased. Those being treated for depression became more depressed, required medication adjustment, and began to come into the office more frequently. What was also apparent was the physician's connectedness to the family as their family physician. As the patient's strength and endurance improved, as his confidence returned, transitioning back to work became an achievable reality. Interestingly, the physician's practice grew because more of the patient's family members began to schedule appointments. As the patient healed and returned to work, the family members improved; smoking decreased, and even ceased, in the case of the patient's spouse. His mother's depression improved and fewer visits to the office were needed. The children felt they could leave home and go to college. Despite having a positive attitude, tremendous family support, employment with a company that valued his skills enough to preserve his job until he could return to work, and excellent short-term and health insurance benefits, the patient still required 4 months of therapy and recovery time before he was ready to resume work for half-days. It took another 3 weeks before he was able to return to an 8-hour day at work.

Chapter 11

His job was sedentary, having primarily cognitive demands and requiring keyboarding skills. There was very limited lifting, and that consisted of lifting computer parts, monitors, and stacks of paper. Initial work limitations and *suggestions* for this patient were general and not specific: "If what you lift bothers you, don't lift it, get help. Avoid strenuous exertional activity. Don't get winded, and stop to rest when you feel fatigued." He was encouraged to walk as far as tolerated, enjoy the companionship of his spouse, take his medication as prescribed, continue cardiac rehabilitation and exercise, and keep scheduled follow-up appointments with his primary care physician and with his cardiologist.

With the start of cardiac rehabilitation, there was a physical and emotional display of progressive improvement in endurance, self-confidence, and mood. Depression was an anticipated reaction to his infarction, but pharmacologic treatment was not required. The family physician reinforced positive progress, gave encouragement, and was careful to avoid defining specific work restrictions and to clarify the patient's unrealistic expectations of functional recovery. The physician consistently set the expectation that the patient would recover the ability to work in his usual job for his employer. Close follow-up, appropriate medical and rehabilitative therapies, avoiding predictions of negative outcomes ("catastrophizing"), providing hope and encouragement, and soliciting hope and encouragement from family all helped to support this man in recovering his life. He became motivated to return to work. Returning to work, to gainful employment, was necessary for full recovery to occur. The primary care physician had the authority to enable prolonged disability or to release the patient back into the workforce. Of paramount importance was the physician taking ownership of his problem and taking the time to listen to his concerns. The physician determined that the patient would be safely capable of returning to his sedentary job and provided the advice to empower him to accept his ultimate level of recovery and quality of life. The patient was willing and able to receive the benefit of a prescription to return to work, and he remained employed at last follow-up.

Conclusions
The healing process of recovery is a shared experience, shared with the whole family and social support system. Illness or injury that impairs and disables someone wounds the entire family. Healing and recovery from such wounds has major impact on the health and well-being of the family. The scars that result from such wounds have the potential to either strengthen or destroy a family. At a basic level, it begins with the absence note.

The absence note and return-to-work prescription are the responsibility of the primary care physician. As inconvenient as the paperwork seems, it becomes the "written word." Thoughtful and accurate communication in the form of the written word is a powerful part of the recovery process. The return-to-work note is a prescription or "physician's order" that gives expressed permission and authorization to transition from disability to being able to return to work. Returning to work is an important part of recovery and needs to occur as soon as it can be safely accomplished. The absence note and return-to-work prescription define restrictions, limitations, and recommendations regarding accommodations. As an essential part of the process, this carries the weighty responsibility of determining whether it is safe for a person to return to a job, knowing certain task demands need to be met. The impact of the physician in directing the patient as to the best course in life should not be minimized. The physician's written word is just that, his or her word, and the physician should make it count.

Case 2: Motor Vehicle Accident (Pelvic Fracture and Closed Head Injury)

A 46-year-old man was behind the wheel of his car when he stopped for a blinking red light at an intersection. He looked left, right, then left again to make sure the coast was clear. Seeing no other cars, he entered the intersection and was struck on the driver's side by a truck traveling at high speed. The next things he remembered were being removed from the passenger side of his demolished car, being placed on a stretcher, and being moved into an ambulance that would carrying him to the local emergency department. The patient's primary care physician was contacted by the emergency department physician at 1 AM to admit the patient to the hospital with an unstable pelvic fracture (orthopedics would consult) and a closed head injury. His blood alcohol level was zero and his urine drug screen was negative. This was anticipated, as he was in recovery and he had been sober for 12 years. Nevertheless, he was given a ticket for failure to yield the right of way and for running a red light. The other driver was not tested for alcohol and was not ticketed. Charged with failure to yield, the patient was responsible not only for his medical expenses, but for the expenses of the other driver. The good news was that he would not lose his driver's license, and that he had medical insurance coverage and short-term disability insurance coverage through his employer. He did not have a long-term disability coverage benefit, but he did have vocational rehabilitation benefits.

The patient worked for a company that built large refrigerated storage units for commercial businesses. His job was to oversee the construction of such units. The job description for this position indicated this was a "heavy" to "very heavy" job according to the *Dictionary of Occupational Titles* criteria.[20] He was a welder by training and had previously worked at a bulk tank manufacturing plant, welding aluminum tanks together. Fortunately he was young enough to learn new skills. He would need to learn new skills to survive; he was single and owned a small house with a mortgage. He did not have any children or a previous spouse to support, but he did have a "significant other" female friend who was committed to helping him recover.

Presumed Disability

The Social Security Administration's criterion for total disability (no job the patient can be expected to do) is as follows[6]:

> The inability to engage in any substantial, gainful activity by reason of any medically determinable physical or mental impairment(s), which can be expected to result in death or which has lasted or can be expected to last for a continuous period of not less than 12 months.

In addition, Social Security considers persons under 50 years of age to be totally disabled if they are not capable of completing any type of job tasks, and persons over the age to 50 disabled if they are unable to complete the job tasks for which they have been trained or have experience performing.

The type of pelvic fractures and the treatment needed affected this patient's duration of disability. His fractures did not involve the acetabulum of either hip, and he did not require surgery (neither internal nor external fixation of these fractures was common when this injury occurred in 1986). There were no complications or injuries to other organ systems. His job demands fell into the heavy to very heavy classification, as listed in Table 11-1. This placed his anticipated work absence between a minimum of 56 to 84 days to a maximum of 140 days.[21]

Risk Assessment

An unstable pelvic fracture at the time this patient was injured required temporary avoidance of weight bearing (standing, walking, and sitting) until sufficient fracture healing had occurred. Premature resumption of standing or sitting during the early recovery phase would cause unnecessary pain and

Table 11-1 Pelvic Fractures Not Including the Acetabulum[21]

Job Classification	Duration, days		
	Minimum	Optimum	Maximum
Sedentary	14	42	56
Light	28	56	84
Medium	42	70	112
Heavy	56	84	140
Very heavy	84	98	140

increased risk of fracture displacement, as well as delayed union or nonunion of the fractures. Obviously, time off work (restriction, based on temporary risk) was necessary until sufficient healing had occurred.[21] The patient's closed head injury resolved quickly and fully and thus did not impose any additional restrictions. Once his fractures had healed, there was no risk of imminent harm with activity, so there was no basis for permanent physician-imposed work restrictions.

Capacity
During early recovery, the patient was placed on bed rest and required assistance with activities of daily living. Safety issues (falls) were of concern, and to ensure optimum safety, he was admitted to a skilled care nursing setting. His medical insurance covered 72 hours of his skilled-care stay even though he had benefit coverage up to 100 days. Despite multiple appeals and a telephone discussion with the insurance medical director, no additional coverage was allowed. This was an additional expense that became the patient's responsibility.

After 6 weeks of bed confinement and nursing assistance with activities of daily living, he was ready and cleared for progressive physical and ambulatory therapy. He was taught the use of first a wheelchair, then a walker, and finally crutches.[21] He was motivated and ambitious, demonstrating the capacity to effectively utilize assistive devices and follow therapy instructions, allowing a steady gain in independence and in functional capacity. Despite his progress, it was apparent that he would not be able to return to his previous job because he would not be able to regain capacity quickly enough to be acceptable to his employer. The Family Medical Leave Act permits only 12 weeks of unpaid leave, and his capacity for work would not be adequate for heavy work tasks until 3 months from the date of injury. His employer was legally permitted to terminate his employment and replace him.

Tolerance
Because of persisting pain and fear of reinjury during heavy work (issues of tolerance), the patient decided to change careers. Vocational rehabilitation benefits were available. The plan was to use these benefits after he left the skilled care setting. Once progressive physical and ambulatory therapy began, functional capacity steadily increased. On light activity, his pain complaints were minimal, and he did not require the use of narcotics for pain control. Heavier activity caused a considerable increase in his pelvic pain. He took his sobriety seriously and refused the use of narcotics. Thus, he chose to change careers on the basis of tolerance. It took him 3 months to recover to a point where he could drive again. Regaining his independence and ability to drive made it easier for him to begin vocational rehabilitation.

He chose to be trained in computer or informational technology because such jobs require specific skills he could learn and the work tasks are at only a sedentary to light duty job demand. At this level of activity, his pain was very tolerable without medication. Through vocational rehabilitation, he was able to return to work and become gainfully employed.

Conclusions
Multiple forces affect the challenge of returning an injured person to work. The astute provider must identify therapeutic interventions needed for recovery, anticipate recovery time frames, and arrange for rehabilitation services needed to meet such time frames. Physicians must know the employer's job requirements, understand the limitations and scope of benefit coverage available, identify needed and available personal and social resources, and understand the actual and potential impact of prolonged disability for their patients. With all of these "needs to know" comes the realization that return to work is not only a goal, but an active part of the recovery process.

An employer uses disability insurance coverage benefits not only to retain employees but to manage the workforce. Even though this patient could not return to his previous job, he did have vocational rehabilitation benefits covering the cost of acquiring new skills needed to return to work at a different job. Interestingly, the patient did not know he had such a benefit until the primary care physician asked him about this possibility. The inquiry prompted him to contact his employer's Human Resources Department to clarify what benefits were available. Knowing he had a way to not only regain function, but return to work, was strategic in preventing long-term disability.

Summary
Primary care physicians are often recruited by the local company to be the company physician. Although confident in their scope of clinical training and ability to treat disease and chronic illness, the challenges accompanying disability can sometime be overwhelming. Obtaining additional training is helpful in allowing the primary care physician to address the return-to-work components of tolerance, capacity, and risk.

References
1. McGrail MP Jr, Lohman W, Gorman R. Disability prevention principles in the primary care office. *Am Fam Physician*. 2001;63:679–684.
2. Kerns WL. Cash benefits for short-term sickness, 1970-94. *Soc Secur Bull*. 1997;60:49–53.

3. Bigos SJ, Battie MC, Spengler DM, et al. A prospective study of work perceptions and psychosocial factors affecting the report of back injury. *Spine*. 1991;16:1–6.

4. Lohmann W. Resources for disability prevention. In: *Occupational Medicine Update: Selected Topics in Occupational Medicine.* St Paul, Minn: Minnesota Medical Association; 1999:72–84.

5. Linton SJ, Hellsing AL, Andersson D. A controlled study of the effects of early intervention on acute musculoskeletal pain problems. *Pain*. 1993; 54:353–359.

6. Social Security Administration. *Disability Evaluation Under Social Security.* (*Blue Book*) SSA Pub. No. 64-039; January, 2003. Available at: www.socialsecurity.gov/disability/professionals/bluebook. Accessed October 27, 2004.

7. Hochman JS, Sleeper LA, Webb JG, et al, for the SHOCK Investigators. Early revascularization in acute myocardial infarction complicated by cardiogenic shock. *N Engl J Med.* 1999;341:625–634.

8. Urban P, Stauffer JC, Khatchatrian N, et al. A randomized evaluation of early revascularization to treat shock complicating acute myocardial infarction: the (Swiss) Multicenter Trail of Angioplasty SHOCK—(S)MASH. *Eur Heart J.* 1999;20:1030–1038.

9. Goldberg RJ, Samad NA, Yarzebski J, et al. Temporal trends in cardiogenic shock complicating acute myocardial infarction. *N Engl J Med.* 1999;340:1162–1168.

10. Hasdai D, Califf RM, Thompson TD, et al. Predictors of cardiogenic shock after thrombolytic therapy for acute myocardial infarction. *J Am Coll Cardiol.* 2000;35:136–143.

11. Danchin N, De Benedetti E, Urban P. Acute myocardial infarction. *Am Fam Physician.* 2003;68:519–521.

12. Urban P, Bernstein M, Costanza M, et al. An internet-based registry of acute myocardial infarction in Switzerland. *Kardiovasc Med.* 2000;3:430–441.

13. Berger PB, Tuttle RH, Holmes DR, et al. One year survival among patients with acute myocardial infarction complicated by cardiogenic shock, and its relation to early revascularization: results of the GUSTO-1 trial. *Circulation.* 1999;99:873–878.

14. Hosteltler M. Shock, cardiogenic. Available at: http://www.emedicine.com/emerg/topic530.htm. Accessed May 24, 2004.

15. Carney RM, Freedland KE, Sheline YI, Weiss ES. Depression and coronary heart disease: a review for cardiologists. *Clin Cardiol.* 1997;20:196–200.

16. Glassman AH, Shapiro PA. Depression and the course of coronary artery disease. *Am J Psychiatry.* 1998;155:4–11.

17. Frasure-Smith N, Lesperance F, Talajic M. Depression following myocardial infarction: impact on 6-month survival. *JAMA.* 1993;270:1819–1825.

18. Lesperance F, Frasure-Smith N, Talajic M. Major depression before and after myocardial infarction: its nature and consequences. *Psychosom Med.* 1996;58:99–110.

Chapter 11

19. Guck TP, Kavan MG, Elasasser GN, Barone EJ. Assessment and treatment of depression following myocardial infarction. *Am Fam Physician.* 2001;64:641–648, 651–652.

20. US Department of Labor. *Dictionary of Occupational Titles.* Rev 4th ed. Washington, DC: US Department of Labor; 1991.

21. Reed P. Fracture, pelvis. In: *Medical Disability Advisor.* 3rd ed. Westminster, Colo: Reed Group, Ltd; 1997.

Working With Common Spine Problems

James B. Talmage, MD, and Robert H. Haralson III, MD, MBA

Spinal conditions are one of the most common reasons physicians are asked by patients, employers, and insurers whether or not a patient can do a particular job. This chapter examines lumbar radiculopathy and mechanical nonspecific low back pain—two spinal conditions that are among the most frequent causes of disability in developed nations. These common conditions will serve as examples of how to think through return-to-work issues related to spinal problems.

Presumed Disability

The Social Security Administration's (SSA's) criteria for total disability due to musculoskeletal impairments include some that are relevant to spinal problems:

> The inability, from a physical standpoint alone, to ambulate effectively on a sustained basis for any reason, including pain, that has lasted for 12 months. To ambulate effectively an individual must be capable of sustaining a reasonable walking pace over a sufficient distance to be able to carry out activities of daily living, including the ability to travel without companion assistance to and from the workplace. Examples of ineffective ambulation include the required use of a walker, two crutches, or two canes, the inability to walk a block at a reasonable pace on rough or uneven surfaces, the inability to use standard public transportation, and the inability to shop and bank, and the inability to climb a few steps at a reasonable pace with the use of a single hand rail. (Section 1.00 B. 2. a. General)[1]

Spinal conditions potentially severe enough to cause the above level of handicap include: herniated nucleus pulposus, spinal arachnoiditis, spinal stenosis, osteoarthritis, degenerative disc disease, facet arthritis, and vertebral fracture resulting in compromise of a nerve root or the spinal cord with one of the following:

A. Evidence of nerve root compression characterized by neuro-anatomic distribution of pain, limitation of motion of the spine, motor loss (atrophy and/or muscle weakness) accompanied by sensory or reflex loss, and if there is involvement of the lower back, positive straight leg raising test (sitting and supine).
B. Spinal arachnoiditis, confirmed by operative note, pathology report, or imaging study (MRI or myelogram), manifest by severe pain resulting in the need for changes in position or posture more than once every two hours.
C. Lumbar spinal stenosis resulting in pseudoclaudification, established by appropriate imaging changes, and manifest by chronic nonradicular pain and weakness, resulting in the inability to ambulate effectively, as defined above. (Section 1.04)[1]

There are individuals who obviously meet these criteria and yet continue to work. Paraplegics who use wheelchairs would be obvious examples. There are others who work daily despite painful conditions severe enough to meet this definition. While these criteria seem reasonable, they are difficult to interpret. Most "poor" results from disk herniation are poor because pain is severe, and the decision not to work despite pain is based in tolerance. Many have significant pain, and yet lack the motor weakness or sensory loss to seem to qualify on the basis of section A of the previous criteria.

Under section B, arachnoiditis, the need to change position or posture more than once every two hours is problematic. Most normal people change position or posture more than once an hour. When typing for this book, the authors would change posture several times an hour, but keep typing.

The definition of ineffective ambulation is hard to relate to a given patient. One aspect is the inability to use public transportation. Taxi cabs are "public transportation." If an individual can enter and ride in a standard car to come to a physician's office, that individual can ride in a taxi cab. A public bus may have a first step located 14 to 18 inches above the street or sidewalk level. Some with bilateral stiff hips and/or stiff knees may not be able to raise a foot far enough off the ground to reach the necessary first step to board the bus. Back problems other than paraplegia would not limit the ability to climb into a bus, but hip or knee comorbid pathology may. A subway station may have an escalator or elevator and no step at all to enter the subway car, and yet a different, less used subway station may require climbing some stairs.

Does "inability to shop" mean inability to stop at a convenience store for a few items, or inability to stay at a mall all day for Christmas shopping with the family? Is "banking" travel to and use of the local branch of a bank, or banking on the Internet? How long is the "city block"? How quickly should one who ambulates effectively be able to walk the block? How rough and how uneven is the surface on which a physician is to evaluate ambulation ability?

Is the use of ambulation aids, such as crutches or canes, a matter of necessity because of capacity, or is it based in symptom tolerance? Does the physician feel the patient's pain or fatigue is really severe enough to require the use of these aids, or does the physician feel the individual may use these aids to come to the office, but not when out in the community? Some individuals use canes or soft cervical collars not for their pain-relieving effect, but rather as a way to communicate to those around them that they are having pain (pain behavior).[2]

Thus, it is difficult for a physician to see a patient with spinal problems and advise the patient as to whether or not an application for disability benefits will be accepted or rejected by the SSA. Some criteria for disability under Social Security, like "amputation of both hands, or of one hand and one lower extremity at or above the tarsal region," are clearly defined. With amputations, it is easier to tell whether a patient will or will not qualify. Even when disability seems obvious, remember, each term in the SSA definition of disability has a precise definition determined by case law. The ambiguity in spinal disorders reflects the fact that there usually will not be objective clinical findings that clearly determine the individual's functional status. Some individuals with mild imaging changes describe severe pain and very limited ability, and yet others with severe imaging changes describe little or no pain and normal function.

How, then, can a physician determine what a patient with a spinal disorder can be expected to do at work? The concepts of risk, capacity, and tolerance will be discussed as they apply to spinal problems.

Lumbar Disk Herniation Resulting in Radiculopathy

Lumbar disk herniation may be an asymptomatic imaging finding.[3] However, this is not what is discussed in this section. Rather, in this section, lumbar disk herniation resulting in nerve root impingement and a recognizable clinical syndrome of radicular pain, numbness, and weakness, with or without bowel and/or bladder control, is discussed.

Risk Assessment

Lumbar disk herniation with radiculopathy is the best example of risk assessment in spinal problems to consider, because risk can be relatively clearly defined and has been studied. Once the condition has stabilized, either with or without surgical treatment, the risk most feared by patients and physicians is recurrent disk herniation. "What if I send this patient back to work and he re-herniates his disk?"

In the past, almost all patients were given permanent work restrictions after successful lumbar diskectomy. The fear was that, without permanent lifting restrictions, re-herniation would occur much more frequently. This fear seems plausible. Because the disk did herniate, and because it required diskectomy, it has already been proven that there is a hole in the annulus of the disk, and that the hole is "aimed" at the nerve root. If any additional disk material (nucleus pulposus) extrudes, it logically will travel directly toward the nerve root to produce recurrent symptoms.

Disk herniation produces a recognizable clinical syndrome and has objective imaging and operative findings, so the re-herniation can be objectively and accurately diagnosed. This scenario of return to work after surgical diskectomy logically is the "worst-case scenario" for return-to-work assessment of individuals with back problems. No other back problem scenario would have as high a risk of a work-related problem that can be objectively documented.

This is the traditional justification for permanent post-operative restrictions after even successful lumbar diskectomy. Historically, with permanent lifting restrictions of somewhere between 20 and 50 pounds, re-herniation occurs in 5% to 12% of cases[4] (surgeons differed markedly on how much these patient should lift).

Recent studies have shown that, with first-operation lumbar diskectomy, patients may be sent back to unrestricted activity, meaning "full duty" work, with no increase in the incidence of re-herniation.[5,6] On the basis of this evidence, spine surgeons are increasingly willing to allow unrestricted activity after successful diskectomy (first operation). Famous athletes, for example, Joe Montana and Steve McNair, who returned to heavy weight lifting and professional football within a few weeks of lumbar diskectomy, have helped make both patients and physicians aware that heavy activity is safe after this surgery.

When permanent restrictions were assigned arbitrarily after lumbar diskectomy, the restrictions most commonly specified only the amount of weight the patient should lift. Current biomechanical and epidemiologic data confirm that lifting is not the most important stress on the back. There are much more data to indicate that sustained static postures, repetitive bending, twisting, and whole-body vibration are risks to the back than there are data to implicate heavy lifting.[7]

The modern post-operative management of lumbar diskectomy patients now includes vigorous exercise or back rehabilitative exercise, frequently under the supervision of a physical therapist. Heavy activity that simulates heavy work and that prepares the individual for heavy work has been shown to be safe and to improve functional status ("current ability" increases toward "capacity").[8]

Individuals with multiple spinal operations are much less common than individuals with first-time lumbar diskectomy. This chapter's discussion does not necessarily apply to individuals with multiple spinal operations. These individuals may be predisposed to disk herniation because of genetic risk factors[9–11] and other risk factors such as smoking.[12] The work ability assessment of these individuals must be individualized, although some of the principles of this discussion may apply.

Capacity

Patients with a lumbar disk herniation often have a decreased exercise capacity (or current ability), both during the acute event (first 3 months after the herniation) and afterward (based on deconditioning). If needed, a formal functional capacity evaluation (FCE) can attempt to quantitate either what the patient is willing to do (tolerance, limited by pain) or able to do (current ability, limited by lack of strength). (See Chapter 7 for more information about FCEs.)

Current ability may be increased by exercise, as noted in studies discussed previously on post-operative physical therapy.[8] In a post-operative therapy program, the exercise intensity increases slowly and gradually. A meta-analysis of studies has concluded that this exercise treatment is both safe and effective.[8] This same gradual return to function can occur without formal physical therapy by returning to work with temporary modified duty that is gradually phased out. Thus, work activity and home exercise can be the "therapy" that improves "current ability."

Tolerance

Pain is usually what determines whether a lumbar diskectomy result is considered to be "good" or "poor." Pain is not currently measurable. There may or may not be a correlation between the amount of pain after a disk herniation and the presence or absence of objective findings on physical examination, imaging studies, and electromyography. As long as Western medicine handles disability issues with a biomedical model in which impairment is expected to correlate with disability, pain accompanied by major objective findings will be the criterion for a disability application to be accepted. The SSA criteria for disability based on spinal problems recognize this. They demand that there be objective evidence of impairment in terms of neurologic deficit or in terms of arachnoiditis or spinal stenosis on imaging.

Thus, for the individual with lumbar radiculopathy with severe complaints of pain and limited activity tolerance who has no or minimal objective findings, current Western medicine would consider this to be an issue of *tolerance*, and not an issue of risk or capacity. Issues of tolerance in the absence of known serious risk are not a basis for physician-imposed work restrictions. Restrictions are to be based on risk. This individual may have a limited current ability to exercise. There is no easy way to quantify how much of a limited exercise ability is due to inactivity-induced deconditioning and how much is due to issues of tolerance of the pain associated with activity. The method of discussing this situation with the patient suggested in Chapter 2 may be utilized here as well:

> You do not appear to meet the Social Security Administration's criteria for total disability. Thus, in our society, there is some job you're expected to be able to do. Because there is no medical evidence that you are at high risk of significant harm by working, I can not certify that you're disabled for this job. There is no basis for work restrictions based on risk. Whether the rewards of working are sufficient for you to choose to remain at work, or whether the pain or fatigue you feel is sufficient for you to choose a different type of work, or not to work at all, is a question only you can answer. I can record what you feel to be your current activity tolerances, but not as work restrictions or work limitations. Your tolerances are not scientifically measurable, and they may change in the future, depending on how active you are.

Disability certification forms usually have a section at the end of the form for "remarks" or "comments," which is the appropriate place to record the individual's comments on tolerances for activity in the absence of significant objective findings.

Tolerance for symptoms such as pain is what usually determines whether or not a patient who has had a lumbar diskectomy will choose to work (whether the rewards of work outweigh the pain). Individuals with "poor" results after lumbar diskectomy may have obvious objective findings that make their decreased *tolerance* for activity, and thus their current decreased "capacity" or "current ability" believable in the Western medicine biomedical model.

As noted earlier, the SSA considers objective radicular neurologic deficit or proven arachnoiditis as confirming that spinal pain can limit performance enough (decrease tolerance) to qualify as disabling. Examples of objective findings that tend to validate a lumbar radiculopathy patient's statements of decreased activity tolerance include leg or calf atrophy, dermatomal sensory loss (decreased sharp vs dull recognition, not just subjectively altered sensation), a consistently positive straight-leg–raising test, a persistent list or sciatic scoliosis, and denervation changes on needle electromyogram. In this circumstance, the physician would record what the patient is willing to tolerate in terms of activity on a disability form as "work limitations" with the addendum that the limitations are based on "believable tolerance with significant objective findings" and not based on actual capacity or ability. Most disability certification forms have sections in which to record work restrictions (based on risk) and work limitations (based on capacity), but no section to record tolerance for activity. Most disability certification forms do not request information about subjective tolerance. They request objective information about risk (restrictions) and capacity (limitations).

Consensus Criteria on Lumbar Disk Herniation

The Medical Disability Advisor from the Reed Group (www.rgl.com) provides consensus return-to-work criteria for *International Classification of Diseases, Ninth Revision* (ICD-9) codes 722.0 (lumbar disk herniation). These criteria indicate that persisting radicular pain is still compatible with function, and that most patients should eventually return to their original type of work. The real-world data that follow in Tables 12-1, 12-2 and 12-3 also indicate that most patients with lumbar radiculopathy do in fact return to work.

Table 12-1 Medical Treatment (Consensus)

Job Classification	Duration, days		
	Minimum	Optimum	Maximum
Sedentary work	1	7	14
Light work	1	14	21
Medium work	1	21	42
Heavy work	1	56	91
Very heavy work	1	91	168

Reproduced with permission from Reed.[13]

Table 12-2 Diskectomy (Consensus)

Job Classification	Duration, days		
	Minimum	Optimum	Maximum
Sedentary work	1	7	28
Light work	7	14	42
Medium work	14	28	56
Heavy work	90	120	Indefinite
Very heavy work	120	150	Indefinite

Reproduced with permission from Reed.[13]

Mechanical Non-specific Low Back Pain

For 85% to 90% of patients with back pain, there is no diagnosis that explains the pain.[14] This problem is called *non-specific low back pain*. Physicians commonly make up diagnostic terms to make our understanding sound more scientific, but with no clear criteria for the diagnosis, and with no medical consensus that a given term should be used.[15] "Mechanical" means the pain is musculoskeletal in origin, and not referred pain from abdominal or retroperitoneal structures. If the pain is not worse with activity and better with rest, the pain is probably not musculoskeletal, and physicians are advised to search for an abdominal or retroperitoneal cause for the pain.

Mechanical back pain is very common. The lifetime prevalence of low back pain is 50% to 80%, and the point prevalence is 15% to 35%.[16] Most back "strains" occur during normal activity the individual is accustomed to doing, and thus most back "strains" are really episodes of acute back pain. A "strain" or "sprain" should indicate the application of major violence to a muscle–tendon unit or to a ligament that results in tearing of fibers of a normal structure. An individual who bends over and experiences acute back pain may be diagnosed as "acute back strain, ICD-9 847.2" by one physician and as "acute back pain, ICD-9 724.5" by a second physician.

Risk Assessment

There are few studies on risk assessment of individuals who are off work and then return to work. Most published studies on risk look at populations at work and the risk of developing back pain problems while continuing to work.

The largest prospective study of American workers' future risk of workers' compensation claims for back pain problems is the Boeing aircraft study.[17]

Table 12-3 Real-world Disability Case Data

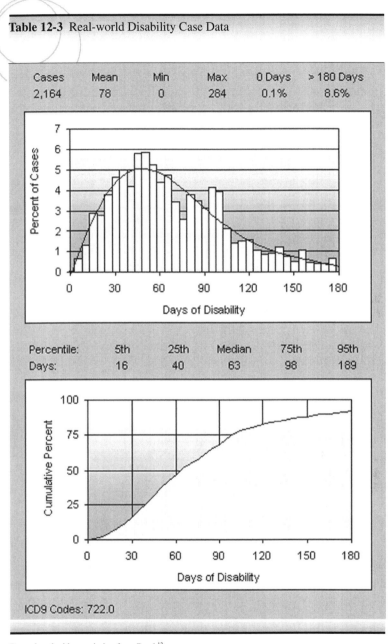

Cases	Mean	Min	Max	0 Days	≥ 180 Days
2,164	78	0	284	0.1%	8.6%

Percentile:	5th	25th	Median	75th	95th
Days:	16	40	63	98	189

ICD9 Codes: 722.0

Reproduced with permission from Reed.[13]

In this study over 3,000 workers were observed prospectively for four years. The greatest risk factors for a future claim were having current back pain or having had previous back pain (relative risk, 1.7) and not enjoying one's job (relative risk, 1.7). The low level of risk was the same regardless of whether the back pain was past pain or current pain, and regardless of whether the individual's job was light or heavy.

Psychological factors have been well documented to predict future chronic back pain.[18] Surprisingly, perhaps, work activity has not been conclusively shown to cause back pain.[16,19-21] It is certainly harder to do heavy work with a back problem than it is to do light work, but this does not mean that heavy work causes back pain. Individuals with back pain and heavy jobs may report their back pain more often than do individuals with back pain and light jobs.

Back pain–induced disability is a multifaceted problem. The largest published prospective study of back disability observed more than 34,000 Norwegians for seven years.[22] Future back disability was predicted to some degree by occupational factors, lifestyle factors, non-spinal comorbidity, and psychosocial factors.

Thus, mechanical back pain does not neatly fit a biomedical model. A biopsychosocial model of illness better explains back pain disability. However, the SSA, private disability insurers, and employers all treat back pain disability as a *biomedical* problem.

Low back pain is commonly treated with "work conditioning," which is progressive exercise under the supervision of a physical therapist. Each day the number of repetitions and the resistance (or weight lifted) is increased. New exercises are added frequently. This includes exercise that directly simulates work activity. This type of exercise treatment that simulates work has been proven to be effective and *safe* for patients with back pain.[23-26]

Physicians may prescribe work conditioning therapy, or they may prescribe return to modified duty work, with permitted work activity increasing gradually over time. In the absence of evidence that this type of treatment is harmful, and with evidence that it benefits the majority of patients, exercise or work is recommended as treatment.[25,27] A comprehensive examination and detailed reassurance that activity (even work) is more likely to be helpful than harmful has been shown to improve recovery and decrease disability in episodes of low back pain.[28-31]

There is only one published randomized study in which patients with acute back pain had FCEs and then were sent back to work at "full duty" despite the FCE frequently saying the patient was not yet capable of full duty.[32] These patients did better than the patients for whom the treating physician wrote work restrictions based on the FCE. (See Chapter 7.)

In conclusion, most patients with back pain will be helped, and not harmed, if the treating physician orders therapeutic exercise that simulates work (work conditioning) and/or advises return to work.

Capacity

Individuals frequently become less active once back pain begins, so decreased "capacity" (current ability) is seen frequently in patients with low back pain. Current ability can be quantitated to a degree by an FCE, although as detailed in Chapter 7, the validity of FCEs is questionable.[32–35] Current ability can be increased up to capacity through activity. Activity may mean formal work conditioning in physical therapy. Activity may be progressive exercise at home, or it may be returning to work at modified duty with restrictions that decease over time while work tasks become progressively more strenuous.[25,36,37] For most patients with low back pain the problem is not capacity, but rather tolerance. It is not that they are physically incapable of activity, but rather that they dislike the pain associated with activity, and thus they choose not to engage in certain activities. Pain is considered a rational reason for *patients to choose* to see physicians, take medications, and undergo hip replacement surgery. Pain thus should logically be a reason for patients to choose not to engage in certain activities. Similarly, the *choice to work despite pain*, or not to work, *is the patient's*. Physicians can describe the choices, the absence of scientific data on risk, and the fact that the discussion is about activities that "hurt to do," meaning that the patient *can do* them.

When patients choose to have medical treatment, Western society is clear that physicians describe treatment options, but the *choice* is the patient's. When patients choose not to work because of pain and to apply for disability benefits, Western society expects physicians to use a *biomedical* model and to be able to somehow discern who is in pain, and whether or not the pain is severe enough to logically preclude the work in question. There is no way to measure pain, and the biomedical model that equates impairment (pathology) with pain is clearly inadequate to explain most failure to function despite pain. However, until society accepts a different model for back pain disability, physicians will be asked to make return-to-work decisions in an impairment-based biomedical model.

There are consistent data in the medical literature indicating that physicians cannot tell who is having back pain, or how severe back pain is, by the use of imaging studies. Other than fracture, infection, tumor, and major disk herniation with obvious nerve root compression, imaging findings do not indicate who is in pain, or how severe pain is.[38–46] Findings such as disk bulges, disk protrusions without nerve compression, and annular tears are equally common in patients with back pain and in the asymptomatic population. Diskography has not been proven to be a reliable and valid way to detect back pain.[47–51] Thus, attributing back pain with failure to function to these imaging findings is illogical.

A common scenario is as follows: Physician A certifies a patient as disabled and uses a "bulging disk" on a magnetic resonance image as the objective evidence. Other physicians who see the same patient state that the patient can choose whether to work, but there is no medical basis for disability certification. These physicians disagree with physician A's opinion and quote the medical literature that bulging disks are not a proven cause of back pain. Thus, physician A appears to be either unscientific or biased in the age of "evidence-based medicine."

As discussed in Chapter 2, when physicians, motivated by the sincere desire to help patients, confuse tolerance for pain with lack of capacity or with risk, and write work limitations (capacity) or work restrictions (risk), they complicate "the system." Because there is no way for any physician to measure pain and/or pain tolerance, no two physicians will have the same opinion on a given patient's work ability despite pain. This leads to "dueling doctors," and confusion and/or anger in the patient, employer, insurer, and attorneys involved.

There is also the problem of the patient whose physician certifies inability to work at a low-paying light job because of back pain, who returns to the same physician with no change in his or her back condition but seeking a "full duty" release to permit working in a much higher-paying but much more physically demanding job. The rewards available for activity despite pain determine the patient's tolerance for the activities in question. This exemplifies the fact that tolerance is subjective, and not measurable. Tolerance is *not* an issue about which physicians can have an objective medical opinion. Thus, separating issues of capacity from issues of tolerance is critical.

Tolerance

Tolerance for activity (including work) despite low back pain is the usual problem facing patients and their physicians when return-to-work decision making must occur. As outlined in Chapter 2 and in the above discussion, tolerance is *not* a basis for physician-imposed work restrictions (risk) or work limitations (capacity). Tolerance issues logically are a *patient choice*, and physicians should decline to certify inability to work on the basis of issues of tolerance in the absence of severe pathology that cannot be medically improved.

The method of discussing this situation suggested in Chapter 2 again can be used:

> You do not appear to meet the Social Security Administration's criteria for total disability. Thus, in our society, there is some job you're expected to be

able to do. Because there is no medical evidence that you are at high risk of significant harm by working, I can not certify that you're disabled for this job. There is no basis for work restrictions based on risk. Whether the rewards of working are sufficient for you to choose to remain at work, or whether the pain or fatigue you feel is sufficient for you to choose a different type of work, or not to work at all, is a question only you can answer. I can record what you feel to be your current activity tolerances, but not as work restrictions or work limitations. Your tolerances are not scientifically measurable, and they may change in the future, depending on how active you are.

The techniques discussed in Chapter 3 are also helpful when discussing return-to-work issues with patients.

Consensus Criteria on Back Pain

The Medical Disability Advisor[13] consensus criteria for ICD-9 codes 846 and 847 are shown in Tables 12-4, 12-5, and 12-6.

Table 12-4 Lumbar or Lumbosacral Spine Strain (Consensus Criteria)

Job Classification	Duration, days		
	Minimum	Optimum	Maximum
Sedentary work	1	3	7
Light work	1	7	14
Medium work	3	14	28
Heavy work	7	21	42
Very heavy work	7	28	56

Reproduced with permission from Reed.[13]

Table 12-5 Thoracic Spine Strain (Consensus Criteria)

Job Classification	Duration, days		
	Minimum	Optimum	Maximum
Sedentary work	1	3	7
Light work	3	7	14
Medium work	7	14	28
Heavy work	7	21	42
Very heavy work	7	28	56

Reproduced with permission from Reed.[13]

Chapter 12

Table 12-6 Real-world Disability Case Data

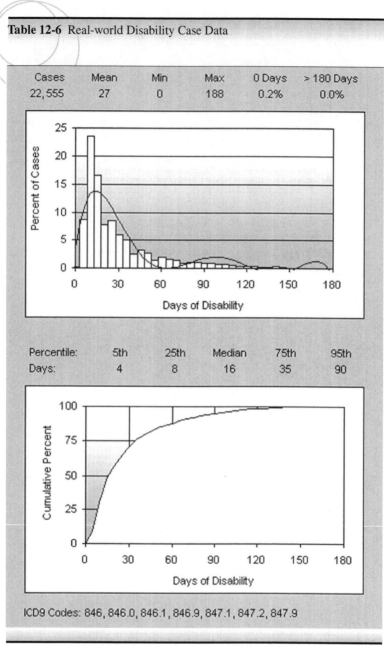

Cases	Mean	Min	Max	0 Days	> 180 Days
22,555	27	0	188	0.2%	0.0%

Percentile:	5th	25th	Median	75th	95th
Days:	4	8	16	35	90

ICD9 Codes: 846, 846.0, 846.1, 846.9, 847.1, 847.2, 847.9

Reproduced with permission from Reed.[13]

Consensus Criteria on Lumbar Disk Herniation

The Medical Disability Advisor[13] provides consensus return-to-work criteria for *International Classification of Diseases, Ninth Revision* (ICD-9) codes 846 and 847 (lumbar strain). These criteria indicate that persisting back pain is still compatible with function, and that most patients should eventually return to their original type of work. The real-world data that appear in Tables 12-3 and 12-4 and in Figure 12-2 also indicate that most patients with lumbar strain do in fact return to work.

Summary

Low back pain and lumbar disk herniations are common problems that illustrate how the principles of risk, capacity, and tolerance can be applied to return-to-work decision making. Most patients with these problems are capable of remaining at work. Even in the "worst-case scenario" of patients who have just had a lumbar diskectomy, return to full duty work is usually possible. Current work ability may increase with recreational activity, formal work conditioning therapy, or with return-to-work with gradually decreasing restrictions.

References

1. Social Security Administration. *Disability Evaluation Under Social Security.* Baltimore, Md: Social Security Administration; January 2003. SSA publication 64-039 (ICN 468600).

2. Andersson GB, Cocchiarella L, eds. *Guides to the Evaluation of Permanent Impairment.* 5th ed. Chicago, Ill: AMA Press; 2001.

3. Deyo RA, Weinstein JN. Low back pain. *N Engl J Med.* 2001;344:363–370.

4. Errico TJ, Fardon DF, Lowell TD. Contemporary concepts in spine care: open discectomy as treatment for herniated nucleus pulposus of the lumbar spine. *Spine.* 1995;20:1829–1833.

5. Carragee EJ, Helms E, O'Sullivan GS. Are postoperative activity restrictions necessary after posterior lumbar discectomy? *Spine.* 1996;21:1893–1897.

6. Carragee EJ, Han MY, Yang B, et al. Activity restrictions after posterior lumbar discectomy: a prospective study of outcomes in 152 cases with no postoperative restrictions. *Spine.* 1999;24:2346–2351.

7. Pope MH, DeVocht JW. The clinical relevance of biomechanics. *Neurol Clin.* 1999;17:17–41.

8. Ostelo RW, de Vet HC, Waddell G, et al. Rehabilitation following first-time lumbar disc surgery: a systematic review within the framework of the Cochrane Collaboration. *Spine.* 2003;28:209–218.

9. Karppinen J, Pääkkö E, Räinä MC, et al. Magnetic resonance imaging findings in relation to the col9a2 tryptohan allele among patients with sciatica. *Spine.* 2002;27:78–83.

10. Paassilta P, Lohiniva J, Göring HH, et al. Identification of a novel common genetic risk factor for lumbar disk disease. *JAMA.* 2001;285:1843–1849.

11. Marini JC. Genetic risk factors for lumbar disk disease. *JAMA.* 2001; 285:1886–1887.

Chapter 12

12. Goldberg MS, Scott SC, Mayo NE. A review of the association between cigarette smoking and the development of nonspecific back pain and related outcomes. *Spine.* 2000;25:995–1014.

13. Reed P. *The Medical Disability Advisor: Workplace Guidelines for Disability Duration.* 5th ed. Westminster, Colo: Reed Group; 2005.

14. Deyo RA, Rainville J, Kent DL. What can the history and physical examination tell us about low back pain? *JAMA.* 1992;268:760–765.

15. Fardon D, Pinkerton S, Balderston R, et al. Terms used for diagnosis by English speaking spine surgeons. *Spine.* 1993;18:274–277.

16. Waddel G. *The Back Pain Revolution.* 2nd ed. London, England: Churchill Livingstone; 2004.

17. Bigos SJ, Battié MC, Spengler DM, et al. A prospective study of work perceptions and psychosocial factors affecting the report of back injury. *Spine.* 1991;16:1–6.

18. Linton SJ. A review of psychological risk factors in back and neck pain. *Spine.* 2000;25:1148–1156.

19. Hadler NM. *Occupational Musculoskeletal Disorders.* 2nd ed. Philadelphia, Pa: Lippincott; 1999:266.

20. Nachemson AL, Jonsson E. *Neck and Back Pain.* Philadelphia, Pa: Lippincott Williams & Wilkins; 2000:118.

21. Videman T, Battié MC. The influence of occupation on lumbar degeneration. *Spine.* 1999;24:1164–1168.

22. Hagen KB, Tambs K, Bjerkedal T. A prospective cohort study of risk factors for disability retirement because of back pain in the general working population. *Spine.* 2002;27:1790–1796.

23. Schonstein E, Kenny DT, Keating J, et al. Work conditioning, work hardening, and functional restoration for workers with back and neck pain. In: *The Cochrane Library, Issue 2, 2004.* Chichester, England: John Wiley & Sons Ltd; 2004. Available at: www.cochrane.org/cochrane/revabstr/AB001822.htm. Accessed May 19, 2004.

24. Van Tulder M, Koes B, Bombardier C. Best practice and research clinical rheumatology: low back pain. *Rheumatology.* 2002;16:761–775.

25. Abenhaim L, Rossignol M, Valat JP, et al. The role of activity in the therapeutic management of back pain: report of the International Paris Task Force on Back Pain. *Spine.* 2000;25:1S–33S.

26. Garcy P, Mayer T, Gatchel RJ. Recurrent or new injury outcomes after return to work in chronic disabling spinal disorders. *Spine.* 1996;21:952–959.

27. Carter JT, Birrell LN, eds. *Occupational Health Guidelines for the Management of Low Back Pain at Work.* London, England: Faculty of Occupational Medicine; 2000. Available at: www.facoccmed.ac.uk/library/index.jsp?ref=383. Accessed October 26, 2004.

28. Indahl A, Velund L, Reikeraas O. Good prognosis for low back pain when left untreated. *Spine.* 1995;20:473–477.

29. Indahl A, Haldorsen EH, Holm S, et al. Five-year follow-up study of a controlled clinical trial using light mobilization and an information approach to low back pain. *Spine.* 1998;23:2625–2630.

30. Hagen EM, Eriksen HR, Ursin H. Does early intervention with a light mobilization program reduce long-term sick leave for low back pain? *Spine.* 2000;25:1973–1976.

31. Karjalainen K, Malmivaara A, Pohjolainen T, et al. Mini-intervention for subacute low back pain: a randomized controlled trial. *Spine.* 2003;28:533–541.

32. Hall H, McIntosh G, Melles T, et al. Effect of discharge recommendations on outcome. *Spine.* 1994;19:2033–2037.

33. King PM, Tuckwell N, Barrett TE. A critical review of functional capacity evaluations. *Phys Ther.* 1998;78:852–866.

34. Gross DP, Battié MC, Cassidy DJ. The prognostic value of functional capacity evaluation in patients with chronic low back pain, part 1: timely return to work. *Spine.* 2004;29:914–919.

35. Gross DP, Battié MC, Cassidy DJ. The prognostic value of functional capacity evaluation in patients with chronic low back pain, part 2: sustained recovery. *Spine.* 2004;29:920–924.

36. van Tulder MW, Koes B, Bombardier C. Low back pain: best practice and research. *Clini Rheumatol.* 2002;16:761–775.

37. Koes BW, van Tulder MW, Ostelo R, et al. Clinical guidelines for the management of low back pain in primary care: an international comparison. *Spine.* 2001;26:2504–2514.

38. van Tulder MW, Assendelft WJ, Koes BW, et al. Spinal radiographic findings and nonspecific low back pain. *Spine.* 1997;22:427–433.

39. Boden SD, Davis DO, Dina TS, et al. Abnormal magnetic-resonance scans of the lumbar spine in asymptomatic subjects: a prospective investigation. *J Bone Joint Surg Am.* 1990;72A:403–408.

40. Jensen MC, Brant-Zawadzki MN, Obuchowski N, et al. Magnetic resonance imaging of the lumbar spine in people without back pain. *N Engl J Med.* 1994;331:69–73.

41. Weishaupt D, Zanetti M, Hodler J, et al. MR imaging of the lumbar spine: prevalence of intervertebral disk extrusion and sequestration, nerve root compression, end plate abnormalities, and osteoarthritis of the facet joints in asymptomatic volunteers. *Radiology.* 1998;209:661–666.

42. Stadnik TW, Lee RR, Coen HL, et al. Annular tears and disk herniation: prevalence and contrast enhancement on MR images in the absence of low back pain or sciatica. *Radiology.* 1998;206:49–55.

43. Jarvik JJ, Hollingworth W, Heagerty P, et al. The longitudinal assessment of imaging and disability of the back (LAIDBACK) study. *Spine.* 2001;26:1158–1166.

44. Beattie PF, Meyers SP, Stratford P, et al. Associations between patient report of symptoms and anatomic impairment visible on lumbar magnetic resonance imaging. *Spine.* 2000;25:819–828.

45. Videman T, Battié MC, Gibbons LE, et al. Associations between back pain history and lumbar MRI findings. *Spine.* 2003;28:582–588.

46. Boos N, Semmer N, Elfering A, et al. Natural history of individuals with asymptomatic disc abnormalities in magnetic resonance imaging: predictors of

Chapter 12

low back pain-related medical consultation and work incapacity. *Spine.* 2000;25:1484–1492.

47. Carragee EJ, Tanner CM, Khurana S, et al. The rates of false-positive lumbar discography in select patients without low back symptoms. *Spine.* 2000;25:1373–1381.

48. Carragee EJ, Chen Y, Tanner CM, et al. Provocative discography in patients after limited lumbar discography: a controlled, randomized study of pain response in symptomatic and asymptomatic subjects. *Spine.* 2000;25:3065–3071.

49. Carragee EJ, Tanner CM, Yang B, et al. False-positive findings on lumbar discography. *Spine.* 1999;24:2542–2547.

50. Carragee EJ, Chen Y, Tanner CM, et al. Can discography cause long-term back symptoms in previously asymptomatic subjects? *Spine.* 2000;25:1803–1808.

51. Block AR, Vanharanta H, Ohnmeiss DD, et al. Discographic pain report: influence of psychological factors. *Spine.* 1996;21:334–338.

Chapter 13

Working With Common Upper Extremity Problems

J. Mark Melhorn, MD

This chapter explores common upper extremity musculoskeletal disorders that may be associated with workplace activities by specific *International Classification of Diseases, Ninth Revision, Clinical Modification* (ICD-9-CM) diagnosis. Work-related injuries continue to be a burden on society and a hardship for the individual employee-patient. In 1998, the Bureau of Labor and Statistics[1,2] reported 1996 data revealing a total of nearly 1.9 million injuries and illnesses in private industry that required recuperation away from work at an estimated $418 billion in direct costs and (using the lower range of estimates) indirect costs of $837 billion.[3]

Although efforts are being made to reduce incidence rates for cumulative trauma disorders (CTDs), disproportionate higher costs are associated with this Occupational Safety and Health Administration (OSHA)-defined illness, commonly described as *musculoskeletal disorders* (MSDs). Feuerstein et al[4] reviewed 185,927 claims in the federal workforce and concluded that upper extremity MSDs had much higher costs for direct and indirect medical care because of the longer duration of treatment and greater work disability. Webster et al[5] found that the mean cost per case for upper extremity MSDs was $8,070 compared to a mean cost of $824 for all other cases. The US Bureau of Labor Statistics found the median number of lost work days for all cases in 1996 was five days, with carpal tunnel syndrome (CTS) at 25 days.[2] As more nations continue to experience an aging workforce, physicians are certain to be confronted with increasing return-to-work and disability determinations.

Presumed Disability

Section 2(a) of the Social Security Administration's criteria for total disability of the upper extremities[6] specifies the inability to perform fine and gross movements effectively on a sustained basis for any reasons, including pain associated with the underlying musculoskeletal impairment that has lasted or is expected to last for at least 12 months. For the purposes of these criteria, the ability to perform these activities must be considered from a physical standpoint alone; subjective complaints do not qualify.

Second, section 2(2)c states that inability to perform fine and gross movements effectively means an extreme loss of function of both upper extremities, ie, an impairment(s) that interferes very seriously with the individual's ability to independently initiate, sustain, or complete activities. To use their upper extremities effectively, individuals must be capable of sustaining such functions as reaching, pushing, pulling, grasping, and fingering to be able to carry out activities of daily living. Therefore, examples of inability to perform fine and gross movements effectively include, but are not limited to, the inability to prepare a simple meal and feed oneself, the inability to take care of personal hygiene, the inability to sort and handle papers or files, and the inability to place files in a file cabinet at or above waist level.

Section 2(2)d states that pain or other symptoms may be an important factor contributing to functional loss. For pain or other symptoms to be found to affect an individual's ability to perform basic work activities, medical signs or laboratory findings must show the existence of a medically determinable impairment(s) that could reasonably be expected to produce the pain or other symptoms. The musculoskeletal listings that include pain or other symptoms among their criteria also include criteria for limitations in functioning as a result of the listed impairment, including limitations caused by pain. It is therefore important to evaluate the intensity and persistence of such pain or other symptoms carefully to determine their impact on the individual's functioning under these listings.

Finally, section 1.05 addresses amputations of both hands due to any cause.

Shoulder: Rotator Cuff Impingement Syndrome

Rotator cuff impingement or rotator cuff syndrome (ICD-9-CM codes 726.1, 726.10, 726.11, 726.2) rarely qualifies for total upper extremity disability. Also known as impingement syndrome, subacromial impingement syndrome, and painful arc syndrome, rotator cuff impingement syndrome occurs when the musculotendinous structure that provides strength and mobility to the shoulder joint (rotator cuff) rubs against the coracoacromial arch (coracoid process, the coracoacromial ligament, the acromion, and the acromioclavicular joint capsule), especially when the shoulder is placed in the forward-flexed and internally rotated position. Impingement is thought to be a precursor to a rotator cuff tear, although the cuff tends to tear near its insertion on the greater tuberosity, and impingement tends to occur a few centimeters further medially. Impingement occurs in three stages and normally increases with age, shoulder laxity, repetitive overhead activity, sleeping with the shoulder abducted, previous injury, osteoarthritis, bone spurs, and anatomic abnormalities.

Risk Assessment

The largest meta analysis of the epidemiologic data for workplace risk factors and the associated development of musculoskeletal disorders by body part was completed in 1997 by the National Institute of Occupational Safety and Health (NIOSH).[7] Workplace risk factors include repetition, force, posture, vibration, and their combination. The analysis cautioned that the development of musculoskeletal disorders is modified by psychosocial factors. For considering risk assessment and capacity, the data can be helpful for constructing return-to-work guides for specific body parts.[8] The tables that follow for each diagnosis in this chapter are based on the criteria outlined in Table 13-1.

Capacity

Chronic cases of impingement may have reduced shoulder motion. This is a limitation in capacity to do activities such as overhead work with the ipsilateral hand. If there is reduced motion, physicians need to describe the work limitations present on the basis of decreased shoulder motion. Other than decreased shoulder motion, there are no issues of capacity for shoulder impingement syndrome. The issue is usually tolerance. Patients can carry out activities involving use of the shoulder, but they dislike doing so because it hurts.

Tolerance

Tolerance is the usual issue when discussions of work ability arise in patients with impingement syndrome. When the degree of impingement is mild on imaging studies, and when limited use of the shoulder is involved, most physicians will agree that patients should be able to work despite pain. When the degree of impingement on imaging studies is severe, when nonoperative treatment has failed, and when the job involved requires significant use of the shoulder, most physicians would recommend surgical treatment. For these patients, most physicians would also give guidance that decreasing the use of the shoulder at work might result in decreased pain.

Chapter 13

Table 13-1 Workplace Risk Factors for Neck and Shoulder Musculoskeletal Pain*

Body Part and Risk Factor	Strong Epidemiologic Evidence (+++)	Epidemiologic Evidence (++)	Insufficient Epidemiologic Evidence (+/0)	No Epidemiologic Evidence (−)
Neck and Neck/Shoulder				
Repetition		X		
Force	X			
Posture	X			
Vibration			X	
Shoulder				
Repetition		X		
Force			X	
Posture		X		
Vibration			X	

*Strong epidemiologic evidence (+++) indicates that the consistently positive findings from a large number of cross-sectional studies, strengthened by the limited number of prospective studies, provide strong evidence of increased risk of work-related musculoskeletal disorders for some body parts based on the strength of the associations, lack of ambiguity, consistency of the results, and adequate control or adjustment for likely confounders in cross-sectional studies and the temporal relationships from the prospective studies, with reasonable confidence levels in at least several of those studies. **Epidemiologic evidence (++)** indicates that some convincing epidemiologic evidence shows a causal relationship when the epidemiologic criteria of causality for intense or long-duration exposure to the specific risk factor(s) and musculoskeletal disorders are used. A positive relationship has been observed between exposure to the specific risk factor and musculoskeletal disorders in studies in which chance, bias, and confounding factors are not the likely explanation. **Insufficient epidemiologic evidence (+/0)** indicates that the available studies are of insufficient number, quality, consistency, or statistical power to permit a conclusion regarding the presence or absence of a causal association. Some studies suggest a relationship to specific risk factors, but chance, bias, or confounding may explain the association. Either there is an insufficient number of studies from which to draw conclusions or the overall conclusion from the studies is equivocal. The absence of existing epidemiologic evidence should not be interpreted to mean that there is no association between work factors and musculoskeletal disorders. **No epidemiologic evidence (−)** indicates that there have been no adequate studies to show that the specific workplace risk factor(s) is not related to development of musculoskeletal disorders.

While this is not a work limitation, the patient's decision not to do certain activities at work would be supported by most physicians. For patients whose degree of impingement falls between the severe and the mild cases described above, there will usually be considerable disagreement among physician evaluators. This is the "How much pain should a person be expected to tolerate?" question, which has no scientific answer.

A temporary period of modified work may be helpful. During this time, shoulder strengthening exercises may be prescribed to improve the impingement, although there is no clear scientific proof of efficacy of this treatment.[9] This is not total cessation of shoulder use, but rather use in a pattern to strengthen specific shoulder muscles. During this time, temporary work guides may be appropriate.

The key is to modify activities but not to have total absence from aggravating activities such as hand use at or above the shoulder. Capacity guides might include limited overhead work (reaching above shoulder) or to shoulder level (90° position); reaching above the shoulder limited to less than 15 to 30 times per hour with up to 15 lb of weight; reaching to shoulder up to 15 to 30 times per hour with up to 25 lb of weight; holding the arm in abduction or flexion limited to up to 15 to 30 times per hour with up to 15 lb of weight; pulling and pushing up to 60 lb 20 to 30 times per hour; lifting and carrying up to 40 lb 15 to 30 times per hour; and climbing ladders up to 60 rungs per hour. An ergonometric evaluation of the workplace may be helpful. Change in job duties, sharing or alternating tasks, reduced work rate, more frequent rest breaks, and limiting the time and frequency of repetitive activities are important accommodations. Work site modifications can include forearm rests for individuals who use computer keyboards frequently, headsets for those who answer telephones, and changing task performance such that repetitive activities can be done with the arms at a lower level of elevation.

Postoperative instructions might include zero to five days with the arm in a sling or support, with the arm used for assist activities only, 10 lb or less maximum, frequent use for 5 lb at waist to chest height, and no arm use at or above shoulder height. At five to 28 days after surgery, light medium to medium work may be permitted (35 to 50 lb maximum, frequent lift and carry of 20 to 25 lb with both arms combined, and no use at or above shoulder height). After 4 weeks, gradual increase in weight is permitted but still with limitation of hands over the shoulder. The ability to return to heavy work and very heavy work may be difficult, and permanent restrictions may be appropriate after surgery.

Tolerance is influenced by the individual's age, occupation, dominant or nondominant arm affected, response to treatment, and compliance with treatment recommendations and rehabilitation programs during the recovery (disability) period. Return to work is often linked to the job category. Job categories include sedentary, light, medium, heavy, and very heavy. The data in Table 13-2 reflect the physician's work guides (capacity), the patient's tolerance, and risk of reinjury. Two groups of data are reported. The first set of data is labeled Target, TMinimum, and TMaximum, representing the "best practice guidelines" as reported by The Hand Center.[10] The second set of data is labeled Optimum, Minimum, and Maximum, representing a composite of recommendations by multiple physicians in multiple states as

Chapter 13

Table 13-2 Suggested Disability Durations (Days)[*†]

Job Classification	The Hand Center			The Medical Disability Advisor		
	Target	TMinimum	TMaximum	Optimum	Minimum	Maximum
Nonsurgical Treatment for Shoulder: Rotator Cuff Impingement Syndrome						
Sedentary	0	0	1	3	0	4
Light	0	0	5	3	0	7
Medium	0	0	7	21	14	42
Heavy	14	0	45	42	28	84
Very Heavy	28	7	56	42	28	84
Arthroscopic Surgery for Shoulder: Rotator Cuff Impingement Syndrome						
Sedentary				10	7	21
Light				10	7	21
Medium				42	28	56
Heavy				70	56	84
Very Heavy				70	56	84
Open Surgery for Shoulder: Rotator Cuff Impingement Syndrome						
Sedentary	5	0	14	42	28	70
Light	5	0	17	56	28	84
Medium	21	7	35	84	42	140
Heavy	42	14	91	84	70	140
Very Heavy	49	21	105	84	70	140

[*] Job classifications are based on the amount of physical effort required to perform the work. The classifications correspond to the Strength Factor classifications described in the *Dictionary of Occupational Titles*,[12] which focus on physical effort only. This may not be relevant to the duration of some disabilities. In addition to pounds of force, other important factors contribute to the definition of an individual's job classification, including posture, biomechanics (size, shape, and manageability of the object being moved), height from and to which the object is lifted, and frequency of exertion. Each of these factors (and any other job-specific requirements) should be considered when determining expected length of disability. The following definitions are quoted directly from the *Dictionary of Occupational Titles*:
Sedentary work indicates exerting up to 10 pounds of force occasionally and/or a negligible amount of force frequently or constantly to lift, carry, push, pull, or otherwise move objects, including the human body. Sedentary work involves sitting most of the time, but may involve walking or standing for brief periods of time. Jobs are sedentary if walking and standing are required only occasionally and other sedentary criteria are met; **light work**, exerting up to 20 pounds of force occasionally and/or up to 10 pounds of force frequently, and/or negligible amount of force constantly to move objects. Physical demand requirements are in excess of those for sedentary work. Light work usually requires walking or standing to a significant degree. However, if the use of the arm and/or leg controls requires exertion of forces greater than that for sedentary work and the worker sits most of the time, the job is rated light work; **medium work**, exerting up to 50 pounds of force occasionally, and/or up to 20 pounds of force frequently, and/or up to 10 pounds of forces constantly to move objects; **heavy work**, exerting up to 100 pounds of force occasionally, and/or in excess of 50 pounds of force frequently, and/or in excess of 20 pounds of force constantly to move objects; **very heavy work**, exerting in excess of 100 pounds of force occasionally, and/or in excess of 50 pounds of force frequently, and/or in excess of 20 pounds of force constantly to move objects.
[†] Data used with permission from Melhorn[10] and Reed.[11]

Chapter 13

reported by *The Medical Disability Advisor.*[11] The best practice guidelines were developed for The Hand Center by the author (J. M. M.), a physician who enthusiastically educates patients and employers about the advantages of early return to work, who assists employers in the development of early-return-to-work programs, and who promotes return to work through educational venues. To reduce unnecessary disability, physicians are encouraged to aim for the target disability day. The minimum and maximum range is provided with the realization that individuals are unique and many factors contribute to early return to work.

The Medical Disability Advisor duration table guidelines outlined in Table 13-2 represent a unique combination of methodologies that have resulted in the development of practical and usable guidelines.[13] Differences may exist between the expected duration tables and the normative graphs. Duration tables provide expected recovery periods based on the type of work performed by the individual. The normative graphs shown in Table 13-3 reflect the actual observed experience of many individuals across the spectrum of physical conditions, in a variety of industries, and with varying levels of case management. Recovery trends (in days) are derived from normative data for cases specifically identified with shoulder rotator cuff syndrome.

Conclusion

For shoulder impingement and rotator cuff syndrome, staying at work or returning to work is primarily based on tolerance. Although the capacity may be limited for a short period after surgery, most individuals can return to pervious employment levels. Capacity may be limited in chronic cases by decreased shoulder motion. Temporary work guides limiting hand-over-shoulder activities may be helpful. Returning to heavy work or very heavy work for extended periods may be difficult after surgery. Believable tolerance of pain in cases of impingement with severe imaging changes may be a basis for physicians to support a patient's decision to choose different work, although the words *work restriction* (based on risk) and *work limitation* (based on capacity) may not apply.

Shoulder: Rotator Cuff Tear

The rotator cuff consists of four muscles that control three basic motions: abduction, internal rotation, and external rotation. The supraspinatus muscle is responsible for initiating abduction, the infraspinatus and teres minor muscles control external rotation, and the subscapularis muscle controls internal rotation. The rotator cuff muscles provide dynamic stabilization to the humeral head on the glenoid fossa, forming a force couple with the deltoid

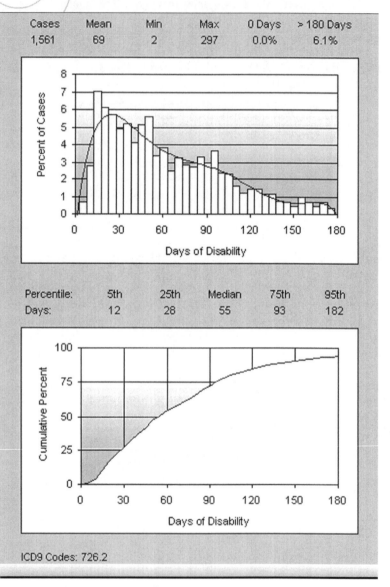

Table 13-3 Recovery Trends (Days) From Normative Data for Cases Specifically Identified With Shoulder Rotator Cuff Impingement

Cases	Mean	Min	Max	0 Days	> 180 Days
1,561	69	2	297	0.0%	6.1%

Percentile:	5th	25th	Median	75th	95th
Days:	12	28	55	93	182

ICD9 Codes: 726.2

Reproduced with permission from Reed.[11]

to allow elevation of the arm. This force couple is responsible for 45% of abduction strength and 90% of external rotation strength. Acromion morphology may contribute to rotator cuff injuries. The risk increases with type 1 flat (17%), type 2 curved (43%), and type 3 anteriorly hooked (40%) acromions.

A rotator cuff injury (ICD-9-CM codes 718.0, 727.61, 840.4) is an injury to one or more of the four tendons attaching muscles to the shoulder. This shoulder injury may come on suddenly and be associated with a specific injury such as a fall (acute), or it may become slowly and progressively worse over time without a specific injury incident. Return to work and outcomes are different for each type. Full-thickness tears are uncommon in individuals younger than 40 years but are present in 25% of individuals older than 60 years. Many of these are asymptomatic.

The Social Security Administration's disability requirements are the same as discussed in the previous section. However, as the size of tear increases and the age increases, the likelihood of disability increases. Therefore, shoulder rotator cuff tear may occasionally qualify for one-sided total upper extremity disability.

Risk Assessment
The risk of rotator cuff tear increases with age and is similar to that of shoulder impingement as outlined earlier. In patients with documented tears, repetitive activity that places major force on the cuff does risk extending the tear (increasing in size). Thus, work restrictions (based on risk) against repetitive lifting of heavier objects into positions requiring significant shoulder motion are appropriate. Similarly, after surgical repair of cuff tears, many surgeons impose restrictions on shoulder activity in the hope of preventing recurrent tears.

Capacity
Capacity may be diminished in patients with rotator cuff tears by decreased motion or decreased strength. The larger the tear, the more it "disconnects" shoulder muscles from their normal bony attachments. Range of motion and strength can be quantified.

In the nonoperative group with small tears, activity modification and functional capacity are similar to those for shoulder impingement. The capacity after surgery is determined by the size of the tear; the quality of the cuff tissue as observed at surgery; whether the cuff could be anatomically repaired; the individual's age, occupation, and overall health; dominant side involvement; and success of rehabilitation. The duration of disability is longer than that for shoulder impingement. The larger the tear, the more likely that permanent

weakness will result, and, therefore, heavy or very heavy work may no longer
be possible. Additionally, there may be permanent disability regarding certain
activities such as hand-over-shoulder movement.

Tolerance
Pain level may limit tolerance. The section on shoulder impingement gives
the specifics. Tables 13-4 and 13-5 are provided as guides.

Conclusion
For rotator cuff tears, staying at work or return to work is primarily based on
size of the tear and whether surgery is performed. Outcomes are better for
acute rotator cuff tears. This is because the injury usually occurs in a younger
patient with better rotator cuff substance. A chronic tear usually represents a
wearing out of the cuff substance with age, and therefore repair is more

Table 13-4 Suggested Disability Durations (Days)[*][†]

Job Classification	The Hand Center			The Medical Disability Advisor		
	Target	TMinimum	TMaximum	Optimum	Minimum	Maximum
Nonsurgical Treatment for Shoulder: Rotator Cuff Tear						
Sedentary	0	0	1	3	0	4
Light	0	0	1	3	0	7
Medium	0	0	8	21	14	42
Heavy	14	0	42	42	28	84
Very Heavy	28	7	49	42	28	84
Arthroscopic Surgery for Shoulder: Rotator Cuff Tear						
Sedentary				10	7	21
Light				10	7	21
Medium				42	28	56
Heavy				70	56	84
Very Heavy				70	56	84
Open Surgery for Shoulder: Rotator Cuff Tear						
Sedentary	5	0	21	42	28	70
Light	5	0	21	56	28	84
Medium	21	7	28	84	42	140
Heavy	56	14	119	84	70	140
Very Heavy	70	28	133	84	70	140

[*] See Table 13-2 for definitions of job classifications.
[†] Data used with permission from Melhorn[10] and Reed.[11]

Table 13-5 Duration Trends From Normative Data for Cases Specifically Identified With Rotator Cuff Tear

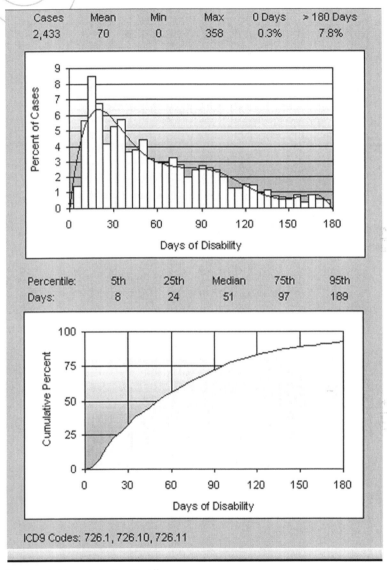

Cases	Mean	Min	Max	0 Days	> 180 Days
2,433	70	0	358	0.3%	7.8%

Percentile:	5th	25th	Median	75th	95th
Days:	8	24	51	97	189

ICD9 Codes: 726.1, 726.10, 726.11

difficult because the remaining tissue is weak. Capacity is further limited for short periods after surgery, and many individuals can return to previous employment levels with permanent work guides limiting hand-over-shoulder movement. Some residual long-term discomfort with activities is likely.

Chapter 13

Elbow: Lateral or Medial Epicondylitis

Epicondylitis (ICD-9-CM codes 726.31, 726.32) occurs when tendons in the elbow develop microscopic tears and inflammation occurs at their attachments on the epicondyles, although the point of maximal pain is usually in the tendon substance just distal to the site of origin of the extensor carpi radialis brevis muscle (lateral) or the origin of the flexor/pronator tendons (medial). This process is known as lateral epicondylitis (tennis elbow) if on the outside, or medial epicondylitis (golfer's elbow) if on the inside. The term *epicondylitis* implies inflammation of the epicondyle or tissue adjoining the epicondyle of the humerus. The current opinion is that the early phase is inflammatory and often responds to anti-inflammatory medications and exercises. In the chronic (late) phase, when tissue biopsy is often done, there are no signs of inflammation, only degeneration. The term *angiofibroblastic degeneration* is consistent with the findings of fibroblastic and vascular response in the tendon at biopsy, which has no evidence of immune cell response.

Although the cause is unknown, epicondylitis may be a result of overuse or overexertion of the forearm and wrist muscles. Many tennis players have had symptoms of epicondylitis. Occupations that involve repetitive and/or stressful use of the forearm may be associated with a higher incidence of epicondylitis; affected groups include cooks, utility workers, secretaries (and others spending a great deal of time using a keyboard), assembly line workers, cashiers, carpenters, plumbers, butchers, and politicians. Individuals participating in tennis, golf, baseball, swimming, racquetball, fly fishing, weight lifting, and track and field sports are at an increased risk of developing epicondylitis. Epicondylitis typically afflicts individuals between the ages of 35 and 50 years. Although men are twice as likely as women to develop medial epicondylitis, lateral epicondylitis afflicts men and women equally. Lateral epicondylitis is common, affecting approximately 2% of the US population, and is eight times more common than medial epicondylitis. The Social Security Administration's disability requirements for epicondylitis are similar and therefore a patient rarely qualifies for one-sided total upper extremity disability.

Risk Assessment

There is no significant risk with epicondylitis. There is no described syndrome of rupture of the involved tendon(s) resulting in disability. One of the surgical options for chronic cases involves removing the already necrotic tendon from its attachment on the epicondyle without reattaching the tendon.

The NIOSH review of the factors that may be involved in producing epicondylitis suggests that only jobs that require repetitive performance of high-force movements in awkward postures are epidemiologically linked to this syndrome. (See Table 13-6.)

Capacity

Capacity is not usually an issue with epicondylitis. Patients can do things, but they dislike doing what they can do because it hurts. If a patient chooses not to use a limb, disuse atrophy may develop, which can be measured. Unlike some other conditions (osteoarthritis of the hip, for example), there is a poor correlation between the severity of imaging findings and the severity of the patient's clinical (pain) problem. Thus, there is not usually "severe objective evidence of pathology" to support physician evaluator agreement.

Tolerance

Tolerance for the pain associated with use of the hand is the issue in epicondylitis. Temporary modification of work activity (work guides) may be helpful while patients are treated with stretching and strengthening exercises, use of a counterforce brace, and perhaps a corticosteroid injection into the area of maximum tenderness.

For chronic cases, temporary work modification is not appropriate. Surgical treatment may decrease the associated pain. Ultimately the patient will need to choose to take a different job or to continue to put up with the pain. In many chronic cases the pain ultimately decreases, but this may require years to occur.

Temporary modification of activities includes limiting exposure to precipitating or exacerbating activity, but not total absence of activity. A change in job duties, sharing or alternating tasks, and limiting time and frequency of repetitive activities are important accommodations. Use of vibrating tools

Chapter 13

Table 13-6 Workplace Risk Factors for Elbow Musculoskeletal Pain[*]

Body Part and Risk Factor	Strong Epidemiologic Evidence (+++)	Epidemiologic Evidence (++)	Insufficient Epidemiologic Evidence (+/0)	No Epidemiologic Evidence (−)
Elbow				
Repetition			X	
Force		X		
Posture			X	
Combination	X			

[*] See Table 13-1 for definitions of levels of evidence.

such as impact wrenches or jackhammers should be minimized. Increasing or decreasing the size of tool grips so the wrist can be held in the neutral position is also helpful. Use of splints, straps, and casts should be limited, as these can affect dexterity and may temporarily limit the individual's ability to lift and carry heavy or bulky objects, operate equipment, or perform other tasks requiring the use of both hands. An ergonometric evaluation of the workplace may be helpful.

Modified light work may be performed the day after surgery (maximum, 20 lb or less lift/carry, with frequent lifting at 10 lb for both arms). Up to 14 days after surgery, a light dressing is applied, no large power or vibratory tools are used, and extremity use on the operated-on side is limited. Work production may initially be decreased in the postoperative period. In general, the individual should gradually increase his or her activities at home and at work.[10]

Tolerance is primarily influenced by pain level and job requirements (use of wrist and forearm with or without power or vibratory tools and intensity of force). Modification of the job on the basis of the risk assessment table is appropriate. Because this diagnosis is described as chronic, some persistent chronic pain with activity is likely even with surgical treatment. Table 13-7 includes suggested disability durations in days for elbow conditions.

Table 13-7 Suggested Disability Durations (Days)[*][†]

Job Classification	The Hand Center			The Medical Disability Advisor		
	Target	TMinimum	TMaximum	Optimum	Minimum	Maximum
Nonsurgical Treatment for Elbow: Lateral or Medial Epicondylitis						
Sedentary	0	0	7	7	0	28
Light	0	0	7	10	1	28
Medium	0	0	14	21	7	56
Heavy	0	0	21	28	14	56
Very Heavy	0	0	28	28	14	56
Surgical Treatment for Elbow: Lateral or Medial Epicondylitis						
Sedentary	0	0	7			
Light	0	0	7			
Medium	7	0	21			
Heavy	14	0	28			
Very Heavy	21	7	32			

[*] See Table 13-2 for definitions of job classifications.
[†] Data used with permission from Melhorn[10] and Reed.[11]

Conclusion

For epicondylitis, risk and capacity are not the issue, and staying at work or returning to work is primarily based on tolerance. There is thus no basis for permanent physician-imposed work restrictions or physician-described work limitations. Symptoms (pain) tend to be chronic with activities, although often not progressive. Although the capacity may be limited for short periods after surgery, most individuals can return to previous employment levels. Temporary work guides limiting combination activities may be helpful. Returning to very heavy work for expanded periods may be difficult, so the patient must decide whether the rewards of work outweigh the pain involved.

Elbow: Ulnar Nerve Entrapment

Ulnar nerve entrapment at the elbow (ICD-9-CM code 354.2) is the second most common entrapment neuropathy in the upper extremity (the first being the median nerve and its branches at the wrist).

The elbow is the most vulnerable point of the ulnar nerve: here it is superficial and fixed and crosses a joint. Because of the anatomic positioning of the ulnar nerve, it is subject to entrapment and injury. Nerves are fragile and can be damaged by pressure, stretching, or cutting. Because of its superficial position at the elbow, the ulnar nerve may be injured either by sustained excessive pressure or by repetitive contusion (bumping). Overstretching of the nerve, either from sustained posturing in near-full elbow flexion or from highly repetitive elbow flexion, can also injure the nerve. The nerve loses its ability to conduct and the small intrinsic muscles of the hand become dysfunctional. Sensory loss may occur, most commonly in the little finger and the ulnar half of the ring finger.

In early cases the symptoms are suggestive, but physical examination and electrodiagnostic tests fail to confirm the diagnosis. Cases that progress to major nerve damage are rare.

The Social Security Administration's disability requirements are the same as discussed earlier in this chapter. Therefore, ulnar nerve entrapment at the elbow rarely qualifies for one-sided total upper extremity disability.

Risk Assessment

Ulnar nerve function can be assessed. Parameters such as two-point sensation testing of the little finger, grip strength, and finger abduction strength can be assessed by physical examination, although these require the cooperation of the patient. Nerve conduction testing can document the conduction

Chapter 13

velocity of the ulnar nerve in the segment crossing the elbow. No patient co-operation is necessary for this test. These tests can be repeated, permitting assessment of change over time. If nerve function is documented at multiple office visits, and if it is clearly worse with continued work activity and sub-sequently improves with temporary work restrictions, it is reasonable to conclude that this work activity is a risk to the patient's ulnar nerve. Either permanent work restrictions or surgical treatment would be indicated. Gen-erally the weight lifted at work is not a problem. Restrictions should address sustained posturing with the elbow in flexion of greater than 90°, highly repetitive elbow flexion, and repetitive contusion of or sustained pressure on the nerve. Ulnar neuropathy can also cause decreased sensation on the ulnar side of the hand. If "protective" sensation (most easily measured as sharp–dull discrimination) is lost, the patient may need restrictions preclud-ing work around hot or sharp objects that would risk cutting or burning skin that lacks its normal protective sensation.

If results of multiple physical examination and nerve conduction tests show that ulnar nerve function is either stable or improving despite continued work activity, the reasonable conclusion is that this work activity does *not* pose a risk to this patient's ulnar nerve. Whether the patient chooses to tol-erate symptoms is then the issue.

Capacity

Capacity may be affected by ulnar neuropathy. Grip strength (due to weak-ness in the flexor profundus) and hand dexterity can be affected, and these deficits can be measured. A Jamar dynamometer can quantitate grip strength, and tests like the Perdue Peg Board Test (available through physi-cal therapists and/or occupational therapists) can assess hand dexterity. These deficits can affect the ability to do routine factory work and can be described by physicians as work limitations.

Tolerance

Tolerance for symptoms such as pain and paresthesias is the most frequent problem. If tests of nerve function confirm that ulnar neuropathy is the cor-rect diagnosis, most physicians would feel the symptoms are believable and the condition is at a level of severity that justifies work restrictions. This is not work restriction based on risk, but rather restriction based on tolerance in the presence of severe, objectively documented pathology. If there is evi-dence of nerve damage, the nerve may well be at risk, as discussed above.

In the early phases of neuropathy, work activity may be a problem based on tolerance of pain, while in late phases capacity is limited by functional loss. All phases are influenced by the individual's age, occupation, dominant or nondominant arm affected, response to treatment, and compliance with

Table 13-8 Suggested Disability Durations (Days)[*†]

Job Classification	The Hand Center			The Medical Disability Advisor		
	Target	TMinimum	TMaximum	Optimum	Minimum	Maximum
Nonsurgical Treatment for Elbow: Ulnar Nerve Entrapment						
Sedentary	0	0	7			
Light	0	0	7			
Medium	0	0	14			
Heavy	0	0	21			
Very Heavy	0	0	28			
Surgical Treatment for Elbow: Ulnar Nerve Entrapment						
Sedentary	0	0	7	21	7	42
Light	0	0	7	28	7	42
Medium	14	0	28	56	28	365
Heavy	21	0	47	98	28	365
Very Heavy	28	0	56	98	42	365

[*] See Table 13-2 for definitions of job classifications.
[†] Data used with permission from Melhorn[10] and Reed.[11]

treatment recommendations and rehabilitation programs during the recovery period. Job modification may be helpful. Ergonometric assessment can help with workplace modifications. Suggested disability durations in days for elbow ulnar nerve entrapment are listed in Table 13-8.

Conclusion

For early ulnar nerve elbow entrapment, staying at work or returning to work is primarily based on tolerance If the diagnosis and treatment (including surgery) are early, before permanent nerve damage occurs, residual functional loss should be minimal. However, if muscle atrophy or weakness is present on physical examination, even with surgery, permanent functional loss and residual disability are more likely. Although the capacity may be limited for a short period after surgery, most individuals can return to previous employment levels with permanent modifications, such as task rotation and limitations of power and vibratory tool exposure.

Wrist: Carpal Tunnel Syndrome

Considerable controversy continues to surround the cause (etiology), definition, diagnosis, and treatment of persons with this disorder. Carpal tunnel syndrome (CTS) (ICD-9-CM codes 354, 354.0), also known as *median nerve compression neuropathy*, is actually a condition (pathophysiology known) and not a syndrome, but the name *carpal tunnel syndrome* has become so well known that *CTS* will be used here rather than median nerve compression neuropathy. It is a condition in which pain, prickling, or tingling (paresthesias) or numbness radiates from the wrist into the palm of the hand and then down into the thumb, index finger, middle finger, and the thumb side of the ring finger. It is caused by elevated pressure on the median nerve. The main (median) nerve and its branches enter the hand through an internal opening (the carpal tunnel) formed by the wrist bones (carpal bones) and the tough membrane that holds the bones together (transverse carpal ligament). The median nerve supplies sensation to the palm of the hand, thumb, and first three fingers. Because this passageway is rigid, inflammation, swelling, or increased fluid retention may compress the nerve (nerve entrapment), causing pain and changes in sensation along the pathways where the nerve runs. Pain may eventually extend to the arm, shoulder, or neck.

Carpal tunnel syndrome may be diagnosed clinically, but it is frequently a difficult diagnosis. There is no pathognomonic test on physical examination, and those physical examination findings that exist have a low sensitivity, specificity, and reliability.[14–16] Nerve conduction testing is the only objective test available, and no national organization defines for CTS what is a normal or an abnormal test result, but practice parameters have been attempted.[17] Each physician performing nerve conduction tests must choose his or her own definition of normal.

Most of the literature on causation of CTS is flawed. Most of the studies are cross sectional, which means that they can generate hypotheses for testing by prospective studies, but by themselves they do not prove causation. Many of the studies use a clinical definition of CTS and not nerve conduction testing for diagnosis, so in studies on the relationship of work activity to CTS, many of the individuals labeled as having CTS do not actually have it.[18] Fifty-nine medical conditions (diseases or injuries) have been reported to be associated with CTS.[19] Thus, in a single individual with CTS, it is impossible to reason from the literature whether work activity was part of the cause of the CTS.

Many countries and the state of Virginia do not accept CTS as work related. The debate on causation is critical to a discussion of risk.[20] The unfounded scientific conclusion is that work is a "toxin" to the carpal tunnel and, therefore, physicians should limit exposure to the toxin by having physician-imposed work restrictions.

The Social Security Administration's disability requirements are the same as discussed earlier in this chapter. Therefore, carpal tunnel syndrome rarely qualifies for one-sided total upper extremity disability.

Risk Assessment

As mentioned earlier, if work is part of the cause of CTS, physicians should limit exposure to the cause by imposed restrictions. The NIOSH review of studies suggested that only in combination of all the ergonomic factors is there strong evidence of causation. (See Table 13-9.)

The only prospective study published in English that did use nerve conduction studies to diagnose CTS concluded that female sex, greater age at baseline, and obesity predict the later development of CTS. Repetition, force, heavy lifting, and keyboard use were not predictive.[16] Thus, in a single individual with CTS, it is impossible to reason from the literature whether work activity was part of the cause of CTS.

Similar to the preceding discussion of ulnar neuropathy, median nerve function can be assessed at multiple office visits. Testing of sensation (for example, by two-point discrimination) and testing of motor function (by thenar atrophy and thenar opposition weakness) can be performed during physical examination. Nerve conduction studies on the median nerve can be repeated (the study of all the nerves in the limb does not need to be repeated; only one or some of the median nerve studies need to be repeated).

If nerve function is documented at multiple office visits, and if median nerve function is clearly worse with continued work activity and subsequently improves with temporary work restrictions, it is reasonable to conclude that this work activity is a risk to this patient's median nerve. Either permanent work restrictions or surgical treatment would be indicated. Generally the weight lifted at work is not a problem. Restrictions should address sustained posturing with the wrist in flexion or extension of greater than 30°, highly repetitive wrist motion, and sustained pressure on the nerve.

Chapter 13

Table 13-9 Workplace Risk Factors for Carpal Tunnel Syndrome[*]

Body Part and Risk Factor	Strong Epidemiologic Evidence (+++)	Epidemiologic Evidence (++)	Insufficient Epidemiologic Evidence (+/0)	No Epidemiologic Evidence (−)
Hand/wrist: Carpal Tunnel Syndrome				
Repetition		X		
Force		X		
Posture			X	
Vibration		X		
Combination	X			

[*] See Table 13-1 for definitions of levels of evidence.

Carpal Tunnel Syndrome can also cause decreased sensation on the radial side of the hand. If protective sensation (most easily measured as sharp–dull discrimination or two-point discrimination of >15 mm) is lost, the patient may need restrictions precluding work around hot or sharp objects that would risk cutting or burning skin that lacks its normal protective sensation.

If results of multiple physical examination and nerve conduction tests show that median nerve function is either stable or improving despite continued work activity, the reasonable conclusion is that this work activity does *not* pose a risk to this patient's median nerve. Whether the patient chooses to tolerate symptoms is then the issue. In the largest published study of the natural course of untreated CTS, patients were most likely to remain un-changed but were more likely to improve than to worsen in terms of electro-diagnostic study class, symptoms, pain, and function.[17] This suggests that short-term risk is not a major issue in most cases of CTS.

Although the popular media suggests that keyboards cause CTS, the science shows otherwise. Nine studies have reviewed this relationship. The results show that keyboards are safe to use and do not cause CTS.[18,21–30] Further-more, keyboard redesign had no effect on incidence of CTS.[31,32] Symptoms may increase with many activities, including the use of keyboards, but key-boards do not cause CTS.

Capacity

Capacity may be affected by CTS. Grip strength is not usually affected, as the nerve compression occurs distal to the forearm muscles involved in grip. Pain may limit grip, but that is an issue of tolerance. Hand dexterity can be affected, and these deficits can be measured with tests like the Perdue Peg Board Test (available through physical therapists and/or occupational thera-pists) that can assess hand dexterity. These deficits can affect the ability to do routine factory work and can be described by physicians as work limitations.

Tolerance

Tolerance for symptoms like pain and paresthesias is the most frequent prob-lem. If tests of nerve function confirm that CTS is the correct diagnosis, many physicians would feel the symptoms are believable and the condition is at a level of severity that justifies work restrictions. This is not work restriction based on risk, but rather restriction based on tolerance in the pres-ence of severe, objectively documented pathology. The problem with this po-sition is that there is no uniformly accepted definition of CTS by nerve con-duction studies. Many cases diagnosed as "mild CTS" by nerve conduction testing are false-positive cases. These cases explain most of the now-frequent scenario of mild "CTS" (false positives) that fail to respond to appropriate treatment. Nonspecific hand and arm pain (ICD-9-CM code 729.5) and

Table 13-10 Suggested Disability Durations (Days)[*†]

Job Classification	The Hand Center			The Medical Disability Advisor		
	Target	TMinimum	TMaximum	Optimum	Minimum	Maximum
Nonsurgical Treatment (Including Injections) for Wrist: Carpal Tunnel Syndrome						
Sedentary	0	0	7	7	0	21
Light	0	0	7	7	0	21
Medium	0	0	12	14	0	28
Heavy	0	0	21	21	0	42
Very Heavy	0	0	28	28	0	63
Surgical (Open or Endoscopic) Treatment for Wrist: Carpal Tunnel Syndrome						
Sedentary	0	0	7	14	1	42
Light	0	0	7	28	1	42
Medium	14	0	28	42	14	56
Heavy	21	0	42	42	28	84
Very Heavy	28	3	61	56	28	84

[*] See Table 13-2 for definitions of job classifications.
[†] Data used with permission from Melhorn[10] and Reed.[11]

numbness (782.0) are common, may be misdiagnosed as CTS, and will fail to respond to carpal tunnel release.

If there is evidence of nerve damage, the nerve may well be at risk, as discussed above. Surgical treatment is logical if there is nerve damage. This is an issue of risk and not of tolerance.

In the early stages of CTS, work activity may be a problem based on tolerance of pain and numbness, while in late stages capacity is limited by nerve function lost. All phases are influenced by the individual's age, occupation, whether the dominant or nondominant arm is affected, the response to treatment, and the compliance with treatment recommendations and rehabilitation programs during the recovery period. Job modification may be helpful. Ergonometric assessment can help with workplace modifications. Suggested disability durations (in days) for CTS are listed in Table 13-10 and the duration trend is listed in Table 13-11.

Conclusion

For early cases of CTS, staying at work or returning to work is primarily based on tolerance of symptoms. If diagnosis and treatment (including surgery) are early, residual functional loss is rare. However, if muscle weakness or atrophy or sensory loss is present on physical examination, even

Table 13-11 Duration Trend From Normative Data for Cases Specifically Identified With Carpal Tunnel Syndrome

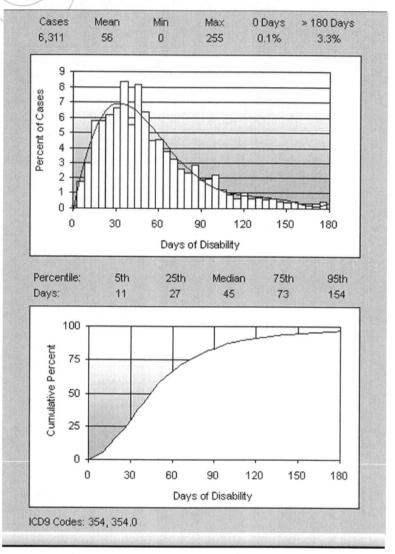

Cases	Mean	Min	Max	0 Days	> 180 Days
6,311	56	0	255	0.1%	3.3%

Percentile:	5th	25th	Median	75th	95th
Days:	11	27	45	73	154

ICD9 Codes: 354, 354.0

Reproduced with permission from Reed.[11]

with surgery, permanent functional loss and residual disability are more likely. Although the capacity may be limited for a short period after surgery, most individuals can return to previous employment levels, but perhaps with permanent modifications or task rotation and limitations of power and vibratory tool exposure.

Wrist: De Quervain's Tenosynovitis

Stenosing tenosynovitis of the extensor pollicis brevis and abductor pollicis longus tendons is a condition where the tendons and their covering tenosynovium, or tendon sheaths, become inflamed. The precise cause of de Quervain's tenosynovitis (ICD-9-CM code 727.04) is unknown. The involved tendons are usually normal, but the tendon covering is inflamed. Because the area within the tunnel for the tendons is confined, any inflammation reduces available space for the tendon-pulley mechanism to function. Pain and increased inflammation are caused when the tendons and their swollen sheaths are pulled through the tighter space. It becomes difficult for the tendons to move and consequently they begin to catch and rub, producing jerky movements and causing more pain and inflammation.

The Social Security Administration's disability requirements are the same as discussed earlier in this chapter. Therefore, de Quervain's tenosynovitis rarely qualifies for one-sided total upper extremity disability.

Risk Assessment

The NIOSH review of published studies suggests the evidence shown in Table 13-12 that work activities cause de Quervain's tenosynovitis.

It is rare for the involved tendons to rupture, so there is no risk of significant harm that is imminent. It is safe (risk) but painful (tolerance) to do work tasks when afflicted with de Quervain's tenosynovitis. Thus, there is no basis for work restrictions.

Chapter 13

Table 13-12 Workplace Risk Factors for Hand or Wrist Tendinitis[*]

Body Part and Risk Factor	Strong Epidemiologic Evidence (+++)	Epidemiologic Evidence (++)	Insufficient Epidemiologic Evidence (+/0)	No Epidemiologic Evidence (−)
Hand/Wrist Tendinitis				
Repetition		X		
Force		X		
Posture		X		
Combination	X			

[*] See Table 13-1 for definitions of levels of evidence.

Capacity

Work capacity is not usually affected by this condition. Wrist range of motion is preserved. Grip strength and function are normal. Moving the wrist into simultaneous flexion and ulnar deviation provokes the pain of this condition, but patients can do what is painful. Thus, there are no work limitations.

Tolerance

For de Quervain's tenosynovitis, staying at work or returning to work is primarily based on tolerance. Symptoms tend to be chronic with activities, although often not progressive. Temporary work modifications (but not total absence from aggravating tasks) while undergoing treatment may help to minimize symptoms and speed recovery. Surgical treatment is usually successful. Although the capacity for work may be limited for a short period after surgery, most individuals can return to previous employment levels. Work guides limiting combination activities (especially repetitive simultaneous wrist flexion and ulnar deviation) may be helpful. In general, the individual should gradually increase activities at home and at work.[10]

Returning to very heavy work for expanded periods may be difficult (painful), resulting in the need for career decisions. Table 13-13 includes suggested disability durations (in days) for de Quervain's tenosynovitis.

Table 13-13 Suggested Disability Durations (Days)[*†]

Job Classification	The Hand Center			The Medical Disability Advisor		
	Target	TMinimum	TMaximum	Optimum	Minimum	Maximum
Nonsurgical Treatment for Wrist: de Quervain's Tenosynovitis Release						
Sedentary	0	0	7			
Light	0	0	7			
Medium	0	0	14			
Heavy	0	0	21			
Very Heavy	0	0	28			
Surgical Treatment for Wrist: de Quervain's Tenosynovitis Release						
Sedentary	0	0	7	7	1	21
Light	0	0	7	14	3	21
Medium	7	0	14	21	7	42
Heavy	14	0	21	28	21	56
Very Heavy	21	0	35	28	21	56

[*] See Table 13-2 for definitions of job classifications.
[†] Data used with permission from Melhorn[10] and Reed.[11]

Chapter 13

Conclusion

For de Quervain's tenosynovitis, staying at work or returning to work is primarily based on tolerance. Symptoms may be chronic with activities, although often not progressive. Although the capacity may be limited for a short period after surgery, most individuals can return to previous employment levels. Work guides limiting combination activities may be helpful. Returning to very heavy work for expanded periods may be difficult (painful, an issue of tolerance), resulting in the need for career decisions.

Finger or Thumb: Trigger

Trigger finger (ICD-9-CM: 727.03) (also known as stenosing tenosynovitis) is the equivalent of de Quervain's tenosynovitis, but affecting a finger or thumb instead of the wrist. *Trigger finger* refers to a sensation in which the fingers or thumb feel stuck or temporarily snagged during efforts to straighten or bend the digit. The condition is caused by swelling often accompanied by inflammation that narrows the hand's tunnels (flexor sheath or A-1 pulley), where tendons glide back and forth to allow movement of the hand and fingers. The tendon itself may develop a knot (nodule) caused by irritation from rubbing against the narrowed tunnel walls of the sheath, similar to a knotted rope repeatedly passing through a constricted area. As the tendon pulls free of any obstacles, a snapping sensation (triggering) accompanied by pain may then be felt. The snapping movement likely will create more damage to the affected area, resulting in even more inflammation and swelling that creates additional narrowing and interference with hand and finger movement. The cycle of damage could result in the finger or thumb becoming stuck or locked, with movement becoming increasingly more painful and difficult. The underlying cause of inflammation creating the condition often is not known, but it can be associated with diseases such as rheumatoid arthritis and diabetes mellitus. Studies indicate that trigger finger is related to certain occupations and repetitive tasks. One Canadian study indicated a 14% prevalence of trigger finger among workers in a meat-packing plant, with the incidence being higher among hand tool users.[13]

The Social Security Administration's disability requirements are the same as discussed earlier in this chapter. Therefore, trigger thumb or finger tenosynovitis rarely qualifies for one-sided total upper extremity disability.

Risk Assessment

The risk for trigger finger or thumb is similar to that of de Quervain's tenosynovitis of the wrist, as outlined above. Even in severe cases it is very rare for the involved tendon to rupture. If the digit becomes locked (unable to flex or unable to extend because the knot in the tendon can no longer

Chapter 13

pass through the constriction), there is a risk of permanent loss of digit motion. Digits that do not move may become permanently stiff. Thus, for the uncommon locked digit, urgent surgical treatment and work restrictions are appropriate.

Capacity
In the common "triggering" or snapping digit scenario, capacity or grip strength and hand dexterity are minimally affected. Trigger finger thus is not generally an issue of capacity.

Tolerance
For trigger finger or thumb, staying at work or returning to work is primarily based on tolerance. Patients can use the involved digit, but to do so is painful. Nonoperative treatment with a brief period of temporary work modification is frequently successful. Comfortable hand function is compromised enough that patients who fail to respond to nonoperative treatment almost always choose to have surgical treatment. Trigger finger release surgery is almost always successful. Thus, trigger finger is rarely a reason for any permanent work problem. Over time, with continued performance of work tasks, additional digits may become involved, but each usually responds to treatment. Table 13-14 contains suggested disability durations in days for trigger digits and the duration and trend data is listed in Table 13-15.

Table 13-14 Suggested Disability Durations (Days)[*][†]

Job Classification	The Hand Center			The Medical Disability Advisor		
	Target	TMinimum	TMaximum	Optimum	Minimum	Maximum
Nonsurgical Treatment (Including Injection) for Finger or Thumb: Trigger						
Sedentary	0	0	7	7	1	21
Light	0	0	7	7	1	21
Medium	0	0	7	7	3	28
Heavy	0	0	14	7	5	35
Very Heavy	0	0	14	7	5	42
Surgical Treatment for Finger or Thumb: Trigger						
Sedentary	0	0	7	14	1	28
Light	0	0	7	14	3	28
Medium	7	0	28	21	7	35
Heavy	21	3	35	28	21	42
Very Heavy	21	7	35	28	21	42

[*] See Table 13-2 for definitions of job classifications.
[†] Data used with permission from Melhorn[10] and Reed.[11]

Table 13-15 Real-world Disability Case Data

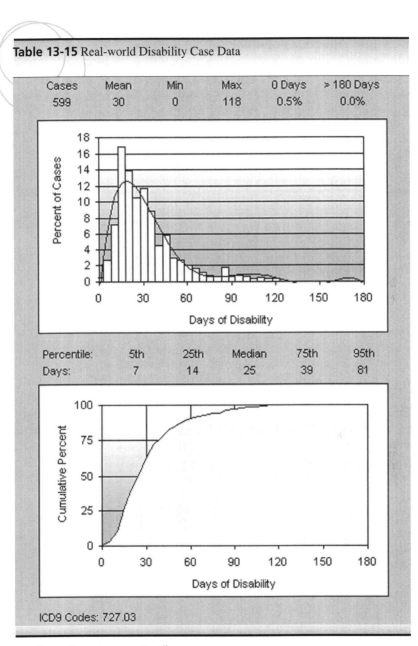

Cases	Mean	Min	Max	0 Days	> 180 Days
599	30	0	118	0.5%	0.0%

Percentile:	5th	25th	Median	75th	95th
Days:	7	14	25	39	81

ICD9 Codes: 727.03

Reproduced with permission from Reed.[11]

Conclusion

For trigger finger or thumb, staying at work or returning to work is primarily based on tolerance. Tolerance is associated with the pain level experienced with movement of the digit. Surgery often results in marked improvement, although the capacity may be limited for a short period after surgery. After surgery, most individuals can return to their previous employment. Temporary work guides limiting combination activities may be helpful.

Nontraumatic Soft-Tissue Disorder

Nontraumatic soft-tissue disorder (ICD-9-CM code 729.5) is used to describe discomfort affecting any part of an extremity (such as an elbow) or the entire limb (arm or leg). The term is general and could be used to describe pain that arises from various causes. Common synonyms include regional arm pain, musculoskeletal disorders, musculoskeletal pain, cumulative trauma disorder, and repetitive strain injury.

The pain may arise from the skin, nerves, muscles, bones, joints, or even the brain (in psychogenic or phantom pain). Typically, the term *pain in the limb* would be used to describe a person's symptoms until a definitive diagnosis is made (such as a broken arm, tendinitis, peripheral neuropathy, etc). In many of these cases, no specific diagnosis is ever possible.

The Social Security Administration's disability requirements are the same as discussed earlier in this chapter. Therefore, nontraumatic soft-tissue disorder or musculoskeletal disorder rarely qualifies for one-sided total upper extremity disability.

Risk Assessment

Although the pain may be associated with physical activities, it is often difficult to establish a reasonable cause and effect: *post hoc ergo propter hoc* (after the fact, therefore because of the fact).[33] Arguments based only on temporal relationships for workers' compensation causation or impairments are logic fallacies, especially in degenerative conditions, as the normal progression of degeneration will lead to worsening in and of itself over time.[34] In the absence of a specific objectively verifiable diagnosis, there is no risk, and thus no basis for physician-imposed work restrictions.

Capacity

Becuase the individual often lacks a specific musculoskeletal diagnosis, unless limited capacity is currently present on the basis of deconditioning, nonspecific hand and/or arm pain does not affect capacity. In general, the goal is to encourage maximum function and limit dysfunction.

Tolerance
Pain is the limiting factor for tolerance of work activities. Pain is a fluid concept and cannot be proved or disproved by a physician.[35] The International Association for the Study of Pain defines pain as an unpleasant sensory and emotional experience associated with actual or potential tissue damage, or described in terms of such damage.[36] At its most basic level, pain is both a physical phenomenon (presence of activity in discrete neural pathways) and a psychological or emotional experience ("it hurts"). Theoretically, pain serves the useful function of prevention of tissue damage. Pain is actually a homeostatic mechanism.[37] It is only when pain becomes chronic, and no longer predictive of possible tissue damage, that it serves no useful function.[38]

Tolerance for pain is the limiting factor for staying at work or returning to work in nonspecific hand and/or arm pain. Symptoms tend to be chronic with activities, although often not progressive. Although work modifi-cations for short periods may be recommended, physicians should encourage increasing tolerance through education and communication and through progressive increases in activity. This can be difficult when the individual reports that any and all activities make the pain worse. Discussions regarding musculoskeletal pain and its relationship to the individual and workplace risk factors may be helpful.[38] General physical conditioning, appropriate diet and sleep habits, and limitation of caffeine and nicotine are helpful.[39] Ergonometric assessment and modification of the workplace may be considered. Suggested disability durations in days for nontraumatic soft-tissue disorders are listed in Table 13-16.

Chapter 13

Table 13-16 Suggested Disability Durations (Days)[*†]

Job Classification	The Hand Center			The Medical Disability Advisor		
	Target	TMinimum	TMaximum	Optimum	Minimum	Maximum
Nonsurgical Treatment for Nontraumatic Soft-Tissue Disorders of the Upper Extremity or Pain in Limb						
Sedentary	0	0	4	0	3	7
Light	0	0	5	0	3	7
Medium	0	0	7	1	3	7
Heavy	0	0	14	1	3	7
Very Heavy	0	0	14	1	3	7

[*] See Table 13-2 for definitions of job classifications.
[†] Data used with permission from Melhorn[10] and Reed.[11]

Conclusion

Patients with nontraumatic soft-tissue disorders or work-related nonspecific musculoskeletal pain are often the most frustrating for the healthcare provider. The response to treatment is often intermittent and inconsistent. Symptoms can remain disproportional to the clinical findings despite appropriate conservative medical care and reasonable modifications to the workplace. Since pain is a plural concept with biological, psychological, and social components, and since its perception is influenced by cognitive, behavioral, environmental, and cultural factors, successful management requires the healthcare provider to go beyond the traditional medical model.[40] Treatment must also address these nonmedical issues to obtain better outcomes.[41-44] Prevention has been the most successful management for this group of patients.[45]

Summary

Musculoskeletal pain may affect any body location. Converting the subjective complaints to a specific pathoanatomic diagnosis can often be challenging. The first step is the traditional medical history and examination. Most individuals can be placed into one of five categories for insight into treatment and outcomes: (1) at risk but without injury or current symptoms, (2) acute traumatic injuries, (3) acute onset of nontraumatic symptoms, (4) chronic symptoms with return to work likely, and (5) chronic symptoms with return to work unlikely (based on severe pathology or psychosocial factors).[46]

When patients are disabled (unable to work), everyone loses. The insurer, employer, and society suffer the economic losses, while the employee and his or her family suffer the individual losses. As a patient advocate, the physician has the best opportunity to encourage staying at work or early return to work. Benefits for the individual include better self-image, improved ability to cope, improved work survivability, and improved ability to be self-sufficient. (See Chapter 1.) Conversely, prolonged time away from work makes recovery and return to work progressively less likely. Benefits for the employer and insurer are financial, while the workers' compensation system lives up to its goal of intended fairness. Severe conditions require the consideration of risk (work restrictions) and capacity (work limitations). Most often, the factor hindering return to work is tolerance.

Returning the individual to work requires a balance between the demands of the job and the capability of the patient. Communication and education are key to addressing tolerance issues. The temporary workplace guides for tolerance must allow for a speedy return to work, with the interests of the patient being the primary responsibility. This approach provides treating physicians with a unique opportunity and obligation to provide reasonable work guides in an effort to reduce work disability, improve the outcome for work-related injuries, and advance the quality of life for their patients.

References

1. US Bureau of Labor Statistics. *Survey of Occupational Injuries and Illnesses, 1996.* Washington, DC, United States Government Printing Office; 1998:1–58.

2. US Bureau of Labor Statistics. BLS issues 1996 lost-worktime injuries and illnesses survey. *Am Coll Occup Environ Med Rep.* 1998;98:6–7.

3. Brady W, Bass J, Royce M, et al. Defining total corporate health and safety costs: significance and impact. *J Occup Environ Med.* 1997;39:224–231.

4. Feuerstein M, Miller VL, Burrell LM, Berger R. Occupational upper extremity disorders in the federal workforce. *J Occup Environ Med.* 1998;40:546–555.

5. Webster BS, Snook SH. The cost of compensable upper extremity cumulative trauma disorders. *J Occup Environ Med.* 1994;7:713–718.

6. Social Security Administration. *Social Security Determination Book for Muscular Skeletal.* Washington, DC: Social Security Administration; 2004:1–45.

7. US Department of Health and Human Services. *Musculoskeletal Disorders and Workplace Factors: A Critical Review of Epidemiologic Evidence for Work-Related Musculoskeletal Disorders of the Neck, Upper Extremity, and Low Back.* Cincinnati, Ohio: National Institute for Occupational Safety and Health; 1997.

8. Melhorn JM. Epidemiology of musculoskeletal disorders and workplace factors. In: Mayer TG, Gatchel RJ, Polatin PB, eds. *Occupational Musculoskeletal Disorders Function, Outcomes, and Evidence.* Philadelphia, Pa: Lippincott Williams & Wilkins; 1999:225–266.

9. Philadelphia Panel evidence-based clinical practice guidelines on selected rehabilitation interventions for shoulder pain. *Phys Ther.* 2001;81:1719–1730.

10. Melhorn JM. *Work Guides, Functional Capacity, Work Restrictions Used by the Hand Center.* Wichita, Kan: Hand Center; 2003.

11. Reed P. *The Medical Disability Advisor.* Boulder, Colo: Reed Group Ltd; 2001.

12. US Department of Labor. *Dictionary of Occupational Titles.* Washington, DC: US Department of Labor; 1991.

13. Reed P. *The Medical Disability Advisor: Workplace Guidelines for Disability Duration.* 5th ed. Westminster, Colo: Reed Group, Ltd; 2005.

14. D'Arcy CA, McGee S. The rational clinical examination: does this patient have carpal tunnel syndrome? *JAMA.* 2000;283:3110–3117.

15. Marx RG, Hudak PL, Bombardier C, et al. The reliability of physical examination for carpal tunnel syndrome. *J Hand Surg.* 1998;23B:499–502.

16. Salerno DF, Franzblau A, Werner RA, et al. Reliability of physical examination of the upper extremity among keyboard operators. *Am J Ind Med.* 2000;37:423–430.

Chapter 13

17. American Academy of Neurology. Practice parameter for electrodiagnostic studies in carpal tunnel syndrome (summary statement). *Neurology.* 1993;43:2404–2405.

18. Hadler NM. *Occupational Musculoskeletal Disorders.* Philadelphia, Pa: Lippincott Williams & Wilkins; 1999.

19. Michelson H, Posner MA. Medical history of carpal tunnel syndrome. *Hand Clin.* 2002;18:257–268.

20. Carrico HL. Virginia declares carpal tunnel not a job injury. *Occup Health Manage.* July 1996:79–80.

21. Nathan PA, Meadows KD, Istvan JA. Predictors of carpal tunnel syndrome: an 11-year study of industrial workers. *J Hand Surg.* 2002;27A:644–651.

22. Padua L, Padua R, Aprile I, Pasqualetti P, Tonali P. Multiperspective follow-up of untreated carpal tunnel syndrome: a multicenter study. *Neurology.* 2001; 56:1459–1466.

23. Andersen JH, Thomsen JF, Overgaard E, et al. Computer use and carpal tunnel syndrome: a 1-year follow-up study. *JAMA.* 2003;289:2963–2969.

24. Clarke Stevens J, Witt JC, Smith BE, Weaver AL. The frequency of carpal tunnel syndrome in computer users at a medical facility. *Neurology.* 2001;56:1568–1570.

25. Nordstrom DL, Vierkant RA, DeStefano F, Layde PM. Risk factors for carpal tunnel syndrome in a general population. *Occup Environ Med.* 1997;54:734–740.

26. Hadler NM. A keyboard for "Daubert." *J Occup Environ Med.* 1996;38:469–476.

27. Egilman D, Punnett L, Hjelm EW, Welch L. Evidence for work-related musculoskeletal disorders. *J Occup Environ Med.* 1996;38:1079–1080.

28. Garland FC, Garland CF, Doyle EJ, et al. Carpal tunnel syndrome and occupation in U.S. Navy enlisted personnel. *Arch Environ Health.* 1996;51:395–407.

29. Lo SL, Raskin K, Lester H, Lester B. Carpal tunnel syndrome: a historical perspective. *Hand Clin.* 2002;18:211–217.

30. Kryger AI, Andersen JH, Lassen CF, et al. Does computer use pose an occupational hazard for forearm pain; from the NUDATA study. *Occup Environ Med.* 2003;60:14.

31. Rempel D, Tittiranonda P, Burastero S, Hudes M, So Y. Effect of keyboard keyswitch design on hand pain. *J Occup Environ Med.* 1999;41:111–119.

32. Lincoln AE, Vernick JS, Ogaitis S, et al. Interventions for the primary prevention of work-related carpal tunnel syndrome. *Am J Prev Med.* 2000;18:37–50.

33. Melhorn JM. Work-related upper extremity musculoskeletal pain: successful disability prevention. In: Genovese E, ed. *First Do No Harm: Medical and Ethical Issues in Disability Management.* Philadelphia, Pa: IMX Medical Management Services Inc; 2004.

34. Melhorn JM. The top 10 most medically controversial or dubious treatments in workers comp. In: *IAIABC 31st International Workers Compensation College.* Madison, Wis: International Association of Industrial Accident Boards and Commissions; 2004.

Chapter 13

35. Melhorn JM. *Employer's Modified Work Program Agreement.* Wichita, Kan: Hand Center; 2003.

36. International Association for the Study of Pain. *Pain Definitions.* Seattle, Wash: International Association for the Study of Pain; 2002. Available at: www.iasp-pain.org/defsopen.html. Accessed November 1, 2004.

37. Melhorn JM. Understanding and managing chronic non-malignant pain for the occupational orthopaedists. In: Melhorn JM, Strain RE Jr, eds. *Occupational Orthopaedics and Workers' Compensation: A Multidisciplinary Perspective.* Rosemont, Ill: American Academy of Orthopaedic Surgeons; 2002.

38. Melhorn JM. Return to work: negotiation strategies. In: Melhorn JM, Strain RE Jr, eds. *Occupational Orthopaedics and Workers' Compensation: A Multidisciplinary Perspective.* Rosemont, Ill: American Academy of Orthopaedic Surgeons; 2002.

39. Melhorn JM. Return to work issues: arm pain. In: Melhorn JM, Strain RE Jr, eds. *Occupational Orthopaedics and Workers' Compensation: A Multidisciplinary Perspective.* Rosemont, Ill: American Academy of Orthopaedic Surgeons; 2002.

40. Melhorn JM, Gardner P. How we prevent prevention of musculoskeletal disorders in the workplace. *Clin Orthop.* 2004;419:285–296.

41. Melhorn JM, Kennedy EM. Musculoskeletal disorders, disability, and return-to-work (repetitive strain): the quest for objectivity. In: Gatchel RJ, Schultz IZ, eds. *At Risk Claims: Predication of Occupational Disability Using a Biopsychosocial Approach.* New York, NY: Kluwer Academic/Plenium; 2004.

42. Melhorn JM. Upper extremities: return to work issues. In: Melhorn JM, Spengler DM, eds. *Occupational Orthopaedics and Workers' Compensation: A Multidisciplinary Perspective.* Rosemont, Ill: American Academy of Orthopaedic Surgeons; 2003:256–285.

43. Melhorn JM. Occupational orthopaedics: evidence-based medicine, HIPAA privacy compliance, and functional capacity evaluations. In: Melhorn JM, Spengler DM, eds. *Occupational Orthopaedics and Workers' Compensation: A Multidisciplinary Perspective.* Rosemont, Ill: American Academy of Orthopaedic Surgeons; 2003:41–80.

44. Talmage JB. Injury healing and maximum medical improvement (MMI): the basic sciences. In: Melhorn JM, Strain RE Jr, eds. *Occupational Orthopaedics and Workers Compensation: A Multidisciplinary Perspective.* Rosemont, Ill: American Academy of Orthopaedic Surgeons; 2002:453–474.

45. Melhorn JM, Wilkinson LK, O'Malley MD. Successful management of musculoskeletal disorders. *J Hum Ecol Risk Assessment.* 2001;7:1801–1810.

46. Melhorn JM. The advantages of early return to work. *IAIABC J.* 2003;41:128–147.

Chapter 13

Working With Common Lower Extremity Problems

Robert H. Haralson III, MD, MBA

Lower extremity injuries are a common cause of the loss of the ability to work, ranking behind only spine injuries and upper extremity injuries. With proper accommodations, however, patients with lower extremity injuries may return to work relatively quickly.

Presumed Disability

The Social Security Administration's (SSA's) criterion for total disability is that the disabling condition must have been present or be expected to be present for at least 12 months. There are very few lower extremity problems that will not have healed sufficiently in 12 months to allow a patient to function at or above the minimum criterion for total disability.

Examples of complications that might lead to total disability include:

- chronic bone infection (osteomyelitis),
- nonunion of fractures,
- recurrent dislocation of a total joint,
- intra-articular fractures that lead to early degenerative arthritis, and
- high-energy injuries that involve bone and significant soft-tissue loss.

In the absence of one of these devastating complications, the most common reason for a patient to be off work is a matter of tolerance, as discussed in

Chapter 2. Pain and lack of tolerance are given by the SSA as a potential reason to be off work[1]:

> In order for pain or other symptoms to be found to affect an individual's ability to perform basic work activities, medical signs or laboratory findings must show the existence of a medically determinable impairment(s) that could reasonably be expected to produce the pain or other symptoms.

This means that there should be objective evidence of severe pathology (the *biomedical* model of disability). Healed fractures and soft-tissue injuries should not cause enough pain to warrant extended periods of non-employment.

The literature on return to work with lower extremity injuries suggests rather long periods before a patient returns to work. This apparently reflects cases that do not include the ability to return an injured worker to modified work. This chapter discusses specifically sprains, strains, fractures, dislocations, total joint arthroplasty, and arthroscopic knee surgery, as these injuries are the most common conditions encountered in the lower extremities in workers.

Risk Assessment
Assessment of risk in the context of returning to work means estimating whether a worker can return to work without high risk of re-injuring the injured part or to another part of the body, slowing the healing process, or otherwise causing an outcome that is less satisfactory than would have occurred if the patient had not returned to work. The main function of the upper extremity is to place the hand in the proper position and then to allow the hand to perform some activity. Limitation of motion, weakness, and pain with motion may well prevent this activity. However, the lower extremity function is mainly to support the body and to allow for locomotion. Many work activities do not require the support of the lower extremities (jobs that can be performed in the sitting position), and locomotion can be assisted by the use of ambulatory aids (walkers, crutches, canes, and/or wheelchairs). In addition, accommodations may be available that limit the amount of locomotion required to get to the work site (eg, handicapped parking) and to perform the required duties (eg, a chair). Therefore, returning to work after lower extremity injuries and surgery is often possible and, as is pointed out in later chapters of this text, is usually preferable to the alternative of long periods of inactivity that allow further deconditioning.

A problem with lower extremity injuries that is not usually encountered in the upper extremity is the risk of thrombophlebitis. With any ambulation, the lower extremity is dependent—a position that predisposes to swelling and venous stasis. Therefore, early return to work may have to include the ability for the patient to spend at least part of the work day elevating the extremity.

Sprains and Strains

Many sprains and strains require nothing but symptomatic treatment. Even the more severe injuries that require some amount of bracing and the limitation of full weight bearing for protection should not prevent early return to work. There is no scientific evidence that there is danger in sending a worker back to work shortly after definitive treatment of a sprain or strain is accomplished. In fact, the evidence is to the contrary: motion and muscular activity are beneficial.[2-5] Even those few injuries that need surgical repair should be amenable to early return to work with proper protection.

Fractures

With the modern methods of treating fractures, early return to work is possible. The goal of treatment of lower extremity fractures is to achieve a stable construct so that axial loading by weight bearing or muscular activity will not deform the fracture. Once that stable construct is achieved, exercise, motion, and at least protected weight bearing are beneficial. Therefore, with proper treatment, proper external support, the use of ambulatory aids if necessary, and limitation of the amount of ambulation, there is little reason to leave a worker off work after the initial period of wound healing and discomfort. In Chapter 10, the authors demonstrated that the use of low doses of opioids for relief of mild discomfort should not preclude a worker from driving or returning to work.

Dislocations

Dislocations are even more amenable to return to work than are fractures. Hip and ankle dislocations are usually stable when reduced, and as a result, range-of-motion exercises are started early. Because both joints are stable due to their configuration, weight bearing to tolerance is allowed. Physicians in the past required a period of non–weight bearing, but there is no evidence that immediate full weight bearing is detrimental. Avascular necrosis of the hip sometimes occurs, especially if reduction was delayed, but weight bearing does not influence the occurrence. Patients should be able to bear weight to tolerance, but should avoid the extremes of motion for periods of three to six weeks.

Knee dislocations are another matter. True knee dislocations usually involve multiple ligament tears and will usually require operative treatment and longer periods of protection.

Total joint replacement is now commonplace, and, though it was done in older patients at first, it is now being performed in the working-age population.

Chapter 14

Once the joint is stable and the early wound healing is complete, there is little reason to remain off work with the proper accommodations. Weight bearing is not detrimental to the stable total joint. However, total joints do not do well with repeated impact loading, so running, heavy lifting, and long periods of walking should be permanently restricted to minimize the chance of loosening of the prosthesis.

Because arthroscopic knee surgery does not injure tissue like the open arthrotomy did, there is little reason to leave patients off work for extended periods of time. If a meniscus was repaired, rather than excised, then a longer period of protection is required to prevent twisting or the extremes of flexion, as both motions will tend to disrupt the repair. However, with proper accommodations, even meniscus repair is amenable to early return to work.

Capacity

As has been stated in previous chapters, *capacity* really means *current ability*, which can usually be increased with rehabilitation. Capacity may be reduced in lower extremity injuries for one of two reasons. First, ambulation with many lower extremity injuries requires the use of ambulatory aids, such as walkers, crutches, and canes. Walking with ambulatory aids is inefficient and requires additional muscular activity and energy. In addition, the patient must use upper extremity muscles that he or she may not be accustomed to using. As a result, the worker may require some limitation of the amount of ambulation required, and fatigue may require less than the usual eight-hour work day.

Second, patients who have had periods of pain before their surgery, such as in the case of chronic knee pain with meniscus tears, and especially arthritis before total joint replacement, may be significantly deconditioned and require a slower return to work. Data show that the longer a patient has been off work before total hip surgery, the less likely he or she will ever return to work.[6] The concomitant occurrence of even minor fractures of the upper and lower extremities might prevent early return to work because the upper extremity fracture may preclude the use of the ambulatory aids required to protect the lower extremity injury.

Tolerance

As is the case much of the time, tolerance will often be the limiting factor for return to work in lower extremity injuries. Many lower extremity injuries are painful at first and remain uncomfortable for weeks, especially if the limb must be dependent. In addition, many patients may be reluctant to spend the added energy required to use ambulatory aids. MacKenzie et al[7,8] suggested that delayed return to work in patients with severe lower extremity injuries was not explained by physical factors. Canelon[9] suggested that job-site analysis facilitated work reintegration.

Strikeleather[10] reported that employer support and degree of flexibility in work, continued health problems, and financial distress affected an injured worker's decision to "push or protect self." Manion and Bartholomew[11] pointed out in their study that people yearn to return to community, seeking a sense of connection with others. Lee[12] suggested that development of explicit criteria for return to work might help in understanding early return to work. This approach has certainly accomplished earlier hospital discharge for total joint replacement recipients through the development of clinical pathways. Van Duijn et al[13] found many barriers to returning to work both from the employee side and the employer side. Most of the literature reports time to full duty, and there is sparse literature on early return to work, that is, to modified duty. This approach would obviate the deconditioning, both physical and psychological, that occurs with extended periods of being off work.

Sprains and Strains

Ligament injuries are called *sprains* and are divided into three classifications, graded I, II, and III. Grade I means that no structure was disrupted and the ligament strength is not altered. Grade II is present if there is partial ligament disruption and the strength of the ligament is altered. This suggests that some level of protection is needed. Grade III represents complete disruption and obviously is the most serious of the three. Some, but not all, grade III ligamentous injuries require operative repair.

Sprains in the knee and ankle are the two most common lower extremity sprains that will be encountered in the workplace. Medial and lateral collateral knee ligament injuries are common, and significant injuries will require some form of protection. Grade III lateral collateral injuries are often treated surgically, while medial collateral injuries can be treated more conservatively. Grade III anterior and posterior cruciate injuries are not amenable to spontaneous healing or direct repair, and are usually treated by reconstruction using a variety of substitutes from autogenous patellar tendon and hamstring tendons to allografts. Most surgeons start these patients on immediate motion with or with out bracing. Ambulation with ambulatory aids and weight bearing to tolerance, with the knee completely extended, is permitted immediately. Formal physical therapy is important, so return-to-work programs must provide for therapy sessions.[14]

Grade I ankle sprains are more of a nuisance than a severe injury, and return to work with bracing should be immediate. Some surgeons prefer to repair grade III lateral ankle sprains, but the tendency now is more conservative.[2,15] Even with operative repair, weight bearing to tolerance with bracing should be permitted within a few days. Activity limitation to eliminate twisting of the foot may be required for several months. College and professional athletes are sometimes hampered for whole seasons by severe ankle sprains, but with bracing and activity modifications, patients should do well.

Strains are injuries to muscles or muscle-tendon units. The most common strains in the lower extremity are the quadriceps, the hamstrings, and the medial head of the gastrocnemius (formerly thought to involve the plantaris). Tears of the gastrocnemius are rarely significant, and treatment is symptomatic. Return to work with weight bearing to tolerance should be immediate. Strains to the quadriceps and hamstrings are usually not serious in a worker, but they can be in a high-performance sprinter. Symptomatic treatment is the norm, and return to work should be based on comfort. A few workers may have complete disruption of the quadriceps at its insertion into the patella, and this uncommon injury requires operative repair and an extended period of immobilization. Tears of the Achilles tendon require several weeks of immobilization in the equinus position (plantar flexion), whether they are treated conservatively or operatively, and this makes walking more difficult, but not impossible.

The Medical Disability Advisor (MDA) from the Reed Group[16] provides consensus return-to-work criteria for *International Classification of Diseases, Ninth Revision, Clinical Modification* (ICD-9-CM) code 845 (sprains and strains of ankle and foot). These criteria indicate that persisting ankle pain is still compatible with function, and that most patients should eventually return to their original type of work. The real-world data that follow also indicate that most patients with ankle sprains do in fact return to work. Table 14-1 lists the MDA consensus criteria for first- or second-degree sprains and strains of the ankle. Table 14-2 illustrates the real-world case data, also from the MDA.

Table 14-1 First- or Second-Degree (Mild to Moderate) Sprain or Strain of the Ankle: Consensus Criteria

Job Classification	Duration, days		
	Minimum	Optimum	Maximum
Sedentary	0	3	7
Light	1	3	7
Medium	3	7	14
Heavy	7	14	28
Very Heavy	7	14	28

Reproduced with permission from Reed.[16]

Table 14-2 First- or Second-Degree (Mild to Moderate) Sprain or Strain of the Ankle: Real-World Case Data

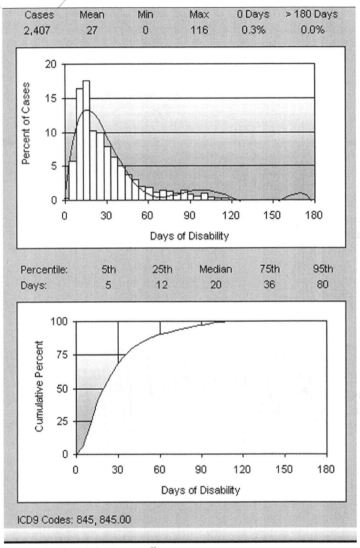

Cases	Mean	Min	Max	0 Days	> 180 Days
2,407	27	0	116	0.3%	0.0%

Percentile:	5th	25th	Median	75th	95th
Days:	5	12	20	36	80

ICD9 Codes: 845, 845.00

Reproduced with permission from Reed.[16]

Fractures

Fractures of the lower extremity are very common, and there are a number of determinants with regard to the ability to return to work. Important are the location of the fracture, the amount of bony and soft-tissue damage, and the stability of the fixation method. The goal of treatment of fractures in the shaft of the femur and tibia is to reestablish alignment and to develop a construct that will prevent shortening. Accordingly, treatment of undisplaced transverse fractures of the tibia may be treated with cast or brace immobilization. Oblique or displaced transverse shaft fractures are usually treated with intramedullary fixation. If the treatment is able to obtain a stable construct, then partial weight bearing and early return to work should be possible.[17,18] Displaced fractures in and around joints will require accurate repositioning and are more likely to require open surgical treatment. The goal of treatment is to accurately reestablish the joint surface and to regain range of motion of the joint. Because the bone adjacent to joints is softer, rigid fixation is often not possible, and thus more protection in the postoperative period may be necessary. And because the fibula does not bear weight and serves mainly for muscle attachment, except at the ankle, fractures of this bone usually require only symptomatic treatment.

Another consideration is the amount of soft tissue and bony damage. Open fractures with significant soft-tissue injury may require multiple trips to the operating theater for debridement, as contaminated wounds are frequently left open initially to prevent infection. Skin grafting or other tissue re-arrangement procedures will preclude early return to work. Significant soft-tissue damage delays fracture healing and causes more swelling. If the fracture is comminuted, preventing a solid construct, and especially if there is actual bone loss, external fixation is sometimes used and long periods of non–weight bearing may be required. Early return to work with these complicated fractures is difficult.[19]

Undisplaced fractures of the lateral malleolus that are stable may be treated nonoperatively with braces.[20] Other fractures in and around the ankle joint can be a problem for return to work. Because unsupported ambulation requires the full weight of the body to be transmitted through the distal tibia and hindfoot bones (talus and calcaneus), fractures in these bones as well as fractures of the distal tibial articular surface may require extended protected ambulation. Displaced fractures of the talus often result in avascular necrosis, and intra-articular fractures of the calcaneus remain difficult to treat. There is controversy over whether calcaneal fractures should be treated open or closed. A study by Tufescu and Buckley[21] suggested that males, multiply injured patients, and heavy laborers may have better outcomes with operative treatment, whereas females and non–workers' compensation patients may do better with non-operative care. Buckley and Meek[22] suggested that in workers, accurate reduction by open methods was superior. Mortelmans et al[23] reported work incapacity lasting an average of 260 days, but this was time to full duty, including working at heights. Naovaratanophas and Thepchatri[24] reported earlier return to work at an average of 3.42 months.

Fractures of the other tarsal bones and the metatarsals are treated closed if they are undisplaced and open if there is significant displacement. Either treatment is followed by cast or brace immobilization, and at least partial weight bearing is allowed.

Fractures in the lower extremity do not usually preclude early return to work if the treatment achieves a rigid construct that allows axial loading to some degree. Sometimes casts or braces are required as adjunctive immobilization, but the tendency now is to prefer braces, because they can be removed for skin care and mobilization of the joints.[25] As long as the job can accommodate for the inability to fully bear weight, and allow periods of extremity elevation, patients can usually be returned to work early.

Table 14-3 lists the MDA consensus return-to-work criteria for ICD-9-CM code 823 (fracture of tibia and fibula) and Table 14-4 illustrates the real-world case data.

Dislocations

Dislocations of lower extremity joints are fairly common, and most are reduced by closed methods. Even if open reduction is required, because the joint configuration is unchanged, most, except for the knee, are relatively stable at the time of reduction. Treatment regimens have changed. Three weeks of immobilization was the norm several years ago, but now immobilization is used only to control discomfort, and most physicians start the patients on range of motion exercises as soon as possible, only limiting the extremes of motion. Schlickewei et al[26] suggested in a 1993 report that early return to work was an advantage of the more active treatment regimen. Dislocations of the hip, ankle, and subtalar joint are the most common, and all three should be stable after reduction. Dislocations of the toe joints are more

Chapter 14

Table 14-3 Tibia Fracture: Consensus Criteria

Job Classification	Duration, days		
	Minimum	Optimum	Maximum
Sedentary	14	28	84
Light	28	42	182
Medium	119	182	224
Heavy	161	224	273
Very Heavy	182	273	Indefinite

Reproduced with permission from Reed.[16]

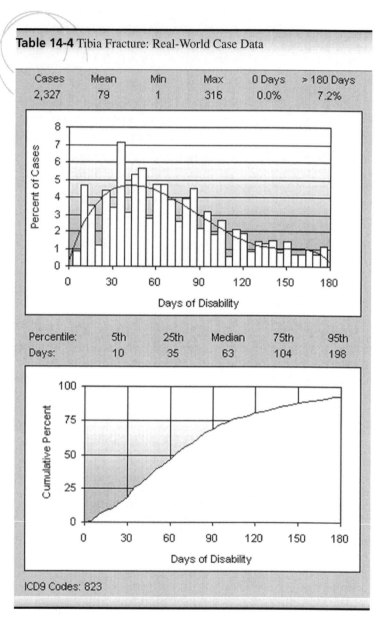

Table 14-4 Tibia Fracture: Real-World Case Data

Cases	Mean	Min	Max	0 Days	> 180 Days
2,327	79	1	316	0.0%	7.2%

Percentile:	5th	25th	Median	75th	95th
Days:	10	35	63	104	198

ICD9 Codes: 823

Reproduced with permission from Reed.[16]

of a nuisance than a serious disorder, and return to work should be immediate (as long as the footwear required at work can fit on the foot). Like the metacarpophalangeal joint of the thumb, dislocations of the metatarsophalangeal joint of the great toe will occasionally require open reduction, but then are stable. Transmetatarsal dislocation, the so-called Lisfranc injury, usually requires pin fixation and casting or bracing but is stable after surgery, and Brinsden et al[27] report successful return to work.

True dislocations of the knee disrupt many of the ligaments, and because the configuration of the knee joint does not make it inherently stable, ligament repair and/or reconstruction is usually necessary. This may require bracing for a period, but Noyes and Barber-Westin[28] have shown that even in these significant injuries, early motion is important.

Table 14-5 lists the MDA consensus return-to-work criteria for ICD-9-CM codes 836.5 and 836.6 (dislocation of knee and other dislocation of knee, open).

The MDA suggests 7 days minimum for return to full duty in sedentary activity. This is probably a little unrealistic if ligament reconstruction wasrequired, which it usually is in true knee dislocation. However, the times for returning to light and medium duty are excessive if accommodations can be afforded and would be in the range of 14 to 28 days. Non-narcotic analgesics and non-steroidal medications should control the discomfort by that time.

Total Joint Arthroplasty

The hip and knee are two joints in the lower extremities that are commonly replaced, and replacement of the ankle is increasing in frequency. As was discussed earlier in this chapter, the stability of the fixation is paramount. There are three considerations regarding stability of total joints. Crucial determinants of early activity are whether the components are cemented in place, or at least one is uncemented and thus time must be allowed for bony ingrowth to produce stability, as well as whether there is ligamentous

Chapter 14

Table 14-5 Knee Dislocation: Consensus Criteria

Job Classification	Duration, days		
	Minimum	Optimum	Maximum
Sedentary	7	14	28
Light	14	21	42
Medium	119	182	224
Heavy	161	224	273
Very Heavy	182	273	Indefinite

Reproduced with permission from Reed.[16]

stability. Cemented components are immediately stable and will withstand weight bearing to tolerance. Uncemented components that will depend on bony ingrowth for stability require a period of partial weight bearing to allow that ingrowth to occur before they are stable.

Because of the ball-and-cup configuration of the artificial hip, once the joint is stable, weight bearing to tolerance is permissible and patients may be allowed to return to modified work. In the hip, patients must avoid the extremes of motion, as those positions are more likely to lead to dislocations. This would mean restrictions on squatting and crawling. If the surgery involved the posterior approach, the position of flexion, adduction, and internal rotation is to be avoided. Rising from a low chair often requires the patient to lean forward, thus flexing the hip more than 90°. Therefore, accommodations should include elevated seating arrangements, including commodes, which are usually lower than most chairs.

Total knee replacements require the same stability parameters as total hip replacements: whether any of the components is uncemented and whether there is ligamentous stability are crucial determinants of early work ability. As in the hip, uncemented components require a period of limited weight bearing. Ligamentous stability is more important in the knee because the joint configuration is not inherently stable. If ligamentous stability is achieved at surgery, then immobilization will be necessary for only a short period and range of motion exercises are started within a few days. Return to work could be within a few weeks with proper accommodations.[29]

The MDA suggests that 28 days is the minimum to return to full sedentary work for total hip replacement and 14 days for total knee replacement, and it is probably unrealistic to expect return to any work before then, even with accommodations.

Chapter 14

Table 14-6 Knee Replacement: Consensus Criteria

Job Classification	Duration, days		
	Minimum	Optimum	Maximum
Sedentary	14	28	42
Light	21	42	84
Medium	84	112	Indefinite
Heavy	Indefinite	Indefinite	Indefinite
Very Heavy	Indefinite	Indefinite	Indefinite

Reproduced with permission from Reed.[16]

Table 14-7 Knee Replacement: Real-World Case Data

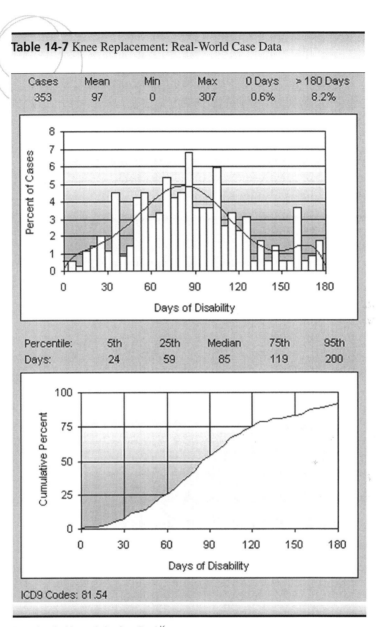

Cases	Mean	Min	Max	0 Days	> 180 Days
353	97	0	307	0.6%	8.2%

Percentile:	5th	25th	Median	75th	95th
Days:	24	59	85	119	200

ICD9 Codes: 81.54

Reproduced with permission from Reed.[16]

Table 14-6 lists the MDA consensus criteria for knee replacement and Table 14-7 illustrates the real-world case data.

Arthroscopic Knee Surgery

Much of knee surgery today is done arthroscopically on an outpatient basis, and this has significantly lessened the recovery time.[30,31] The most common arthroscopic knee surgery involves either repair or excision of a meniscus or cartilage. Anterior and posterior cruciate ligament surgery was discussed earlier. Meniscectomy requires no major incision and only a few arthroscopic portals (very small incisions). As a result, there is very little reason not to return to limited work within a week. Ambulatory aids may be required for comfort for a week or two, but proper accommodations should allow early return to work.

If a meniscus is repaired, rather than excised, protection for a longer period of time is indicated. Some surgeons use braces for 4 to 6 weeks while others use none, but in either case, protection from twisting and extreme flexion of the knee is necessary until the repaired meniscus heals. Return to modified duty, however, should take place within 1 to 2 weeks with the proper accommodations.

There are some new and innovative procedures to repair injuries to the articular cartilage in young patients that require long periods of extended non–weight bearing. These will be uncommon, and return to work would be possible if accommodations are available to allow mostly sedentary activity.

Tables 14-8 and 14-9 list the MDA consensus criteria for arthroscopic meniscectomy and meniscus repair, respectively. The tables suggest times to full duty. Return to limited duty after arthroscopic meniscectomy or meniscus repair could be within a few days with proper accommodations.

Table 14-8 Arthroscopic Meniscectomy: Consensus Criteria

Job Classification	Duration, days		
	Minimum	Optimum	Maximum
Sedentary	7	14	28
Light	7	14	35
Medium	14	21	56
Heavy	21	42	84
Very Heavy	28	42	126

Reproduced with permission from Reed.[16]

Chapter 14

Table 14-9 Meniscus Repair: Consensus Criteria

	Duration, days		
Job Classification	Minimum	Optimum	Maximum
Sedentary	7	14	42
Light	14	21	84
Medium	28	35	91
Heavy	42	84	140
Very Heavy	56	91	182

Reproduced with permission from Reed.[17]

Summary

Lower extremity injuries are amenable to early return to work. Most jobs require use of the upper extremity to perform a task. This means that residual stiffness and soreness may be aggravated by the activity. The lower extremities are mainly used for locomotion, and it is easy to compensate for that activity by allowing the use of ambulatory aids and minimizing the amount of locomotion. A job can be designed so that once a worker gets to his or her work site, he or she can sit or stand to do the job. There is a huge body of scientific information that proves that early return to work is beneficial and that being off work merely leads to further deconditioning, making return to work at any time more difficult. Being off work certifies disability and furthers the disability cascade, often leading to a worker who never returns to work. Because data show that it is less expensive in the long run to have a worker at work than doing nothing at home, and because ambulatory aids and limitation of locomotion should be readily available in the work place, there seems to be little reason to keep workers with most lower extremity injuries off work for extended periods.

Chapter 14

References

1. *Disability Evaluation Under Social Security.* Baltimore, Md: Social Security Administration; January 2003. SSA publication 64–039.

2. Balduini FC, Vegso JJ, Torg JS, Torg E. Management and rehabilitation of ligamentous injuries to the ankle. *Sports Med.* 1987;4:364–380.

3. Eiff MP, Smith AT, Smith GE. Early mobilization versus immobilization in the treatment of lateral ankle sprains. *Am J Sports Med.* 1994;22:83–88.

4. Kerkhoffs GM, Handoll HH, de Bie R, Rowe BH, Struijs PA. Surgical versus conservative treatment for acute injuries of the lateral ligament complex of the

later ligament complex of the ankle in adults. In: *The Cochrane Library, Issue 3, 2002*. Chichester, England: John Wiley & Sons Ltd; 2002. CD000380.

5. Kerkhoffs GM, Rowe BH, Assendelft WJ, Kelly KD, Struijs PA, van Dijk CN. Immobilisation for acute ankle sprain: a systematic review. *Arch Orthop Trauma Surg*. 2001;121:462–471. Review.

6. Nevitt MC, Epstein WV, Masem M, Murray WR. Work disability before and after total hip arthroplasty: assessment of effectiveness in reducing disability. *Arthritis Rheum*. 1984;27:410–421.

7. MacKenzie EJ, Morris JA Jr, Jurkovich GJ, et al. Return to work following injury: the role of economic, social, and job-related factors. *Am J Public Health*. 1998;88:1630–1637.

8. MacKenzie EJ, Cushing BM, Jurkovich GJ, et al. Physical impairment and functional outcomes six months after severe lower extremity fractures. *J Trauma*. 1993;34:528–539.

9. Canelon MF. Job site analysis facilitates work reintegration. *Am J Occup Ther*. 1995;49:461–467.

10. Strikeleather L. An older worker's decision to "push or protect self" following a work-related injury. *Work*. 2004;22:139–144.

11. Manion J, Bartholomew K. Community in the workplace: a proven retention strategy. *J Nurs Adm*. 2004;34:46–53.

12. Lee RH. Length of sickness absence from work after minor fractures. *Int J Rehabil Res*. 1982;5:499–506.

13. van Duijn M, Miedema H, Elders L, Burdorf A. Barriers for early return-to-work of workers with musculoskeletal disorders according to occupational health physicians and human resource managers. *J Occup Rehabil*. 2004;14:31–41.

14. Stanitski CL. Rehabilitation following knee injury. *Clin Sports Med*. 1985;4:495–511.

15. Lynch SA, Renstrom PA. Treatment of acute lateral ankle ligament rupture in the athlete: conservative versus surgical treatment. *Sports Med*. 1999;27:61–71.

16. Reed P. *The Medical Disability Advisor: Workplace Guidelines for Disability Duration*. 5th ed. Westminster, Colo: Reed Group, Ltd; 2005.

17. Hooper GJ, Keddell RG, Penny ID. Conservative management or closed nailing for tibial shaft fractures: a randomised prospective trial. *J Bone Joint Surg Br*. 1991;73:83–85.

18. Bednar DA, Ali P. Intramedullary nailing of femoral shaft fractures: reoperation and return to work. *Can J Surg*. 1993;36:464–466.

19. Arangio GA, Lehr S, Reed JF III. Reemployment of patients with surgical salvage of open, high-energy tibial fractures: an outcome study. *J Trauma*. 1997;42:942–945.

20. Brink O, Staunstrup H, Sommer J. Stable lateral malleolar fractures treated with aircast ankle brace and DonJoy R.O.M.-Walker brace: a prospective randomized study. *Foot Ankle Int*. 1996;17:679–684.

21. Tufescu TV, Buckley R. Age, gender, work capability, and worker's compensation in patients with displaced intraarticular calcaneal fractures. *J Orthop Trauma*. 2001;15:275–279.

22. Buckley RE, Meek RN. Comparison of open versus closed reduction of intra-articular calcaneal fractures: a matched cohort in workmen. *J Orthop Trauma.* 1992;6:216–222.

23. Mortelmans LJ, Du Bois M, Donceel P, Broos PL. Impairment and return to work after intra-articular fractures of the calcaneus. *Acta Chir Belg.* 2002;102:329–333.

24. Naovaratanophas P, Thepchatri A. The long term results of internal fixation of displaced intra-articular calcaneal fractures. *J Med Assoc Thai.* 2001;84:36–44.

25. Egol KA, Dolan R, Koval KJ. Functional outcome of surgery for fractures of the ankle: a prospective comparison of management in a cast or a functional brace. *J Bone Joint Surg Br.* 2000;82:264–269.

26. Schlickewei W, Elsasser B, Mullaji AB, Kuner EH. Hip dislocation without fracture: traction or mobilization after reduction? *Injury.* 1993;24:27–31.

27. Brinsden MD, Smith SR, Loxdale PH. Lisfranc injury—surgical fixation facilitates an early return to work. *J R Nav Med Serv.* 2001;87:116–119.

28. Noyes FB, Barber-Westin SD. Reconstruction of the anterior and posterior cruciate ligaments after knee dislocation: use of early protected postoperative motion to decrease arthrofibrosis. *Am J Sports Med.* 1997;25:769–778.

29. Jorn LP, Johnsson R, Toksvig-Larsen S. Patient satisfaction, function and return to work after knee arthroplasty. *Acta Orthop Scand.* 1999;70:343–347.

30. St-Pierre DM. Rehabilitation following arthroscopic meniscectomy. *Sports Med.* 1995;20:338–347.

31. Pettrone FA. Meniscectomy: arthrotomy versus arthroscopy. *Am J Sports Med.* 1982;10:355–359.

Chapter 14

Chapter 15

Working With Common Cardiopulmonary Problems

Mark H. Hyman, MD

This chapter explores the common cardiopulmonary problems encountered in clinical return-to-work evaluations. Heart disease and associated vascular conditions continue to dominate Western society as the number one cause of death and medical expenditures.[1] Lung difficulties are also rising in prevalence. The estimated prevalence of asthma in the US population is 7.2%, and at least 11 million people have a chronic lung disease.[2,3] As industrialized nations continue to experience an aging workforce, physicians are certain to be confronted with disability determinations in patients with these cardiopulmonary conditions that accompany aging.

General Considerations in Cardiopulmonary Assessment

The key to cardiopulmonary evaluations is understanding the use of exercise treadmill testing, echocardiography, and pulmonary function testing. A brief explanation here of these procedures will allow a better understanding of the illnesses discussed in this chapter. More comprehensive reviews, summaries, and studies are available.[4–8]

In treadmill testing, exercise (or work) capacity is measured. There are different treadmill testing protocols, including the Bruce, Balke, Naughton, and Ellestad tests. These tests vary in how fast patients walk and how steep an incline the patient must work against. The most common protocol is the Bruce, which changes these parameters every three minutes.

Adequate testing usually means a patient achieved at least 85% of his or her maximum predicted heart rate (MPHR). There are normal tables of target heart rate based on patient age, an example of which is shown in Table 15-1.[9] There are also tables of the expected duration of exercise capacity for individuals of varying ages, as shown in Table 15-2.[10]

An important concept in treadmill testing is the metabolic equivalent (MET) system. One MET equals the oxygen cost of, or the oxygen consumed in, sitting at rest in a room of normal temperature and humidity. The numerical value of 1 MET is 3.5 mL of oxygen per kilogram per minute. Each activity to be performed requires a unique or specific amount of energy (or oxygen). Physicians can estimate the maximum exercise ability of patients as the maximum number of METs expended on a treadmill (Tables 15-3 and 15-4). The number of METS an individual should be capable of achieving on the basis of age and sex is shown in Table 15-5. The objective test outlined in Table 15-6 may be used to identify an individual's functional capacity.

Several factors must be considered when exercise performance is interpreted. The most important is effort. This can be assessed subjectively by a

Table 15-1 Maximal Predicted Heart Rate Averages for Exercise

	Maximal Predicted Heart Rate, beats/min								
Age, y	Maximum	95%	90%	85%	80%	75%	70%	65%	60%
25	190	180	171	162	152	143	133	124	114
30	186	177	167	158	149	140	130	121	112
35	182	173	164	155	146	137	127	118	109
40	181	172	163	154	145	136	127	118	109
45	179	170	161	152	143	134	125	116	107
50	175	166	158	149	140	131	123	114	105
55	171	162	154	145	137	128	120	111	103
60	168	160	151	143	134	126	118	109	101
65	164	156	148	139	131	123	115	107	98
70	160	152	144	135	128	120	112	104	96
75	156	148	140	131	125	117	109	101	94
80	152	144	137	130	122	114	106	99	91
85	148	140	133	126	118	111	104	96	89

Adapted from Sheffield.[9]

Table 15-2 Cardiorespiratory Fitness Classification for Bruce Protocol

| Age, y | Classification by Expected Duration of Exercise Capacity, min | | | | |
	Low	Fair	Average	Good	High
Males					
20–29	<6	8	11	14	>15
30–39	<5	7	10	13	>14
40–49	<4	6	9	12	>13
50–59	<3	4	8	11	>12
60–69	<3	4	8	10	>12
Females					
20–29	<6	7	9	11	>13
30–39	<4	5	8	10	>12
40–49	<3	4	7	9	>11
50–59	<3	3	5	8	>10
60–69	<2	3	4	7	>9

Adapted from Bruce et al.[10]

physician watching the patient's performance during testing. If the testing was done previously by someone else, and no comment on patient effort during testing was recorded, the decision to accept the previous test result or to repeat treadmill testing can be difficult. If the patient's condition seems "too good" for the reported exercise ability on a previous treadmill test, retesting may be indicated.

A patient who achieves 85% of his or her MPHR, but at an early stage of testing (low work load), is probably deconditioned. Deconditioning means that the individual is usually sedentary and thus currently has a low exercise capacity, but this capacity may be increased with an activity program. This activity program may mean cardiac rehabilitation (supervised, medically safe progressive exercise), or progressive home-based exercise like walking, or it may mean return to work with work limitations that progressively decrease over time as work assignments become progressively more strenuous.

If a patient terminates treadmill testing because of nonspecific symptoms such as fatigue at a low work load with a heart rate far below the MPHR and without any worrisome ischemic, hemodynamic, or arrhythmic changes,

Chapter 15

Chapter 15

Table 15-3 Relationship of METs and Functional Class According to Five Treadmill Protocols*

METs	1.6	2	3	4	5	6	7	8	9	10	11	12	13	14	15	16
Treadmill tests																
Ellestad																
Miles per hour					1.7	3.0			4.0						5.0	
% grade					10	10			10						10	
Bruce																
Miles per hour					1.7		2.5		3.4				4.2			
% grade					10		12		14				16			
Balke																
Miles per hour				3.4	3.4	3.4	3.4	3.4	3.4	3.4	3.4	3.4	3.4	3.4	3.4	3.4
% grade				2	4	6	8	10	12	14	16	18	20	22	24	26
Balke																
Miles per hour			3.0	3.0	3.0	3.0	3.0	3.0	3.0	3.0	3.0	3.0				
% grade			0	2.5	5	7.5	10	12.5	15	17.5	20	22.5				
Naughton																
Miles per hour	1.0	2.0	2.0	2.0	2.0	2.0	2.0									
% grade	0	0	3.5	7	10.5	14	17.5									
METs	1.6	2	3	4	5	6	7	8	9	10	11	12	13	14	15	16
Clinical status																
Symptomatic patients	←————→															
Diseased, recovered		←——————————————→														
Sedentary healthy					←——————————————→											
Physically active									←——————————————→							
Functional class	IV	←—— III ——→				←II→				I and Normal						

*Adapted from: Fox et al.[11]

Table 15-4 Energy Expenditure in METs During Bicycle Ergometry

Body Weight		Work Rate on Bicycle Ergometer, kg m^{-1} min^{-1} (Watts)												
kg	(lb)	75	150	300	450	600	750	900	1050	1200	1350	1500	1650	1800
(12)	(25)	(50)	(75)	(100)	(125)	(150)	(175)	(200)	(225)	(250)	(275)	(300)		
20	(44)	4.0	6.0	10.0	14.0	18.0	22.0							
30	(66)	3.4	4.7	7.3	10.0	12.7	15.3	17.9	20.7	23.3				
40	(88)	3.0	4.0	6.0	8.0	10.0	12.0	14.0	16.0	18.0	20.0	22.0		
50	(110)	2.8	3.6	5.2	6.8	8.4	10.0	11.5	13.2	14.8	16.3	18.0	19.6	21.1
60	(132)	2.7	3.3	4.7	6.0	7.3	8.7	10.0	11.3	12.7	14.0	15.3	16.7	18.0
70	(154)	2.6	3.1	4.3	5.4	6.6	7.7	8.8	10.0	11.1	12.2	13.4	14.0	15.7
80	(176)	2.5	3.0	4.0	5.0	6.0	7.0	8.0	9.0	10.0	11.0	12.0	13.0	14.0
90	(198)	2.4	2.9	3.8	4.7	5.6	6.4	7.3	8.2	9.1	10.0	10.9	11.8	12.6
100	(220)	2.4	2.8	3.6	4.4	5.2	6.0	6.8	7.6	8.4	9.2	10.0	10.8	11.6
110	(242)	2.4	2.7	3.4	4.2	4.9	5.6	6.3	7.1	7.8	8.5	9.3	10.0	10.7
120	(264)	2.3	2.7	3.3	4.0	4.7	5.3	6.0	6.7	7.3	8.0	8.7	9.3	10.0

Adapted from American College of Sports Medicine.[12]

Chapter 15

Table 15-5 Normal MET Values for Men and Women

	Men			Women		
Age, y	10th Percentile	Mean	90th Percentile	10th Percentile	Mean	90th Percentile
20–29	9.0	11.0	13.5	6.2	8.6	10.8
30–39	8.6	10.5	13.2	6.2	8.6	10.2
40–49	7.8	10.0	12.8	6.0	7.6	10.0
50–59	7.0	9.4	12.4	5.0	7.0	9.4
60+	5.7	8.2	11.7	4.5	6.2	8.6

Adapted from Pollock et al.[13]

then a poor tolerance for exercise exists despite adequate capacity. If a patient terminates treadmill testing because of nonspecific symptoms at a very low work load, and by history that patient routinely performs activities of daily living that require exertion to higher work loads, either malingering or unconscious symptom magnification should be suspected.

Studies and guidelines suggest that a person has the capacity to perform sustained work, ie, an eight-hour workday with typical breaks, to at least 40% of his or her maximal MET level. He or she could also be expected to perform for 15-minute intervals, once or twice a day, at 80% of the maximal MET level.[15–17] Certain occupations, while generally having low demands, could at times be associated with a sudden increase in either physical or psychological demands. Examples include police officer, firefighter, airline pilot, air traffic controller, and commercial vehicle driver.[17] Estimates of the oxygen cost of many jobs and activities (in METs) have been published.[17,18]

For example, if a patient can exercise to 10 METs safely on the treadmill and the job in question requires sustained exertion of 2.5 METs and brief periods of exertion to 5 METs, then the patient should be safe in this job (2.5 METs is less than 40% of 10 METs, and 5 METs is less than 80% of 10 METs).

Another important measure of cardiopulmonary disability estimation comes from the ejection fraction.[4] This measure of systolic heart function appears to be a more reliable indicator of disability than diastolic dysfunction, the latter being harder to measure.[19] Both systolic and diastolic function are measured by the gold standard of angiographic left ventriculography with pressure measurements. For disability investigation, radionuclide angiography can be used, although transthoracic echocardiography with Doppler is non-invasive, less expensive, useful with associated valvular disease, and

Table 15-6 Physical Demand, Energy Requirements, and Activities

Demand Level	Energy Required (METs)	Work Lifting Demand, lb			Sample Occupations	Home Activity	Recreational Activity	Physical Conditioning
		Occasional (0%–33% of Work Day)	Frequent (34%–66% of Work Day)	Constant (67%–100% of Work Day)				
Sedentary	1.5–2.1	10	None	None	Clerical, store clerk, bartender, truck driver, crane operator	Washing, shaving, dressing, writing, washing dishes, driving car	Shuffleboard, horse-shoes, billiards, archery, golf with cart	Walking 2 mph, stationary bicycle, very light calisthenics
Light	2.2–3.5	20	10	None and/or operating controls while seated	Light welding, car-pentry, auto repair, machine assembly	Raking leaves, weeding, painting, cleaning windows, waxing floor	Dancing, golf walking, sailing, horseback riding, doubles tennis	Walking 3–4 mph, cycling 6–8 mph, light calisthenics
Medium or Moderate	3.6–6.3	20–50	10–25	10	Carpentry, shoveling, pneumatic tools	Gardening, lawn mowing, slow climbing of stairs	Badminton, singles tennis, skiing down-hill, basketball, football, ice skating, light backpacking	Walking 4–5 mph, cycling 9–10 mph, swimming breaststroke
Heavy	6.4–7.5	50–100	25–50	10–20	Ditch digging, pick and shovel	Sawing wood, heavy shoveling	Canoeing, mountain climbing, fencing, paddleball	Jogging 5 mph, cycling 12 mph, swimming crawl, rowing
Very Heavy	>7.5	>100	>50	>20	Lumberjack, heavy labor	Heavy snow shovel-ing, fast stairs	Handball, squash, cross-country skiing	Running ≥6 mph, cycling ≥13 mph, jumping rope

Adapted from Haskell[14] and Astrand.[15]

equally acceptable.[20,21] The general rule is that a systolic ejection fraction greater than 50% is normal, 40% to 50% is a mild or slight impairment or dysfunction, 30% to 40% is a moderate impairment or dysfunction, and less than 30% is a severe or total impairment or dysfunction.

Pulmonary function testing provides similar helpful functional information. As seen in treadmill testing, different protocols are used in evaluating a patient's performance, the most common probably being that of Morris et al.[22] Once again, patient effort is the cornerstone for test interpretation. The American Thoracic Society has identified standards for assessing patient effort and interpreting results.[23] Every pulmonary function test must follow these standards to be fully interpretable. The test should indicate the data obtained as well as the best of three trials a patient performed. There should be a clear section on the report of reproducibility measures. Sample reports and their basic interpretation are shown in Tables 15-7, 15-8, 15-9, and 15-10.

Risk in Cardiopulmonary Disease

Later sections of this chapter briefly explore what little is known about the *risk of working* with a condition. In contrast, when discussing cardiopulmonary disease *risk*, it is often helpful to consider the known risk factors that may have contributed to the disease formation in the first place. If there are identified risk factors that have not been modified, then progression of the disease will be expected.

Coronary Artery Disease

Presumed Disability

The Social Security Administration (SSA) estimates that, in general, if a patient has a treadmill study with an exercise capacity of at most 5 METs of work, *or* an ejection fraction of at most 30%, *or* significant angiographic coronary artery disease, then total disability is presumed to exist.[24] The treadmill would be limited on the basis of at least 1mm (mV) ST segment change, failure to increase systolic blood pressure by 10 mm Hg, or significant reversible ischemic defect on imaging. The angiographic disease must be associated with typical angina or dyspnea limitations (Tables 15-11 and 15-12) and must meet or exceed criteria for significant narrowing (Table 15-13). Some individuals with sedentary jobs work despite meeting these criteria.

Table 15-7 Sample Pulmonary Function Test Results for a Normal 37-Year-Old Patient

		Spirometry				
		Pre-Results 05/03/2004 14:35		**Post-Results** 05/03/2004 14:56		
Parameter	**Predicted**	**Best: #2**	**% Predicted**	**Best: #3**	**% Predicted**	**% Difference**
FVC	2.86	3.09	107.94	3.06	106.89	-0.97
$FEV_{.5}$	1.93	2.17	112.63	2.14	111.08	-1.38
FEV_1	2.45	2.67	109.00	2.66	108.60	-0.37
FEV_3	2.79	2.98	106.65	2.99	107.01	-0.34
PEFR	5.17	7.06	136.58	7.01	135.61	-0.71
FEF 25%–75%	2.90	3.28	113.03	3.09	106.48	-5.79
FEV_1/FVC	0.85	0.86	100.77	0.87	101.94	1.16
FEV_3/FVC	0.97	0.96	98.64	0.98	100.69	2.08
FET		5.29		5.58		5.48

MVV	87.46	87.00	99.48					
Reproducibility:	**%**	**Volume**	**Criteria Met**	**%**	**Volume**	**Criteria Met**		
FVC (5%/200 mL)	1.29	0.04	Y	0.33	0.01	Y		
FEV_1 (5%/200 mL)	1.12	0.03	Y			Y		
PEFR (15%/300 mL)	10.06	0.71	Y	2.28	0.16	Y		

Lung Volumes			05/03/2004 14:44
Parameter	**Predicted**	**Test 1**	**% Predicted**
TLC	4.12	4.03	97.82
FRC	2.23	1.75	78.48
RV	1.26	1.11	88.10
RV/TLC	0.30	0.28	93.33
SVC	2.86	2.92	102.10
IC	1.90	2.27	119.47
ERV	0.97	0.64	65.98
TV		0.91	
FRCT		2.47	

(Continued)

Chapter 15

Table 15-7   (*Continued*)

Diffusion Capacity		05/03/2004	14:50
Notice: DLco results are based on the following values: Hb = 14.6 g/dL, COHb = 0 g/dL			
Parameter	**Predicted**	**Test 1**	**% Predicted**
DLco	23.68	24.81	104.77
VA	4.15	4.02	96.87
DLco/VA	5.90	6.17	104.58
IV		2.94	
BHt		9.64	
Sample Volume		0.94	

BHt indicates breath hold time; COHb, carboxyhemoglobin; DLco, carbon monoxide diffusion capacity; ERV, end residual volume; FEF, forced expiratory flow; FET, forced expiratory time; $FEV_{.5}$, forced expiratory volume for .5 second; FEV_1, forced expiratory volume for 1 second; FEV_3, forced expiratory volume for 3 seconds; FRC, functional residual capacity; FRCT, functional residual capacity time (also called helium equilibration time); FVC, forced vital capacity; Hb, hemoglobin; IC, inspiratory capacity; IV, inspiratory volume; MVV, maximal voluntary ventilation; PEFR, peak expiratory flow rate; RV, residual volume; SVC, slow vital capacity; TLC, total lung capacity; TV, tidal volume; VA, alveolar ventilation.

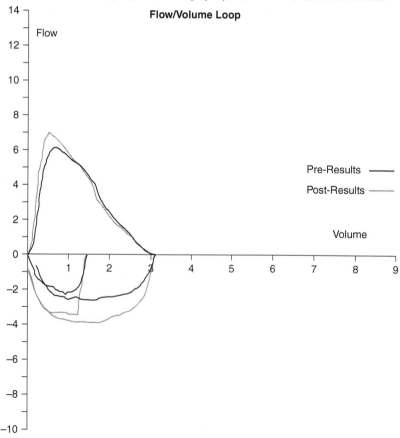

Table 15-8 Sample Pulmonary Function Test Results for a 44-Year-Old Patient With Chronic Obstructive Pulmonary Disease

		Spirometry				
		Pre-Results 02/05/2004 12:37		**Post-Results** 02/05/2004 12:54		
Parameter	Predicted	Best: #3	% Predicted	Best: #1	% Predicted	% Difference
FVC	5.23	5.72	109.39	5.73	109.59	0.17
FEV_1	4.20	3.45	82.09	3.68	87.57	6.67
FEV_3	4.94	4.86	98.31	4.91	99.32	1.03
PEFR	9.42	9.08	96.40	9.06	96.19	−0.22
FEF 25%–75%	4.14	1.66	40.10	2.02	48.79	21.69
FEV_1/FVC	0.80	0.60	74.67	0.64	79.64	6.67
FEV_3/FVC	0.94	0.85	90.04	0.86	91.10	1.18
FET		10.29		8.99		−12.63

MVV	141.33	148.88		104.72			
Reproducibility:	%	Volume	Criteria Met	%	Volume	Criteria Met	
FVC (5%/200 mL)	2.62	0.15	Y	0.52	0.03	Y	
FEV_1 (5%/200 mL)	0.29	0.01	Y	0.54	0.02	Y	
PEFR (15%/300 mL)	3.41	0.31	Y	6.73	0.61	Y	

Lung Volumes		02/05/2004 12:43	
Parameter	Predicted	Test 1	% Predicted
TLC	7.23	8.84	122.27
FRC	3.58	4.94	137.99
RV	2.05	3.15	153.66
RV/TLC	0.28	0.36	128.57
SVC	5.23	5.68	108.60
IC	3.64	3.89	106.87
ERV	1.53	1.79	116.99
TV		2.05	
FRCT		2.80	

Chapter 15

(*Continued*)

Table 15-8   *(Continued)*

Diffusion Capacity		02/05/2004	12:50
Notice: DLco results are based on the following values: Hb = 14.6 g/dL, COHb = 0 g/dL			
Parameter	**Predicted**	**Test 1**	**% Predicted**
DLco	38.39	28.28	73.67
VA	7.28	8.15	111.95
DLco/VA	5.48	3.47	63.32
IV		5.55	
BHt		10.30	
Sample Volume		1.02	

BHt indicates breath hold time; COHb, carboxyhemoglobin; DLco, carbon monoxide diffusion capacity; ERV, end residual volume; FEF, forced expiratory flow; FET, forced expiratory time; FEV_1, forced expiratory volume for 1 second; FEV_3, forced expiratory volume for 3 seconds; FRC, functional residual capacity; FRCT, functional residual capacity time (also called helium equilibration time); FVC, forced vital capacity; Hb, hemoglobin; IC, inspiratory capacity; IV, inspiratory volume; MVV, maximal voluntary ventilation; PEFR, peak expiratory flow rate; RV, residual volume; SVC, slow vital capacity; TLC, total lung capacity; TV, tidal volume; VA, alveolar ventilation.

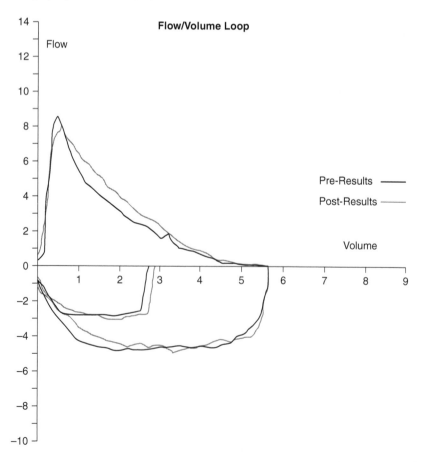

Table 15-9 Sample Pulmonary Function Test Results for a 61-Year-Old Patient With Restrictive Lung Disease

		Spirometry				
		Pre-Results 10/07/2002 16:34		Post-Results 10/07/2002 16:48		
Parameter	Predicted	Best: #2	% Predicted	Best: #3	% Predicted	% Difference
FVC	4.52	2.47	54.60	2.35	51.95	−4.86
FEV$_5$	2.81	1.25	44.49	1.22	43.43	−2.40
FEV$_1$	3.49	1.73	49.60	1.64	47.02	−5.20
FEV$_3$	4.16	2.26	54.36	2.01	48.35	−11.06
PEFR	8.11	3.94	48.59	3.91	48.22	−0.76
FEF 25%–75%	3.10	1.13	36.43	0.94	30.30	−16.81
FEV$_1$/FVC	0.77	0.70	91.17	0.70	91.17	
FEV$_3$/FVC	0.91	0.91	99.50	0.86	94.03	−5.49
FET		5.44		6.59		21.14

MVV	116.06	39.00	33.60			
Reproducibility:	%	Volume	Criteria Met	%	Volume	Criteria Met
FVC (5%/200 mL)	6.07	0.15	N	16.17	0.38	N
FEV$_1$ (5%/200 mL)	3.47	0.06	Y	17.07	0.28	N
PEFR (15%/300 mL)	1.02	0.04	Y	2.30	0.09	Y

Lung Volumes		10/07/2002 16:41	
Parameter	Predicted	Test 1	% Predicted
TLC	6.70	4.68	69.85
FRC	3.48	2.69	77.30
RV	2.19	2.51	114.61
RV/TLC	0.33	0.54	163.64
SVC	4.52	2.17	48.01
IC	3.22	1.99	61.80
ERV	1.29	0.18	13.95
TV		0.67	
FRCT		1.55	

Chapter 15

(Continued)

Table 15-9   *(Continued)*

Diffusion Capacity		10/07/2002	16:45
Notice: DLco results are based on the following values: Hb = 14.6 g/dL, COHb = 0 g/dL			
Parameter	Predicted	Test 1	% Predicted
DLco	32.25	22.32	69.21
VA	6.71	5.25	78.24
DLco/VA	4.92	4.25	86.38
IV		2.76	
BHt		10.01	
Sample Volume		0.43	

BHt indicates breath hold time; COHb, carboxyhemoglobin; DLco, carbon monoxide diffusion capacity; ERV, end residual volume; FEF, forced expiratory flow; FET, forced expiratory time; $FEV_{.5}$, forced expiratory volume for .5 second; FEV_1, forced expiratory volume for 1 second; FEV_3, forced expiratory volume for 3 seconds; FRC, functional residual capacity; FRCT, functional residual capacity time (also called helium equilibration time); FVC, forced vital capacity; Hb, hemoglobin; IC, inspiratory capacity; IV, inspiratory volume; MVV, maximal voluntary ventilation; PEFR, peak expiratory flow rate; RV, residual volume; SVC, slow vital capacity; TLC, total lung capacity; TV, tidal volume; VA, alveolar ventilation.

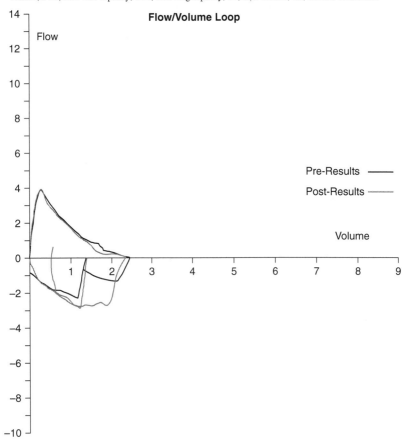

Table 15-10 Sample Pulmonary Function Test Results for a 23-Year-Old Patient With Nonphysiologic Test*

		Spirometry				
		Pre-Results 05/05/2004 16:13		Post-Results 05/05/2004 16:24		
Parameter	Predicted	Best: #3	% Predicted	Best: #2	% Predicted	% Difference
FVC	2.99	2.88	96.24	3.41	113.95	18.40
$FEV_{.5}$	2.09	1.62	77.69	2.69	129.01	66.05
FEV_1	2.66	2.49	93.46	3.15	118.23	26.51
FEV_3	2.99	2.23	74.70	3.37	112.88	51.12
PEFR	5.34	3.74	70.04	8.53	159.75	128.07
FEF 25%–75%	3.41	2.38	69.81	4.94	144.89	107.56
FEV_1/FVC	0.89	0.86	96.10	0.92	102.81	6.98
FEV_3/FVC	1.00	0.77	77.08	0.99	99.11	28.57
FET		1.70		4.56		168.24

MVV						
Reproducibility:	%	Volume	Criteria Met	%	Volume	Criteria Met
FVC (5%/200 mL)	2.08	0.06	Y	0.29	0.01	Y
FEV_1 (5%/200 mL)	18.07	0.45	N	0.32	0.01	Y
PEFR (15%/300 mL)	40.11	1.50	N	0.70	0.06	Y

Lung Volumes		05/05/2004 16:15	
Parameter	Predicted	Test 1	% Predicted
TLC	3.96	3.86	97.47
FRC	2.10	1.64	78.10
RV	0.97	0.74	76.29
RV/TLC	0.24	0.19	79.17
SVC	2.99	3.12	104.35
IC	1.87	2.22	118.72
ERV	1.13	0.90	79.65
TV		0.52	
FRCT		2.36	

(Continued)

Chapter 15

Table 15-10   (*Continued*)

Diffusion Capacity		05/05/2004	16:20
Notice: DLco results are based on the following values: Hb = 14.6 g/dL, COHb = 0 g/dL			
Parameter	**Predicted**	**Test 1**	**% Predicted**
DLco	24.81	20.82	83.92
VA	3.98	3.66	91.96
DLco/VA	6.30	5.69	90.32
IV		2.09	
BHt		9.64	
Sample Volume		0.41	

*Note the poor prebronchodilator effort resulting in irregular flow/volume loop, failed reproducibility, large apparent reversibility, and low MVV.

BHt indicates breath hold time; COHb, carboxyhemoglobin; DLco, carbon monoxide diffusion capacity; ERV, end residual volume; FEF, forced expiratory flow; FET, forced expiratory time; FEV$_{.5}$, forced expiratory volume for .5 second; FEV$_1$, forced expiratory volume for 1 second; FEV$_3$, forced expiratory volume for 3 seconds; FRC, functional residual capacity; FRCT, functional residual capacity time (also called helium equilibration time); FVC, forced vital capacity; Hb, hemoglobin; IC, inspiratory capacity; IV, inspiratory volume; MVV, maximal voluntary ventilation; PEFR, peak expiratory flow rate; RV, residual volume; SVC, slow vital capacity; TLC, total lung capacity; TV, tidal volume; VA, alveolar ventilation.

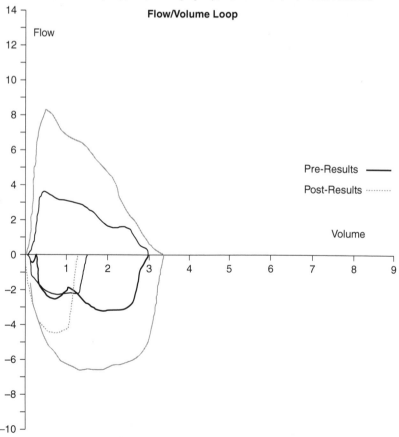

Flow/Volume Loop

Table 15-11 New York Heart Association Functional Classification of Cardiac Disease

Class	Description
I	Individual has cardiac disease but no resulting limitation of physical activity; ordinary physical activity does not cause undue fatigue, palpitation, dyspnea, or anginal pain.
II	Individual has cardiac disease resulting in slight limitation of physical activity; is comfortable at rest and in the performance of ordinary, light, daily activities; greater than ordinary physical activity, such as heavy physical exertion, results in fatigue, palpitation, dyspnea, or anginal pain.
III	Individual has cardiac disease resulting in marked limitation of physical activity; is comfortable at rest; ordinary physical activity results in fatigue, palpitation, dyspnea, or anginal pain.
IV	Individual has cardiac disease resulting in inability to carry on any physical activity without discomfort; symptoms of inadequate cardiac output, pulmonary congestion, systemic congestion, or anginal syndrome may be present, even at rest; if any physical activity is undertaken, discomfort is increased.

Adapted from Criteria Committee of the New York Heart Association.[25]

Table 15-12 American Thoracic Society Functional Classification of Dyspnea[*]

Severity	Definition and Question
Mild	Do you have to walk more slowly on the level than people of your age because of breathlessness?
Moderate	Do you have to stop for breath when walking at your own pace on the level?
Severe	Do you ever have to stop for breath after walking about 100 yards or for a few minutes on the level?
Very Severe	Are you too breathless to leave the house, or breathless on dressing or undressing?

[*] The person's lowest level of physical activity and exertion that produces breathlessness denotes the severity of dyspnea.
Adapted from Cocchiarella and Andersson.[4]

Table 15-13 Social Security Listing for Significant Angiographic Disease

Percent Narrowing	Involved Coronary Vessel
50	Left main
70	Any vessel
50	Any vessel where narrowing is >1 cm in length
50	Any 2 vessels
100	Any previously bypassed graft vessel

Adapted from the US Social Security Administration.[24]

Risk Assessment

There is little information about workers with documented ischemic heart disease and specific occupations they can not perform. Certain occupations have been identified in the literature that place a worker at risk of developing cardiovascular morbidity and mortality. Depending on the study, examples of these can include workers in metal processing, paper, chemicals, plastics, air traffic control, bus operation, assembly, nursing, and waiting tables.[26–28] If chemical exposure at work is thought to play a role in the development of an individual's heart disease, a physician should prevent further potentially harmful exposure to that substance by work restrictions (restrictions are based on risk). When work ability is assessed in patients with coronary artery disease, the risks to consider are angina, myocardial infarction, and hemodynamically significant arrhythmias.

Angina

Angina is the chest pain syndrome associated with reversible myocardial ischemia. With angina of short duration, eg, less than 15 to 30 minutes, there is no heart muscle damage; thus, no change in impairment has occurred. The frequency and severity of angina can identify a patient who is at risk for further cardiac difficulties. Thus, if a patient is developing angina and if one is certain that the chest pain or anginal equivalent is truly cardiac in origin, then the symptom of angina can be used as a gauge to restrict a work activity. This should be supported by an evaluation of exercise capacity as discussed below. If there is doubt about whether or not angina is occurring at work, the patient can wear a Holter monitor during a work day. This permits evaluation of heart rate and ST segment change at the times when chest pain occurred at work.

In a patient who is out of work, if the job demands of potential employment are below the exercise level that provokes angina on treadmill testing, a trial of return to work is very reasonable.

Myocardial Infarction

A second risk concern is myocardial infarction (or acute unstable angina). Patients and physicians are concerned that the work environment will precipitate an acute coronary syndrome. Yet, most episodes of acute coronary syndrome occur in the early morning hours before work, at rest or with minimal physical exertion.[29] Stress and heavy physical exertion appear to be identifiable in only 10% to 15% of cases. Further, studies support that exercise capacity is predictive of the risk of death in "normal" subjects, as well as in patients with coronary artery disease and many noncardiac conditions, including chronic lung disease, diabetes, hypertension, elevated body mass index, hypercholesterolemia, and cigarette smoking.[30,31] Physical exertion becomes a stronger predictor when patients are inactive, male, hyperlipidemic, and cigarette smokers.[32] The exercise experienced at work may thus be protective against future coronary events.

While there are many well-known risk factors that predict who will ultimately develop coronary artery disease,[4,5,33–42] these risk factors do *not* predict who will experience problems on returning to work. Perhaps the best study on the risk of returning to work after myocardial infarction was done in Israel.[43] Two hundred sixteen patients were evaluated for return-to-work ability after myocardial infarction. Of the 168 who attempted to return to work, 150 successfully did so and were followed up for 2 years. Six sustained a second infarction, but only two of these occurred while the patient happened to be at work. Thus, returning to work did not pose a significant risk to these patients.

Because the medical literature contains few studies on the risk of working despite known heart disease, following consensus guidelines may be rational and may provide some medical–legal protection for physician opinion. One excellent source of consensus guidelines for activity is to use the analogy of athletes. Studies have been done on athletic competition requirements and the risks of competition-induced cardiovascular complications for the athletes. A good summary of presumably safe exercise levels for various cardiovascular conditions, known as the 26th Bethesda Conference, has been published by the American College of Cardiology. One section discusses the risk of competitive athletics with known coronary artery disease.[44] The approach promulgated is to assess each sport's activity in terms of its dynamic/isotonic endurance requirement along with its static/isometric lifting requirements. Parallels can be drawn between a worker's Bethesda static requirement and the work demands estimate listed in Table 15-6.

Capacity

Measuring current capacity in cardiopulmonary conditions has been described above. In general, if a patient has simple chronic stable angina, a normal stress treadmill study, and normal ejection fraction, there has been no change in his or her work capacity. If one or more measures of heart function are altered, then Table 15-6 offers parameters for work limitation. If the measured safe exercise capacity is less than the job demands (sustained exertion exceeds 40% of treadmill-determined maximum ability or infrequent exertion exceeds 80% of capacity), then the individual is not currently safely capable of performing the job in question, and there is a medically determined work limitation (limitations are based on capacity).

A useful analogy may be the Department of Transportation criteria for commercial drivers.[45] The criteria are adequate cardiac function despite coronary artery disease to permit commercial driving, which is most often light work with occasional periods of heavy work, ejection fraction of at least 40%, exercise capacity of 6 METs or better (finish stage II on the Bruce protocol, achieving at least 85% of MPHR without evidence of ischemia while systolic blood pressure increases at least 20 mm Hg from its resting level), and tolerance of medications without orthostatic symptoms (systolic blood pressure, 95 mm Hg or greater with less than a 20 mm Hg drop in BP when the patient arises to a standing position).

Cardiac rehabilitation is an important ischemic heart disease intervention. Many studies have shown that cardiac rehabilitation will increase a patient's physical capacity and survival but not necessarily translate into return to work.[46–48] The fact that improved work capacity does not often result in return to work raises the issue of tolerance.

Tolerance

Many factors explore why a patient with ischemic heart disease may not want to tolerate his or her job when work capacity appears more than adequate. Risk factors for refusal to work (due to tolerance) despite adequate capacity include lower socioeconomic class, poor social network, high psychosocial stressors, shift work, low job satisfaction, anger, hostility, and excessive fatigue. These components of a job and personal psychosocial factors are helpful to consider when patients are looking at returning to work. As an example, one study found that while angioplasty returned patients to work sooner than coronary artery bypass grafting, non-medical factors predominated in determining long-term employment.[49] Many studies from various countries and across medical disciplines have concurred that these non-medical findings are predictive, and different models have been developed to explain these findings.[50–55] A good summary of this area is available.[56] Unfortunately, attempts at treating the more well-recognized psychosocial factors have not translated into a reduction in future cardiovascular events.[57] The American College of Cardiology has advocated that patients should undergo psychological assessment when their capacity seems sufficient for their job yet they claim intolerance. This is especially true when the claim is primarily stress related. "Stress" can influence the underlying ischemic symptoms, but rarely to a degree that changes capacity or places the patient at significant risk.[17,58]

Disability Duration

Expected disability duration for patients with more commonly used *International Classification of Diseases, Ninth Revision, Clinical Modification* (ICD-9-CM) codes for ischemic heart disease is shown in Table 15-14. In comparing an individual patient with these normative data, variances can be explained by the factors outlined in this section. In particular, effort on objective testing, identified risk factors or comorbid conditions, and psychosocial factors would be the areas to pursue in a patient falling below these expected outcomes.

Table 15-14 Disability Duration for Coronary Artery Disease[*][†]

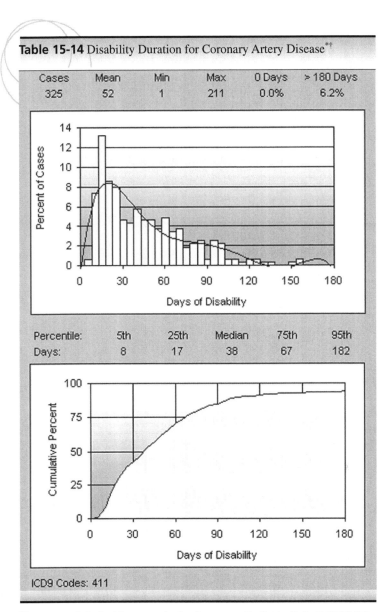

Cases	Mean	Min	Max	0 Days	> 180 Days
325	52	1	211	0.0%	6.2%

Percentile:	5th	25th	Median	75th	95th
Days:	8	17	38	67	182

ICD9 Codes: 411

[*]Recovery trends (in days) from normative data for cases specifically identified with ICD-9-CM codes 414.0, 414.8, and 414.9.

[†]Differences may exist between the expected duration tables and the normative graphs. Duration tables provide expected recovery periods based on the type of work performed by the individual. The normative graphs reflect the actual observed experience of many individuals across the spectrum of physical conditions, in a variety of industries, and with varying levels of case management.

Reproduced with permission from Reed.[59]

Hypertension and Hypertensive Heart Disease

Screening and treatment benefits for high blood pressure are one of the strongest societal recommendations.[60,61] The most important first step in hypertension evaluation is a correct diagnostic method. Many resources have advocated proper methods for measuring blood pressure.[62,63] A growing trend, supported by the literature, is using 24-hour ambulatory blood pressure monitoring to permit more accurate diagnosis and prognosis, and to measure the response to intervention.[64–67] The cornerstone of all studies and recommendations is that blood pressure must be measured with good technique in the office and, ideally, supplemented with measures taken from the home and work environments.

Presumed Disability

The presumed criteria for disability from hypertension or hypertensive heart disease are the same as outlined earlier for coronary artery disease. Complications of hypertension (eg, stroke, renal failure) may be severe enough to constitute evidence of presumed disability by SSA criteria.

Risk Assessment

The complications of long-standing untreated or poorly treated hypertension include retinopathy, nephropathy, peripheral vascular disease, coronary artery disease, cerebrovascular disease, and left ventricular hypertrophy. The presence of these complications might influence the risk of a particular occupation independent of blood pressure measures.

Blood pressure is easily measured, and the consequences of hypertension are rarely immediate. Thus, a trial of return to work with blood pressure monitoring at work is almost always indicated. A most important focus for long-term risk is left ventricular hypertrophy. Left ventricular hypertrophy is primarily genetic until adulthood, when male gender and workload become the predominant risk factors.[68] If patients have regular heavy isometric lifting, arterial hypertension, or obesity, they are at risk for developing an increase in their left ventricular mass.[69] The presence of left ventricular hypertrophy increases cardiovascular morbidity and mortality.[69] This argument parallels other known risk factors, their time to cause secondary effects, and stabilization or regression of end-organ damage with treatment.[70] There is a lot of literature that places lifestyle as a central cause of hypertension and documents the benefits of nonpharmacologic as well as more standard medication interventions.[71–75]

Psychological stress can influence blood pressure and left ventricular mass.[76] However, stress would need to be present on a fairly constant basis for many months to years to produce left ventricular hypertrophy through hypertension. There is no job that has been described in the medical literature as "free of stress."

Blood pressure that is acceptable at rest, but that increases to unacceptable levels with exercise, represents undertreatment of hypertension. Exercise is contraindicated only until a change in treatment brings the blood pressure with exercise under control. Exercise is recommended as treatment because sustained endurance exercise leads to increasing aerobic fitness, resulting in decreased blood pressure. Similarly, blood pressure that increases to unacceptable levels at work does not usually mean that work is contraindicated. Rather, it reflects undertreatment. When a change in blood pressure treatment has occurred, two or three weeks may be required for blood pressure stabilization. Patients most commonly can continue to work during this period, except if there is accelerating or severe elevation in their reading. Adequate blood pressure treatment permits exercise or work and can be determined by measuring blood pressure at work intermittently, by ambulatory blood pressure monitors, or by treadmill testing. Decreasing blood pressure translates to increased measures of cardiopulmonary function as well as diminished secondary complications, and would be associated with greater job capacity.

The risks of commercial driving despite hypertension have been extensively reviewed by the Department of Transportation (DOT).[45] The DOT criteria for commercial drivers permit continued work (one-year medical certification) for drivers with a blood pressure of 140 to 159 mm Hg systolic and 90 to 99 mm Hg diastolic. The DOT criteria still permit continued work, but with only a three-month certification, for drivers with blood pressures of 160 to 179 mm Hg systolic and 100 to 109 mm Hg diastolic. In both of these scenarios, the examining physician is to refer the driver for treatment so that the blood pressure is lowered during the certification interval. A blood pressure of greater than 180 mm Hg systolic or greater than 110 mm Hg diastolic is considered disqualifying for commercial drivers, but only until treatment results in lower blood pressure. These criteria are expected to protect the general public from risk, while the stated treatment goal of a resting blood pressure of less than or equal to 140/90 mm Hg is expected to protect the driver from long-term personal health risk. By analogy, even in "safety-sensitive" jobs, the above consensus criteria can be applied and individuals can be considered safe to work while treatment is begun or modified. Physicians may modify the goal of treatment to less than 130/80 mm Hg if the patient has concomitant diabetes or kidney disease.

When treadmill testing is performed, most protocols demand that the test be stopped before target work loads are achieved if the blood pressure exceeds 250 mm Hg systolic (220 mm Hg if there has been a prior infarction) or 120 mm Hg diastolic. If work activity results in blood pressures near these levels, such work should not be performed. This would be a basis for physician-imposed work restrictions *until* a change in therapy results in improved blood pressure control.

Capacity

For purposes of capacity, hypertension is viewed as being associated with hypertensive heart disease. In other words, the tests for capacity center on not just the absolute blood pressure reading, but also whether there is any effect on cardiopulmonary function. Cardiopulmonary evaluation is pursued by means of the methods outlined in the introduction to this chapter. If the individual has adequate capacity for work at acceptable risk by treadmill testing, work should be recommended.

Tolerance

Hypertension does not usually cause symptoms. Few individuals are able to predict their own blood pressure measurements. The fear that one's blood pressure may be elevated with work activity can be addressed by arranging for self-monitoring or professional monitoring of blood pressure during work activities.

Disability Duration

Table 15-15 shows the expected duration of disability from this condition. The area of discrepancy between objective capacity measures and ability to return to work in hypertensive disease parallels the findings in coronary artery disease. In particular, stress may influence both conditions as discussed previously. Literature from different studies suggests that stress predicts hypertension.[77–79] Long-standing efforts at using psychotherapy and alternative medicine to control hypertension have had mixed results.[80]

Table 15-15 Disability Duration for Hypertension or Hypertensive Heart Disease

Job Classification	Duration, days		
	Minimum	Optimum	Maximum
Sedentary	0	3	5
Light	0	3	5
Medium	0	3	5
Heavy	0	3	5
Very Heavy	0	3	5

Reproduced with permission from Reed.[59]

Reactive Airway Disease/Chronic Obstructive Pulmonary Disease

Presumed Disability

The presumed level of disability for reactive airway disease/chronic obstructive pulmonary disease (COPD) as outlined by the SSA is shown in Table 15-16. Note that this figure contains less detail than impairment tables normally used in disability evaluation.[4]

Risk Assessment

The potential risk of working despite lung disease occurs if the disease is either caused or aggravated by exposure to a chemical or substance encountered in the workplace. Examples include occupational asthma, hypersensitivity pneumonitis, pneumoconiosis, and reactive airways dysfunction syndrome.[81–84] Material safety data sheets can be very helpful in elucidating this history. In addition, a history of cigarette use, air pollution, asthma, or allergies makes all these conditions more likely to occur.[81,85,86] There are jobs that carry a higher incidence of occupational lung troubles. This can include the fields of plastic, print, metal, baking, milling, farming, grain elevator, drugs, and detergents. An exhaustive review is beyond the scope of this chapter, though good sources are available.[81,85,87]

There are many forms of lung disease that a physician may confront in disability assessments. The most common are asthma and COPD. The diagnosis of these conditions as occupational diseases is beyond the scope of this text. If a patient's lung disease is clearly recognized as work related, then the physician evaluating the individual's work ability has the responsibility to prevent further exposure to the involved substance through work restrictions (restrictions are based on risk).

Capacity

If a patient's lung disease is not caused by work exposure, then risk is not the issue. Whether the patient has the capacity to do the job in question is determined by exercise stress testing. At times cardiopulmonary stress testing is useful to determine the work load at which the patient crosses the anaerobic threshold and to determine whether arterial oxygen desaturation occurs with exercise (or work). Many resources exist to aid in test interpretation.[8,88,89]

If the patient's symptoms have a suspected occupational component, then testing at the worksite, or at a quickly accessible nearby facility, may be necessary. This would allow documentation of a more severe impairment than is being appreciated by the current testing.

Chapter 15

Table 15-16 Social Security Administration Presumed Disability
in Pulmonary Conditions

3.01 Category of Impairments, Respiratory System

3.02 *Chronic Pulmonary Insufficiency*

A. Chronic obstructive pulmonary disease due to any cause, with the FEV_1 equal to or less than the values specified in Table I corresponding to the person's height without shoes. (In cases of marked spinal deformity, see 3.00E.)

Table I

Height Without Shoes (cm)	Height Without Shoes (in)	FEV_1 Equal to or Less Than (L, BTPS)
154 or less	60 or less	1.25
155–160	61–63	1.35
161–165	64–65	1.45
166–170	66–67	1.55
171–175	68–69	1.65
176–180	70–71	1.75
181 or more	72 or more	1.85

Or

B. Chronic restrictive ventilatory disease, due to any cause, with the FVC equal to or less than the values specified in Table II corresponding to the person's height without shoes. (In cases of marked spinal deformity, see 3.00E.)

Table II

Height Without Shoes (cm)	Height Without Shoes (in)	FEV_1 Equal to or Less Than (L, BTPS)
154 or less	60 or less	1.25
155–160	61–63	1.35
161–165	64–65	1.45
166–170	66–67	1.55
171–175	68–69	1.65
176–180	70–71	1.75
181 or more	72 or more	1.85

Or

C. *Chronic impairment of gas exchange due to clinically documented pulmonary disease.* With:

1. Single breath DLCO (see 3.00F1) less than 10.5 mL/min/mm Hg or less than 40% of the predicted normal value. (Predicted values must either be based on data obtained at the test site or published values from a laboratory using the same technique as the test site. The source of the predicted

Table 15-16   (*Continued*)

values should be reported. If they are not published, they should be submitted in the form of a table or nomogram); or

2. Arterial blood gas values of PO_2 and simultaneously determined PCO_2 measured while at rest (breathing room air, awake, and sitting or standing) in a clinically stable condition on at least two occasions, three or more weeks apart within a six-month period, equal to or less than the values specified in the applicable Table III-A or III-B:

Table III-A

(Applicable at test sites less than 3,000 feet above sea level)

Arterial PCO_2 (mm Hg)	Arterial PO_2 Equal To or Less Than (mm Hg)
30 or below	65
31	64
32	63
33	62
34	61
35	60
36	59
37	58
38	57
39	56
40 or above	55

Table III-B

(Applicable at test sites 3,000 through 6,000 feet above sea level)

Arterial PCO_2 (mm Hg)	Arterial PO_2 Equal To or Less Than (mm Hg)
30 or below	60
31	59
32	58
33	57
34	56
35	55
36	54
37	53
38	52
39	51

FEV_1 indicates forced expiratory volume for 1 second; FVC, forced vital capacity; PO_2, partial pressure of oxygen; PCO_2, partial pressure of carbon dioxide.

Adapted from Social Security Administration.[24]

Table 15-17 Disease Duration for Occupational Asthma Acute Disability

Job Classification	Duration, days		
	Minimum	Optimum	Maximum
Sedentary	1	3	7
Light	1	3	7
Medium	1	3	7
Heavy	1	3	7
Very Heavy	1	3	7

Reproduced with permission from Reed.[59]

Tolerance

Dyspnea at low work loads, not accompanied by subjective signs like tachypnea or deoxygenation, suggests that psychosocial factors and tolerance, not risk or capacity, are the issues. As seen above, psychosocial factors like job satisfaction impact a patient's decision to work. Patient and physician ability to base work recommendations on tolerance are poor, especially when seen in an emergency setting.[90,91] There are descriptions of psychological factors precipitating acute asthmatic attacks, perpetuation of symptoms in the face of gastroesophageal reflux disease, and women in the perimenstrual period having transient worsening of symptoms.[92]

Disability Duration

Disability durations for a classic simple acute occupational asthma reaction are shown in Table 15-17.

Summary

Cardiopulmonary conditions are common, and cases of return-to-work assessment in individuals with these conditions are challenging. Using what information is available will help physicians think through the issues of risk, capacity, and tolerance. As with other body system problems, patients with cardiopulmonary disease are rarely harmed by a return-to-work recommendation. The considerable benefits of returning to work usually significantly outweigh the risk.

References

1. American Heart Association. *Heart Disease and Stroke Statistics—2004 Update.* Dallas, Tex: American Heart Association; 2003.

2. American Lung Association. *Trends in Asthma Morbidity and Mortality; Trends in Chronic Bronchitis and Emphysema: Morbidity and Mortality—April 2004.* New York, NY: American Heart Association; 2004.

3. Centers for Disease Control and Prevention. Behavioral Risk Factor Surveillance System (BRFSS): 2002 Asthma Data: Prevalence Tables and Maps. Available at: www.cdc.gov/asthma/brfss/02/brfssdata.htm. Accessed: November 1, 2004.

4. Cocchiarella L, Andersson GBJ, eds. *AMA Guides to the Evaluation of Permanent Impairment.* 5th ed. Chicago, Ill: AMA Press; 2001:62–63, 112–114.

5. American College of Cardiology Guidelines, 2004. Available at: www.acc.org/clinical/guidelines/exercise/summary%5Fmodification3.htm. Accessed: November 1, 2004.

6. Fuster V, Alexander RW, O'Rourke RA, et al, eds. *Hurst's The Heart.* 10th ed. Columbus, Ohio: McGraw Hill; 2001.

7. Beers MH, Berkow R, eds. *The Merck Manual of Diagnosis and Therapy.* Whitehouse Station, NJ: Merck & Co; 2004.

8. Barreiro TJ, Perillo I. An approach to interpreting spirometry. *Am Fam Physician.* 2004;69:1107–1114.

9. Sheffield LH. Exercise stress testing. In: Braunwald E, ed. *Heart Disease: A Textbook of Cardiovascular Medicine.* 3rd ed. Philadelphia, Pa: WB Saunders Co, 1988:227.

10. Bruce RA, Kusumi F, Hosmer D. Maximal oxygen intake and nomographic assessment of functional aerobic impairment in cardiovascular disease. *Am Heart J.* 1973;85:546.

11. Fox SM III, Naughton JP, Haskell WL. Physical activity and the prevention of coronary artery disease. *Ann Clin Res.* 1971;3:404–432.

12. American College of Sports Medicine. *Guidelines for Graded Exercise Testing and Exercise Prescription.* Philadelphia, Pa: Lea and Febiger; 1975:17.

13. Pollock ML, Wilmore JH, Fox SM. *Health and Fitness Through Physical Activity.* New York, NY: John Wiley & Sons Inc; 1978.

14. Haskell WL. Design and implementation of cardiac conditioning programs. In: Wenger NK, Hellerstein H, eds. *Rehabilitation of the Coronary Patient.* New York, NY: John Wiley & Sons Inc; 1978.

15. Astrand PO, Rodahl K. *Textbook of Work Physiology.* New York, NY: McGraw-Hill Co; 1977.

16. Cotes JE, Zejda J, King B. Lung function impairment as a guide to exercise limitation in work-related lung disorders. *Am Rev Respir Dis.* 1988;137:1089–1093.

17. Haskell W, Brachfeld N, Bruce RA, et al. Task Force II: determination of occupational working capacity in patients with ischemic heart disease. *J Am Coll Cardiol.* 1989;14:4:1025–1034.

18. Ainsworth BE, Haskell WL, Leon AS, et al. Compendium of physical activities: classification of energy costs of human physical activities. *Med Sci Sports Exerc.* 1993;25:71–80.

19. Nishimura RA, Tajik AJ. Evaluation of diastolic filling of left ventricle in health and disease: Doppler echocardiography is the clinician's Rosetta Stone. *J Am Coll Cardiol.* 1997;30:8–18.

Chapter 15

20. Jaffe WM, Roche AG, Coverdale HA, et al. Clinical evaluation versus Doppler echocardiography in quantitative assessment of valvular heart disease. *Circulation*. 1988;78:267–275.

21. Fleischmann KE, Hunink MG, Kuntz KM, et al. Exercise echocardiography or exercise SPECT imaging? A meta-analysis of diagnostic test performance. *JAMA*. 1998;280:913–920.

22. Morris AH, Kanner RE, Crapo RO, et al. *Clinical Pulmonary Function Testing: A Manual of Uniform Laboratory Procedure*. 2nd ed. Denver, Colo: Intermountain Thoracic Society; 1984.

23. American Thoracic Society. Standardization of spirometry: 1994 update. *Am J Respir Crit Care Med*. 1995;152:1107–1136.

24. Social Security Administration. *Disability Evaluation Under Social Security*. Baltimore, Md: Social Security Administration; January 2003. SSA publication 64-039.

25. Criteria Committee of the New York Heart Association. *Diseases of the Heart and Blood Vessels: Nomenclature and Criteria for Disease*. 6th ed. Boston, Mass: Little Brown & Co; 1964.

26. Hammar N, Alfredsson L, Smedberg M, et al. Differences in the incidence of myocardial infarction among occupational groups. *Scand J Work Environ Health*. 1992;18:178–185.

27. Karasek RA, Brisson C, Kawakani N, et al. The job content questionnaire (JCQ): an instrument for internationally comparative assessments of psychosocial job characteristics. *J Occup Health Psychol*. 1998;3:322–355.

28. Karasek RA, Theorell T. *Healthy Work*. New York, NY: Basic Books; 1990.

29. American Heart Association. *Advanced Cardiac Life Support*. Dallas, Tex: American Heart Association; 1997.

30. Myers J, Prakash M, Froelicher V, et al. Exercise capacity and mortality among men referred for exercise testing. *N Engl J Med*. 2002;346:793–801.

31. Goroya T, Jacobsen S, Pellikka P, et al. Prognostic value of treadmill exercise testing in elderly persons. *Ann Intern Med*. 2000;132:11:862–870.

32. Giri S, Thompson P, Kiernan F, et al. Clinical and angiographic characteristics of exertion-related acute myocardial infarction. *JAMA*. 1999;282:18:1731–1736.

33. National Cholesterol Education Program. Risk Assessment Tool for Estimating 10-Year Risk of Developing Hard CHD (Myocardial Infarction and Coronary Death). Available at: http://hin.nhlbi.nih.gov/atpiii/calculator.asp?usertype=prof. Accessed: November 1, 2004.

34. Mosca L. Novel cardiovascular risk factors: do they add value to your practice? *Am Fam Physician*. 2003;67:264.

35. Zhang R, Brennan ML, Fu X, et al. Association between myeloperoxidase levels and risk of coronary artery disease. *JAMA*. 2001;286:2136–2142.

36. Heeschen C, Dimmeler S, Fichtlscherer S, et al. Prognostic value of placental growth factor in patients with acute chest pain. *JAMA*. 2004;291:435–441.

37. Peters RJG, Boekholdt SM. Gene polymorphisms and the risk of myocardial infarction: an emerging relation. *N Engl J Med*. 2002;347:1963–1965.

Chapter 15

38. Ridker PM. Evaluating novel cardiovascular risk factors: can we better predict heart attacks? *Ann Intern Med.* 1999;130:933–937.

39. Pischon T, Girman CJ, Hotamisligil GS, et al. Plasma adiponectin levels and risk of myocardial infarction in men. *JAMA.* 2004;291:1730–1737.

40. Ansell BJ, Navab M, Hama S, et al. Inflammatory/anti-inflammatory properties of high-density lipoprotein distinguish patients from control subjects better than high-density lipoprotein cholesterol levels and are favorably affected by simvastatin treatment. *Circulation.* 2003;108:2751–2756.

41. Grundy SM, Brewer HB, Cleeman JI, et. al. NHLBI/AHA Conference Proceedings. Definition of metabolic syndrome: report of the National Heart, Lung, and Blood Institute/American Heart Association Conference on Scientific Issues Related to Definition. *Circulation.* 2004;109:433–438.

42. Bonow RO. Prognostic applications of exercise testing. *N Engl J Med.* 1991;325:805.

43. Froom P, Cohen C, Rashcupkin J, et al. Referral to occupational medicine clinics and resumption of employment after myocardial infarction. *J Occup Environ Med.* 1999;41:943–947.

44. Thompson PD, Klocke FJ, Levine BD, et al. 26th Bethesda Conference: recommendations for determining eligibility for competition in athletes with cardiovascular abnormalities. Task force 5: coronary artery disease. *J Am Coll Cardiol.* 1994;24:888–892.

45. Blumenthal R, Connolly H, Gersh BJ, Braunstein J, Epstein A, Wittels EH. *Cardivascular Advisory Panel Guidelines for the Medical Examination of Commercial Motor Vehicle Drivers.* Washington, DC: US Department of Transportation; 2003. Available at: www.fmcsa.dot.gov/pdfs/cardio.pdf. Accessed May 18, 2004.

46. Fletcher G, Oken K, Safford R. Comprehensive rehabilitation of patients with coronary artery disease. In: Braunwald E, ed. *Heart Disease: A Textbook of Cardiovascular Medicine.* 6th ed. Philadelphia, Pa: WB Saunders Co; 2001:1406–1417.

47. Dorn J, Naughton J, Imamura D, et al. Results of a multicenter randomized clinical trial of exercise and long-term survival in myocardial infarction patients: The National Exercise and Heart Disease Project (NEHDP). *Circulation.* 1999;100:1764–1769.

48. Agency for Healthcare Research and Quality. *Cardiac Rehabilitation.* Washington, DC: US Department of Health and Human Services; October 1995. Publication 96-0672.

49. Hlatky MA, Boothroyd D, Horine S, et al. Employment after coronary angioplasty or coronary bypass surgery in patients employed at the time of revascularization. *Ann Intern Med.* 1998;129:543–547.

50. Schnall PL, Landsbergis PA, Baker D. Job strain and cardiovascular disease. *Ann Rev Public Health.* 1994;15:381–411.

51. Siegrist J. Adverse health effects of high effort–low reward conditions. *J Occup Health Psychol.* 1996;1:27–41.

52. Williams RB, Barefoot JC, Schneiderman N. Psychosocial risk factors for cardiovascular disease: more than one culprit at work. *JAMA.* 2003;290:2190–2192.

Chapter 15

53. Bunker SJ, Colquhoun DM, Esler MD, et al. Stress and coronary heart disease: psychosocial risk factors. *Med J Aust.* 2003;178:272–276.

54. Bigos SJ, Battie MC, Spengler DM, et al. A prospective study of work perceptions and psychosocial factors affecting the report of back injury. *Spine.* 1991;16:1–6.

55. Cats-Baril WL, Frymoyer JW. Identifying patients at risk of becoming disabled because of low-back pain: the Vermont Rehabilitation Engineering Center predictive model. *Spine.* 1991;16:6:605–607.

56. Williams C, ed. *Social Factors, Work, Stress and Cardiovascular Disease Prevention in the European Union.* Brussels, Belgium: European Heart Network; July 1998.

57. ENRICHD Investigators. Effects of treating depression and low perceived social support on clinical events after myocardial infarction: the Enhancing Recovery in Coronary Heart Disease Patients (ENRICHD) randomized trial. *JAMA.* 2003;289:3106–3116.

58. 20th Bethesda Conference: insurability and employability of the patient with ischemic heart disease. *J Am Coll Cardiol.* 1989;14:1003–1044.

59. Reed P. *The Medical Disability Advisor: Workplace Guidelines for Disability Duration.* 5th ed. Westminster, Colo: Reed Group Ltd; 2005.

60. Berg AO, chair; US Preventive Services Task Force. Screening for high blood pressure: recommendations and rationale. *Am J Prev Med.* 2003;25:159–164.

61. Sheridan S, Pignone M, Donahue K. Screening for high blood pressure. *Am J Prev Med.* 2003;25:151–158.

62. Chobanian AV, Bakris GL, Black HR, et al. The seventh report of the Joint National Committee on the Detection, Evaluation, and Treatment of High Blood Pressure: the JNC 7 report. *JAMA.* 2003;289:2560–2572.

63. Jones DW, Appel LJ, Sheps SG, et al. Measuring blood pressure accurately: new and persistent challenges. *JAMA.* 2003;289:1027–1030.

64. Clement DL, De Buyzere ML, De Bacquer DA, et al. Prognostic value of ambulatory blood-pressure recordings in patients with treated hypertension. *N Engl J Med.* 2003;348:2407–2415.

65. White WB. Ambulatory blood pressure monitoring in clinical practice. *N Engl J Med.* 2003;348:2377–2378.

66. Ernst ME, Bergus GR. Ambulatory blood pressure monitoring: technology with a purpose. *Am Fam Physician.* 2003;67:2262–2270.

67. Bobrie G, Chatellier G, Genes N, et al. Cardiovascular prognosis of masked hypertension detected by blood pressure self-measurement in elderly treated hypertensive patients. *JAMA.* 2004;291:1342–1349.

68. de Simone G, Devereux RB, Kimball TR. Interaction between body size and cardiac workload: influence of left ventricular mass during body growth and adulthood. *Hypertension.* 1998;31:1077–1082.

69. Palmieri V, de Simone G, Arnett DK, et al. Relation of various degrees of body mass index in patients with systemic hypertension to left ventricular mass, cardiac output, and peripheral resistance (the Hypertension Genetic Epidemiology Network Study). *Am J Cardiol.* 2001;88:1163–1168.

Chapter 15

70. Devereux RB. Therapeutic options in minimizing left ventricular hypertrophy. Cardiac protection: the evolving role of ARBS. *Am Heart J.* 2000;139:S9–S14.

71. Carethon MR, Gidding SS, Nehgme R, et al. Cardiorespiratory fitness in young adulthood and the development of cardiovascular disease risk factors. *JAMA.* 2003;290:3092–3100.

72. Stevens VJ, Obarzanek E, Cook NR, et al. Long-term weight loss and changes in blood pressure: results of the Trials of Hypertension revention phase II. *Ann Intern Med.* 2001;134:1–11.

73. Pickering TG. Lifestyle modification and blood pressure control: is the glass half full or half empty? *JAMA.* 2003;289:16:2131–2132.

74. Whelton PK, He J, Appel LJ, et al. Primary prevention of hypertension: clinical and public health advisory from the National High Blood Pressure Education Program. *JAMA.* 2002;288:1882–1888.

75. August P. Initial treatment of hypertension. *N Engl J Med.* 2003;348:610–616.

76. Blood pressure responses to acute stress and left ventricular mass (the Hypertension Genetic Epidemiology Network Study). *Am J Cardiol.* 2002;89:536–540.

77. Markovitz JH, Matthews KA, Kannel WB, et al. Psychological predictors of hypertension in the Framingham study. *JAMA.* 1993;270:2439–2443.

78. Pickering TG, Devereux RB, James GD, et al. Environmental influences on blood pressure and the role of job strain. *J Hypertens.* 1996;14(suppl): S179–S185.

79. Yan LL, Liu K, Matthews KA, et al. Psychosocial factors and risk of hypertension: the Coronary Artery Risk Development in Young Adults (CARDIA) study. *JAMA.* 2003;290:2138–2148.

80. Stone RA, DeLeo J. Psychotherapeutic control of hypertension. *N Engl J Med.* 1976;294:80–84.

81. Harber P, Schenker MA, Balmes J, eds. *Occupational and Environmental Respiratory Disease.* St Louis, Mo: Mosby-Year Book; 1996.

82. Chan-Yeung M, Malo JL. Occupational asthma. *N Engl J Med.* 1995;333:107–112.

83. Bone RC, ed. Occupational asthma and related respiratory disorders. *Dis Mon.* 1995;41:146–199.

84. Youakim S. Work-related asthma. *Am Fam Physician.* 2001;64:1839–1848.

85. Murray JF, Nadel JA, eds. *Textbook of Respiratory Medicine.* 3rd ed. Philadelphia, Pa: W.B. Saunders Co; 2000.

86. Thurston GD, Bates DV. Air pollution as an underappreciated cause of asthma symptoms. *JAMA.* 2003;290:1915–1917.

87. Demeter SL, Cordasco EM. Occupational asthma. In: Zenz C, ed. *Occupational Medicine.* 3rd ed. St Louis, Mo: Mosby-Year Book; 1994.

88. Hansen JE, Wasserman K. Integrated cardiopulmonary exercise testing. In: Demeter SL, Andersson GBJ, Smith GM, eds. *Disability Evaluation.* St Louis, Mo: Mosby-Year Book; 1996.

89. Townsend MC. Technique and equipment pitfalls in spirometry testing: serious threats to your respiratory surveillance program. In: NORA Medical Surveillance

Chapter 15

Workshop. Available at: www.cdc.gov/niosh/sbw/osh prof/townsendhandout. html. Accessed May 18, 2004.

90. Nowak RM. National and international guidelines for the emergency management of adult asthma. In: Brenner BE, ed. *Emergency Asthma*. New York, NY: Marcel Dekker Inc; 1999.

91. Edmond SD, Camargo CA, Nowak RM. Advances, opportunities, and the new asthma guidelines. *Ann Emerg Med*. 1998;31:590–594.

92. Nowak R, Tokarski G. Asthma. In: Marx J, ed. *Rosen's Emergency Medicine: Concepts and Clinical Practice*. 5th ed. St Louis, Mo: CV Mosby; 2002:938–956.

Chapter 16

Working With Common Neurologic Problems

Edwin H. Klimek, MD

Advances in general health have resulted in long-term survival of individuals burdened with central nervous system disorders. This chapter addresses return to work and risks to individuals and workplaces among persons of working age (arbitrarily designated 16 to 65 years) for conditions including primary and secondary headache syndromes, epilepsy (recurrent seizures vs first-time witnessed seizure), acquired brain injury, and progressive neurodegenerative conditions (eg, multiple sclerosis [MS] and hereditary neuropathies).

Physician-Certified Absenteeism for Neurologic Illness

Physician-certified absenteeism for neurologic illness may arise out of occupational health evaluations or within ongoing attending care without compromising the patient care relationship or casting doubt upon the advocacy role of the physician. This certification both arises from and is limited by the following circumstances:

- The patient stops work when he or she feels that illness or injury justifies absence.
- The physician certifies illness or injury, deciding when the patient is fit to return to work.
- The patient returns to work when sufficiently recovered.
- Management attempts to provide accommodation and work autonomy.
- Insurers support this system by providing economic benefits for partial disability.

Patients confound this model by endorsing pain as a sign of a serious injury. Some are unprepared to attempt to return to work until all indicators of illness have resolved. They express a belief that the presence of pain or manifestations of neurologic illness is inconsistent with returning to work. The "enabling philosophy" of care by the certifying physician may also discount the therapeutic affiliation of work-related activities with the hazards of daily life. Some certifying physicians fear that any increased risk of injury during the attempt to return to work places the onus on the certifying physician to disprove the risk. In all cases this is a misleading, if not an erroneous, assertion. The physician and individual should be reminded that the decision is not whether a return to work imposes a risk, but rather whether a return to work imposes a risk unacceptably greater than that of not returning to work.

For most musculoskeletal illnesses, guidelines for injury-specific recovery times are available from medical and scientific literature or are developed through consensus opinion of medical experience.[1] These guidelines frequently are based on return to work in job classifications of sedentary, light, medium, heavy, and very heavy activities. Unfortunately, the performance characteristics affected by neurologic illness related to motor coordination, sensation, and mental competence manifest in measurement of speed, accuracy, and reproducibility of the task are not as readily available.

This chapter intends to assess capacity to undertake *gainful employment*, which is regular attendance in a non-sheltered environment requiring competitive employment with or without accommodations that are feasible and realistic. Return to work may be possible through either modifications to the workplace or work autonomy.

The concept of work *autonomy*, or the ability of the worker to pace the work to suit the limitations of a continuing illness or injury, is slightly different from (although related to) workplace modifications. This concept of return to modified work presumes residual work capacity and availability of workplace alterations. The employer establishes the minimum performance reasonably necessary to accomplish a legitimate work-related purpose. To show that the standard is reasonably necessary, it must be demonstrated that, without it, it would be impossible to accommodate individual employees sharing the characteristics of the claimant without imposing undue hardship on the employer or a serious safety risk to the individual, coworkers, or the general public. Patients are also assumed to be mentally competent despite neurologic illness and have primary responsibility to be informed enough about their condition to thoughtfully consider modified work opportunities available from the employer. The employer and patient should accept and understand the philosophy of "partial disability" and rapid return to work, as well as the role of modified work opportunities in achieving this goal.

Neurologic Illness: General

In general terms, persistent neurologic illness may be static or slowly deteriorating. In most situations, determination, motivation, and effort overcome established neurologic handicaps. This results in opportunities for reevaluation of evolving symptoms causally related with confidence to the original injury. If the presence of newly identifiable organic changes is entirely explained by the persisting neurologic illness, the trial of return to work is reassessed and encouraged. However, if a clear link to the workplace can be established for the worsening of the neurologic condition (risk), a continued return to work with or without suitable accommodation to reduce the risk of recurrence is a matter for informed discussion. Shift work and sleep cycle alteration, which may normally elicit fatigue, may be a cause of unavoidable deterioration. In the latter case, medical advice against a return to work may be given.

The best prediction of non return is offered by a combination of medical, sociodemographic, and psychological variables. Fear-avoidance variables, taken alone, provide a 70% correct prediction of continuing sick leave for patients with back pain at 12 months after treatment.[2] Intercurrent employment-related factors associated with poor outcome of a trial of return to work include a job in the public sector, a longer time in the occupation, and multiple job changes and periods of unemployment. Failure to return to work may also be associated with work factors, eg, job dissatisfaction.[3–5] Some patients with low back pain may not return to work simply because it is more rewarding not to work, both financially and psychologically.[6–8] Self-determination and the will to be sick remain powerful predictors of an unsuccessful trial of return to work.

Headache

Persistent daily non-debilitating headaches are likely to be tension type or mixed headaches, including migraine. *Migraine* is a common, chronic, incapacitating neurovascular disorder, characterized by attacks of severe headache, autonomic nervous system dysfunction, and, in some patients, an aura involving neurologic symptoms. This characteristic pattern of stereotypical recurrence is required to support the diagnosis.

Persistent debilitating daily headache is rare in clinical neurologic practice outside of infectious illness, abnormality of cerebrospinal fluid pressure, temporal arteritis, or head trauma. The hallmark of these conditions is abnormality of rheumatologic serology, cerebrospinal fluid contents, or opening pressure obtained by lumbar puncture after neuroimaging studies. The clinical characteristics of the headache are insufficient to rule out the possibility of intracranial disease.[9] Neuroimaging studies should be considered in all adult patients with headache of recent onset or in previously headache-free individuals in whom a trial of return to work is being considered. This is a defensive position consistent with practice guidelines of professional organizations, which suggest that there is insufficient evidence to make recommendations in patients for headaches other than migraine.[10,11]

Typically, not only is the neurologic examination entirely normal in headache syndromes such as migraine, but studies suggest the incidence of clinically important findings on neuroimaging studies to be low (between 0.4% and 2.4%) in patients with acute headaches without head trauma.[10] How such data might be generalizable to the occupational health setting is not well established in light of the known 18% rate of false-positive findings on magnetic resonance (MR) imaging screening of self-declared normal volunteers.[12] This results in a large part from the white-matter hyperintensities present in at least 13% of asymptomatic individuals.[13]

Plausible theories abound to account for how migraine is initiated and for the phases of complete migraine: the prodrome, the aura, the headache, the headache termination, and the postdrome. However, the initial diagnostic evaluation of all headache syndromes including posttraumatic headaches rests on a carefully obtained history including pain character, location, onset, precipitants, aura, other associated symptoms, duration, frequency, and time course followed by a focused neurologic examination to identify the red flags that warrant intensive or invasive investigations.[14]

Headache associated with head trauma may be considered either acute posttraumatic headache (PTH) or chronic PTH. Chronic PTHs, the headaches that persist for more than 8 weeks, occur infrequently. These often difficult cases may persist for months or years. The preceding head injury may vary from minimal to severe and does not correlate with the duration or intensity of headache.[15] By the definition put forth by the International Headache Society, headaches must start within two weeks of the injury itself or within two weeks of the time of termination of posttraumatic amnesia.

Chronic PTH has no special features but is symptomatically identical to other headaches such as chronic tension-type headache or migraine without aura.[16,17] This suggests that PTHs are generated by the same processes that cause the natural headaches, not by intracranial derangement from head blows or jolts.[18] The incidence of this entity is not clearly defined, with advocates indicating that it is found in most patients with postconcussional syndrome and skeptics suggesting it is nearly nonexistent in countries where possibilities for monetary compensation are minimal.[19]

Chapter 16

Posttraumatic headache is often seen as part of the post-concussion syndrome.[20] Post-concussion syndrome refers to a large number of symptoms and signs usually following mild traumatic brain injury (MTBI).[21] The most common complaints are headaches, dizziness, fatigue, irritability, anxiety, insomnia, loss of consciousness and memory, and noise sensitivity.[22] While some proportion of difficult-to-manage cases may be malingerers or frauds or have compensation neurosis, most patients nevertheless have genuine complaints, in part resembling depression or dissociative phenomena, not all of which are cured by a verdict or any recommended treatment.[23–26]

Antipodal schools of thought exist to explain the mechanism of PTH. Some suggest that plausible mechanisms for chronic PTH exist, with circumstantial support for the neurobiological legitimacy of PTH. Others suggest that chronic PTHs are most often a myth attributable in large measure to rebound or treatment-induced headaches with neuropsychiatric disorders (epilepsy, major affective and anxiety disorders) showing increased comorbidity with migraine.[27] Some agree with the *Diagnostic and Statistical Manual of Mental Disorders, Fourth Edition,*[28] which outlines circumstances in which malingering should be strongly suspected.

Advocates of all sides seem to accept a bona fide presentation of an initial isolated migraine or an increased frequency of previously existing migraine headaches subsequent to an injury.[29] Essentially this accords with the belief that anyone may have a migraine attack occasionally without necessarily being a migraine patient. In the absence of trait markers specific to migraine or its subtypes, the classification of migraine headache is guided by diagnostic criteria.[30] That PTH is a diagnostic challenge may be inferred from the extreme frequency of headaches in the general population, affecting about eight of nine people at some time in their life, thereby diluting the presentation.[31]

Risk
In primary headache syndromes, risk is not an issue. Headaches secondary to structural disease are uncommon and are beyond the scope of this chapter.

Capacity
Capacity is rarely an issue in headache patients. They can perform activities, but they dislike doing so because of symptoms (pain, nausea, fatigue).

Tolerance
Tolerance for activity despite symptoms is the problem for patients with primary headache syndromes. In keeping with the philosophy outlined in Chapters 1 and 2, physicians should typically work with patients to minimize

the frequency and severity of headaches, and certify disability only for the specific days of severe headache. Many migraine patients work despite migraine. There is no objective way for a physician to determine, and thus certify, that a given headache is severe enough to justify missing work on a given day.

Sample Case: Headache

A middle-aged woman employed as a front desk receptionist for a large commercial enterprise feels unable to return to work as a result of debilitating headaches subsequent to a thyroid operation (tolerance). Headaches occur on a daily basis, with a severe headache that is described as a migraine about once a week. When a severe headache occurs, she is effectively housebound and chooses not "to do anything" because of severe pain. Before the surgery, a similar very bad headache occurred about once a year. For this problem she has been referred to a neurologist, who injected botulinum toxin on four occasions for headaches.

At the time of the encounter, the patient is having one of her daily headaches, for which she took two tablets of oxycodone before coming to the office. No other medication is taken regularly.

The history confirms that family members had headaches. The general medical and neurologic examination are unremarkable. Neuroimaging studies are normal. Serologic evaluation including thyroid function studies are normal.

Indicators of superimposed depression or traits of avoidant personality are not found. Although the patient accepts a trial of interval therapy to reduce the frequency and severity of the migraine, she does not wish to reduce daily analgesic use. A trial of increased activity and progressive return to work is obstructed by family commitments to childcare.

In this case the diagnosis of daily headaches and common migraine was supported. Daily analgesic use raised the possibility of medication-induced rebound headaches. Maximal medical therapy was not established. While continuing to advocate for a trial of return to work and compliance with treatment, her attending physician was **not** able to certify her as disabled for her usual occupation.

To prepare for a return to work for patients who report chronic disabling headache, a challenge of graded activity and exercise while keeping a headache diary or using a headache scale is advisable.[32] The failure to adhere to a graded increase in exercise allows social and personal barriers to emerge and be addressed without being complicated by workplace stressors. Identification of the benefits of increased activity on most headaches is underscored.

Debilitating chronic headache rarely occurs without amplification of other normal body sensations. Patients who experience chronic headache also seem to confuse responsible therapeutic drug use with drug misuse for symptoms common to everyday life, which they misunderstand as warning signs of serious disease. Some thereby express emotional distress constrained only by cultural and familial rules.

Although "central activation" to account for pain with non-physiologic features of psychological origin has been suggested to account for pain amplification, this is difficult to distinguish from the behavior noted by others as somatization. Clinical experience and existing research on diagnostic criteria for the more severe forms of somatization suggest that two features are necessary to establish the presence of somatization. The first is several (more than three) vague or exaggerated symptoms in, often, different organ systems. The other is a chronic course (ie, a history of such symptoms for more than 2 years).[33]

There are more reviews of treatment options in the literature than original clinical research outlining the incidence, characteristics, and effectiveness of therapy for PTH. At the time of this writing, only one study with adequate evidence was found.[34] This may be in part because the clinical distinction between PTH and other headache subtypes is obscured by the substantial degree of overlap in the symptoms, by the ways in which these headache subtypes evolve over time, and by the use of retrospective symptom histories to assign clinical diagnosis.[35,36] This is further blurred when diagnostic suspicion and acumen are focused on existing criteria for diagnosis of headache that may in themselves not be adequate in either primary or post-traumatic headaches.[37]

Responses to therapeutic intervention are diagnostically unreliable, since there may be an undue lag in response that may be contaminated by external events and by the natural course of headaches and underlying medical illness.[38,39] The risk to the workplace of a trial of return to work in headache is typically limited to lack of productivity attributable to unreliable or unpredictable attendance rather than damage of product or hazard to coworkers.

Chapter 16

Epilepsy

Epilepsy is distinct among diseases for fleeting yet severe impact on employment, social life, and the sense of well-being. It is complicated by the balance between a person's right to manage his or her seizures and guard his or her confidentiality against the employer's knowledge. In the United Kingdom, 53% of employed people with epilepsy chose to conceal their illness.[40] The employer is often reluctant to allow these individuals to continue at the workplace, fearing workplace disruption or repercussion of potential workplace injury. A difficulty commonly encountered in epilepsy is that employers are hesitant to recognize that employees, despite having epilepsy, are able to return to work if reasonable accommodations can be made. The "reasonableness" of the accommodation is not a medical issue.

Sample Case: Seizure

A factory worker has a witnessed first-time seizure without focal onset or prolonged post ictal period. It is unaccompanied by indication of substance misuse, or previous childhood or family history of seizure. Physical examination limited to the neurologic system reveals no abnormality. Magnetic resonance imaging and electroencephalography (EEG) are unremarkable. After discussion of the options, anticonvulsant therapy is not initiated. The employer is keen to temporarily provide employment alternatives ensuring no use of machinery and no work activities that could result in injury if a seizure occurred during work.

Although in many such presentations confirmation of the diagnosis may be medically and ethically challenging,[41,42] the crux of this problem is prognostication of recurrence so that work tasks can be addressed. Prognosis and treatment of the first seizure depend on diagnostic accuracy in identification of a specific epilepsy syndrome, yet patients with first seizures are generally falsely regarded as a homogeneous group.[43] Studies of seizure recurrence after a first tonic-clonic seizure give conflicting predictions of recurrence, with a meta-analysis suggesting a two-year risk of recurrence as high as 40%.[44]

Assessment of adults should comprise rigorous clinical evaluation with explicit questions about previous minor epileptic symptoms, early EEG (ideally within 24 hours of the seizure), sleep-deprived EEG if the first EEG is non-diagnostic, and MR imaging for all patients except those for whom idiopathic generalized epilepsy is confirmed on their EEG or those with benign rolandic epilepsy.[45]

In part this extensive emphasis on investigations reflects the uncertainty and unreliability of the investigation in prognostication. Electroencephalography is most useful in the management of patients with suspected epilepsy. In patients without a diagnosis, the EEG presence of "epileptiform" activity does not establish the diagnosis beyond doubt because similar activity may be found in about 2% of individuals who have never had a seizure.[46] Similarly, in patients with undoubted epilepsy, multiple recordings may fail to demonstrate epileptiform activity in 8%.

A problematic issue sometimes confused with the capacity to work is the privilege to drive. Patients who should not be driving or who should be driving only under certain circumstances should be so advised. This does not preclude them from gainful employment, except employment as the operator of a motor vehicle. Most physicians have a standard warning letter about driving (or a form providing advice for multiple risks, including driving) and many provide the patient with a copy.

While the confidential nature of the physician-patient relationship is of the utmost importance, some jurisdictions have an explicit reporting requirement, which the physician should call to the patient's attention. These requirements generally state that any physician who diagnoses or treats a person with epilepsy must report that person's name, age, and address to a central state agency, usually the Department of Motor Vehicles or Department of Public Safety. Some statutes grant physicians immunity for their opinions and recommendations to the state Department of Motor Vehicles.

In planning a return to work for patients with seizures, one should consider the predictability of the disorder and aura that may precede the loss of consciousness. Spudis et al[47] suggested that idiopathic isolated attacks should be treated more favorably than recurrent attacks with abnormal investigations. These might include a breakthrough seizure due to physician-directed medication change, an isolated seizure where the medical examination indicates that another episode appears unlikely, a seizure related to a temporary illness, a seizure due to an isolated incident of not taking medication, an established pattern of nocturnal seizures, an established pattern of seizures that do not impair driving ability, or an established pattern of an extended warning aura.

The major risk to the workplace of a trial of return to work in seizures is probably productivity reduction attributable to unreliable or unpredictable attendance. The risk to the patient from a seizure is similar to the risk were it to occur in a non-workplace setting. It is rare for damage of product or hazard to coworkers to be found during the ictus.

Chapter 16

A common error in evaluating patients with a seizure disorder is misattribution of persistent concurrent cognitive impairment to seizures, rather than drug-induced side effects. Drowsiness in the workplace may be cause for work restriction. Shift work not only makes seizures more likely as a result of sleep deprivation but has the potential to intensify the drowsiness induced by therapy.

Risk

Typical work restrictions for patients with seizures include no driving, no climbing to heights, and no working with machinery or under conditions where significant injury to self or others is predictable if a seizure occurred. Drowsiness from medications may be an additional issue of risk.

Capacity

Capacity in patients with seizure disorders is not affected. As long as risk is adequately addressed, these patients work *without* limitations.

Tolerance

Patients with seizure disorders may dislike working, fearing that seizures in the workplace will be embarrassing, but this is an issue of patient choice (to work or not to work) and *not* a reason for physician-certified work absence or disability.

Brain Injury

Brain injuries vary in severity. Severe traumatic brain injury is obvious to the layperson and is seldom misdiagnosed by health professionals.[48] Severe head injury may result in partial or complete paralysis, speech problems, impaired cognitive functioning, disability from employment, long periods of coma, and long-term care requirements. The injury will be apparent in changes on computed tomography, MR imaging, and other brain imaging. Disability after closed head injury varies depending on the injury mechanism, neuropathology, and other factors, such as medical complications.[48]

Patients with mild traumatic brain injury (MTBI) describe a similar constellation of post-injury complaints. Symptoms may include headaches,[49] dizziness, lethargy, memory loss, irritability, personality changes, cognitive deficits, and/or perceptual changes. These symptoms have been characterized under various names, including minor head injury,[50] mild head injury,[51] closed head injury,[52] post concussive syndrome,[53] post concussional syndrome,[54] post concussional disorder,[55] minor traumatic brain injury,[56] traumatic cephalgia, post brain injury syndrome, and posttraumatic syndrome. The variability in neurobehavioral outcome after MTBI may be, in part, attributed to ascertainment bias, giving a wide variance to severity and dysfunction in individuals after MTBI.

Research studies show a wide variability in the degree and duration of disability after MTBI. For example, some clinical observations show that patients with MTBI (Glasgow Coma Scale score, 13–15), who are able to follow commands less than one hour after injury, demonstrate no long-term persistent neuropsychological impairments.[57] Other research indicates that only 49% had a "good recovery."[58]

Individuals who were productive before injury may become unproductive after a MTBI. Patients with fractures of the skull, severe cerebral contusions, or large intracranial hematomas that are successfully treated can make uneventful and complete recoveries,[59] but patients with stable pre-accident psychological and work histories with no prior complaints may apparently develop functional impairments after MTBI. This is the "MTBI paradox": a so-called mild injury can result in apparently serious problems. Evidence indicates that 1 year after injury most patients (73%) return to work, even thought 84% report having complaints.[60]

Although patients with MTBI report similar clusters of symptoms and complaints, the precise etiology of symptoms is elusive, and many health professionals take an aggressive treatment approach and treat all reported symptoms. Others advise that the majority of symptoms will resolve within 90 days of the injury. In some cases, "expectation" may be the cause of these early symptoms.[61–63]

Risk
Patients with head injury, mild or severe, are not at risk of harm with work activities for which they have appropriate intellect and motor skills. The brain does not become injured or get worse with activity. There is no basis for work restrictions, unless posttraumatic seizures are present.

Capacity
Individuals with severe brain injury may lack the intellectual or motor skills to perform essential work functions. Their work limitations may preclude a return to employment. Functional testing or a trial of supervised work activity may be helpful in determining work ability.

Tolerance
Tolerance for symptoms like headache, malaise, and fatigue may be reasons cited by patients with brain injury for choosing not to work. These symptoms are not measurable or verifiable, and are infrequently a basis for physician certification of work absence. Commonly, such symptoms can be

Chapter 16

satisfactorily addressed by work autonomy, in which the pace and rate of work are modified. Personality changes found in severe TBI may become significant obstacles to return to work through changes in motivation and effort.

Multiple Sclerosis

In 1983, the Kurtzke Expanded Disability Status Scale (EDSS), shown in Table 16-1, considered eight functional systems intended to be independent of each other and that in combination reflect all the manifestations of neurologic impairment in multiple sclerosis (MS).[64] These functional groups or functional systems were pyramidal (P), cerebellar (Cll), brain stem (BS), sensory (S), bowel and bladder (BB), visual (V), cerebral or mental (Cb), and other or miscellaneous (O).

Within the EDSS, the principle of objective abnormality with no impairment of function is accepted, with step 3.0 being mild impairment without impeding normal functions except in rare individuals (steeplejacks or concert pianists). The lowest grades (up to step 4.0) presume the ability to ambulate fully for 500 m and carry out full daily activities. The EDSS correlates with the MR imaging–defined volume of plaque burden most closely for the pyramidal subscores. This probably reflects that factors other than volumetrically determined lesion load are important determinants for disability.[65]

Sample Case: Multiple Sclerosis

A 30-year-old female laboratory technician with known clinically definite MS presents with a flare of optic neuritis in the left eye and ataxia. She has an EDSS score of 4.0 at the time of relapse. She has worked for 10 years with the disorder. She and her husband have made a conscious decision not to inform her employer and her family of the disorder so that she will not be treated "differently." She has been on immunomodulating therapy for much of the time.

In this case a temporary medical absence for suppression of the relapse is undertaken. A remission is expected and occurs, with resumption of full-time work in three weeks.

In planning a return to work for patients with established MS, the temporal profile of the disorder can predict future recurrence and loss of ability. Early in the course of the disorder the presentation is less reliable; however, patients with prominent cerebellospinal signs have a less favorable prognosis.

Table 16-1 Kurtzke Extended Disability Status Scale

0.0	Normal neurologic examination (all grade 0 in all functional system [FS] scores)
1.0	No disability, minimal signs in one FS (ie, grade 1)
1.5	No disability, minimal signs in more than one FS (more than 1 grade 1)
2.0	Minimal disability in one FS (one FS grade 2, others 0 or 1)
2.5	Minimal disability in two FSs (two FSs grade 2, others 0 or 1)
3.0	Moderate disability in one FS (one FS grade 3, others 0 or 1) or mild disability in three or four FSs (three or four FSs grade 2, others 0 or 1) though fully ambulatory
3.5	Fully ambulatory but with moderate disability in one FS (one grade 3) and one or two FSs grade 2; or two grade 3 (others 0 or 1) or five grade 2 (others 0 or 1)
4.0	Fully ambulatory without aid, self-sufficient, up and about some 12 hours a day despite relatively severe disability consisting of one FS grade 4 (others 0 or 1), or combination of lesser grades exceeding limits of previous steps; patient should be able to walk >500 m without assist or rest
4.5	Fully ambulatory without aid, up and about much of the day, may otherwise require minimal assistance; characterized by relatively severe disability usually consisting of one FS grade 4 (others 0 or 1) or combinations of lesser grades exceeding limits of previous steps; walks >300 m without assist or rest
5.0	Ambulatory without aid for at least 200 m; disability severe enough to impair full daily activities (eg, working a full day without special provision) (usual FS equivalents are one grade 5 alone, others 0 or 1; or combinations of lesser grades); patient walks >200 m without aid or rest
5.5	Ambulatory without aid for at least 100 m; disability severe enough to preclude full daily activities (usual FS equivalents are one grade 5 alone, others 0 or 1; or combinations of lesser grades). Enough to preclude full daily activities. (Usual FS equivalents are one grade 5 alone, others 0 or 1; or combinations of lesser grades).
6.0	Intermittent or unilateral constant assistance (cane, crutch, brace) required to walk at least 100 m (usual FS equivalents are combinations with more than one FS grade 3)
6.5	Constant bilateral assistance (canes, crutches, braces) required to walk at least 20 m (usual FS equivalents are combinations with more than one FS grade 3)
7.0	Unable to walk at least 5 m even with aid, essentially restricted to wheelchair; wheels self and transfers alone; up and about in wheelchair some 12 hours a day (usual FS equivalents are combinations with more than one FS grade 4+; very rarely pyramidal grade 5 alone)
7.5	Unable to take more than a few steps; restricted to wheelchair; may need aid in transfer; wheels self but cannot carry on in wheelchair a full day (usual FS equivalents are combinations with more than one FS grade 4+; very rarely pyramidal grade 5 alone)
8.0	Essentially restricted to chair or perambulated in wheelchair, but out of bed most of day; retains many self-care functions; generally has effective use of arms (usual FS equivalents are combinations, generally grade 4+ in several systems)
8.5	Essentially restricted to bed most of day; has some effective use of arm(s); retains some self-care functions (usual FS equivalents are combinations, generally 4 in several systems)
9.0	Helpless, bed-ridden patient; can communicate and eat (usual FS equivalents are combinations, mostly grade 4+)
9.5	Totally helpless, bed-ridden patient; unable to communicate effectively or eat or swallow (usual FS equivalents are combinations, almost all grade 4+)
10.0	Death due to MS

Chapter 16

The benefits of established disease predicting future response to therapy are fortunately present in the previous case example. Chronic progressive MS with an EDSS score of 4.0 is often inconsistent with regular competitive employment.

Significant temporary relapses treated with intravenous corticosteroid infusions are likely inconsistent with workplace attendance during the relapse. Corticosteroids are also a psychoactive stimulant, and a withdrawal depression may be noted that may prolong the work absence.

The risk to the workplace of a trial of return to work in MS is dependent on the extent of the incoordination and corticospinal involvement. Unilateral visual dysfunction is rarely relevant except when strict binocular vision is a rigid task prerequisite. Damage to product or hazard to coworkers may ensue from incoordination. Therapeutic intervention including self-injection of immunomodulating therapy is unlikely to produce disabling side effects. Transient influenza-like reactions and local soreness may occur.

Disability From Multiple Sclerosis

The US Social Security Administration's criteria for total disability from MS are as follows:

A. Disorganization of motor function, meaning significant and persistent disorganization of motor function in two extremities, resulting in sustained disturbance of gross and dexterous movements, or gait and station

B. Significant visual impairment (as described in the vision criteria) or significant mental impairment (as described in the mental illness criteria)

C. Significant, reproducible fatigue of motor function with substantial weakness on repetitive activity, *demonstrated on physical examination* (not just by patient history), resulting from neurologic dysfunction in areas of the central nervous system known to be pathologically involved by the MS process

Risk

Patients with MS are not at risk of harm with work activities for which they have appropriate intellect and motor skills. The brain does not become injured or get worse with activity. There is no basis for work restrictions.

Capacity

Patients with MS may be deconditioned from inactivity, but their current exercise ability, although measurable by treadmill testing, may be capable of increasing with progressive exercise or with progressively more difficult work. Fatigue or muscle weakness that can be documented on physical examination (and not merely reported by the patient) is an issue of work limitation based on capacity. If patients lack the necessary visual, auditory, sensory, motor, or intellectual function for the job in question, they usually have appropriate lesions on MR images. This loss of neurologic function, "objectified" by the presence of appropriate lesions on MR images, may be the basis for physician certification of disability based or work limitations (due to capacity).

Magnetic resonance images do not predict disability. The plaque burden affecting the coritcospinal tract approximates the EDSS score. Ataxia or incoordination may result in work limitations. Typically this is seen in older males presenting with spasticity who have a predominance of spinal and cerebellar involvement. They tend to have a gradually progressive downhill course.

The EDSS is intended to reflect all manifestations of MS in a hierarchical fashion; however, the arithmetic appearance may be misleading, since an EDSS score of 4 is not "twice as bad" as an EDSS score of 2. Chronic progressive MS with an EDSS score of 4.0 is often inconsistent with regular competitive employment (based on capacity).

Tolerance

Tolerance for symptoms like headache, malaise, weakness, and fatigue may be reasons cited by patients with MS for choosing not to work. These symptoms are not measurable or verifiable, and are infrequently a basis for physician certification of work absence. The common complaint of fatigue in MS is of practical significance with impaired motor function, since there is typically no "mental fatigue" in the early stages of MS. Fatigue or weakness that cannot be documented on physical examination, but is reported by the patient, is an issue of tolerance and not capacity. As such, it is not generally a reason for physician-imposed work limitations. The choice to work or not to work despite subjective fatigue is the patient's.

Commonly such symptoms can be satisfactorily addressed by work autonomy, in which the pace and rate of work are modified. Personality changes found in MS may become significant obstacles to return to work through changes in motivation and effort. Without a limitation of walking (manifest with an EDSS score of 4.0), this is rarely an obstacle to function.

Polyneuropathy

Diabetes is the most common disorder presenting with prominent signs and symptoms of neuropathy. The police officer at the practice range who discharges his weapon accidentally because he is unable to sense the trigger of the revolver poses a great hazard to himself and others. Driving skills are unlikely to be affected by diabetic neuropathy, although the concomitant hypoglycemia of overmedication and visual disturbance of retinal disease must be considered.

Sample Case: Polyneuropathy

A 35-year-old carpenter presents for evaluation with Charcot-Marie-Tooth disease, a familial polyneuropathy. He notes that he is unable to ascend or descend ladders because his plantar flexion at the ankle is weak (capacity) and the perception of the rungs through his steel-toe and steel-shank work boots is unreliable (risk). He has inexplicably dropped windows carried in the grip of the hand (capacity). Although he enjoys his job, he is concerned that he may not be able to drive because of foot pedal miscue (risk).

In the case given, the worker has a mismatch of occupational and personal expectations with the medical illness. He should be considered for retraining as the requirements of his job are inconsistent with personal safety (risk).

In planning a return to work for patients with established polyneuropathy, the temporal profile of the disorder can predict the loss of ability. Early in the course of the disorder, the neuropathic symptoms may be distracting but of limited functional importance. As the disease progresses, difficulty manipulating objects, such as starting threaded connections, is a common complaint of tradesmen.

Therapeutic interventions in familial polyneuropathies are generally of limited benefit. If the cause is diabetes, the systemic medical illness must be considered.

The risk to the workplace of a trial of return to work in polyneuropathy is dependent on the extent of the incoordination and motor weakness that develops late in the disease. The damage to product or hazard to coworkers ensues from the incoordination.

Risk

The risk to patients with peripheral neuropathy relates to the sensory deficit and to the motor deficit. If gait and coordinated activity are impaired, the individual may be at risk climbing to heights, walking on narrow surfaces, and working with hazardous equipment. These factors would be a basis for physician-imposed activity restrictions. Prolonged standing or walking on feet that lack sensation may lead to skin ulceration and is a basis for work restrictions on standing, walking, and carrying.

Capacity

Individuals with peripheral neuropathy may no longer be capable of the walking or coordinated activity required to meet the essential functions of the job in question. This would be the basis for a work limitation. Functional testing or a trial of supervised work activity may be helpful in determining work ability.

Tolerance

There are usually no issues of work tolerance in individuals with peripheral neuropathy. If they have the capacity to work at acceptable risk, they may work. If the neuropathy is painful, the decision to work or not to work despite pain is the patient's. Pain is not measurable and thus is not a basis for a physician to impose work restrictions or work limitations.

Summary

Persistent neurologic illness may be remitting-relapsing, static, or slowly deteriorating. This results in opportunities for reevaluation of evolving concerns causally related with confidence to the original injury or illness. In most situations, determination, motivation, and effort overcome established neurologic handicaps. Temporary work absence to permit treatment or convalescence may be required. Permanent work restriction may allow the worker to continue productive activity. Prohibiting return to work should consider the risk of workplace attendance to the individual. A trial of supervised work activity may be helpful in determining work ability.

References

1. Reed P. Workplace guidelines for disability duration. In: *The Medical Disability Advisor.* 3rd ed. Boulder, Colo: Reed Group Ltd; 2001.

2. Klenerman L, Slade PD, Stanley M, et al. The prediction of chronicity in patients with an acute attack of low back pain in a general practice setting. *Spine.* 1995;20:478–484.

3. Deyo RA. Practice variations, treatment fads, rising disability: do we need a new clinical research paradigm? *Spine.* 1993;18:2153–2162.

4. Deyo RA, Andersson G, Bombardier C, et al. Outcome measures for studying patients with low back pain. *Spine.* 1994;19(suppl):S2032–S2036.

5. Nachemson A. Newest knowledge of low back pain: a critical look. *Clin Orthop.* 1992;279:8–20.

Chapter 16

6. Eaton MW. Obstacles to the vocational rehabilitation of individuals receiving workers' compensation. *J Rehabil.* 1979;45:59–63.

7. Lamb HR, Rogawski AA. Supplemental security income and the sick role. *Am J Psychiatry* 1978;35:1221–1224.

8. McIntosh G, Melles T, Hall H. Guidelines for the identification of barriers to rehabilitation of back injuries. *J Occup Rehabil.* 1995;5:195–201.

9. Duarte J, Sempere AP, Delgado JA, Naranjo G, Sevillano MD, Claveria LE. Headache of recent onset in adults: a prospective population-based study. *Acta Neurol Scand.* 1996;94:67–70.

10. Quality Standards Subcommittee of the American Academy of Neurology. Practice parameter: the utility of neuroimaging in the evaluation of headache in patients with normal neurologic examinations [summary statement]. *Neurology.* 1994;44:1353–1354.

11. Solomom GD, Cady RG, Klapper JA, Ryan RE. National Headache Foundation: standards of care for treating headache in primary care practice. *Cleve Clin J Med.* 1997:64;373–383.

12. Katzman GL, Dagher AP, Patronas NJ. Incidental findings on brain magnetic resonance imaging from 1000 asymptomatic volunteers. *JAMA.* 1999; 282:36–39.

13. Lindgren A, Roijer A, Rudling O, et al. Cerebral lesions on magnetic resonance imaging, heart disease, and vascular risk factors in subjects without stroke: a population-based study. *Stroke.* 1994;25:929–934.

14. Kaniecki R. Headache assessment and management: contempo update. *JAMA.* 2003;289:1430–1433.

15. Warner JS. Posttraumatic headache: a myth? *Arch Neurol.* 2000;57:1778–1780.

16. Couch JR, Bearss C. Chronic daily headache in the posttrauma syndrome: relation to extent of head injury. *Headache.* 2001;41:559–564.

17. Radanov BP, Di Stefano G, Augustiny KF. Symptomatic approach to posttraumatic headache and its possible implications for treatment. *Eur Spine J.* 2001;10:403–407.

18. Haas DC. Chronic post-traumatic headaches classified and compared with natural headaches. *Cephalalgia.* 1996;16:486–493.

19. Mickeviciene D, Schrader H, Surkiene D, Kunicka R, Stovner LJ, Sand T. A historical cohort study on posttraumatic headache outside the medicolegal context. *Cephalgia.* 2001;21:524.

20. Packard RC. Epidemiology and pathogenesis of posttraumatic headache. *J Head Trauma Rehabil.* 1999;14:9–21.

21. Evans RW. The postconcussion syndrome and the sequelae of mild head injury. *Neurol Clin.* 1992;10:815–847.

22. Consensus conference from the National Institutes of Health: rehabilitation of persons with traumatic brain injury. *JAMA.* 1999;282:974–983.

23. Binder LM, Rohling ML. Money matters: a meta-analytic review of the effects of financial incentives on recovery after closed-head injury. *Am J Psychiatry.* 1996;153:7–10.

24. Rosenthal M, Christensen BK, Ross TP. Depression following traumatic brain injury. *Arch Phys Med Rehabil.* 1998;79:90–103.

25. Mittenberg W, DiGiulio DV, Perrin S, Bass AE. Symptoms following mild head injury: expectation as aetiology. *J Neurol Neurosurg Psychiatry.* 1992; 55:200–204.

26. Mooney G, Peed JS. The association between mild traumatic brain injury and psychiatric conditions. *Brain Inj.* 2001;15:865–877.

27. Lipton RB, Stewart WF. Epidemiology and comorbidity of migraine. In: Goadsby PJ, Silberstein SD, eds. *Headache.* Boston, Mass: Butterworth-Heinemann, 1997:75–97.

28. American Psychiatric Association. *Diagnostic and Statistical Manual of Mental Disorders.* 4th ed. Washington, DC: American Psychiatric Association; 2000:739.

29. Rasmussen BK, Jensen R, Schrod M, Olesen J. Epidemiology of headache in a general population: a prevalence study. *J Clin Epidemiol.* 1991;44:1147–1157.

30. Pryse-Phillips WE, Dodick DW, Edmeads JG, et al. Guidelines for the diagnosis and management of migraine in clinical practice. *CMAJ.* 1997;156:1273–1287.

31. Stewart WF. Epidemiology of migraine. *Am J Manage Care.* 1999;5(suppl): S63–S72.

32. Goadsby PJ, Lipton RB, Ferrrari MD. Migraine: current understanding and therapy. *N Engl J Med.* 2002;346:257–270.

33. Kroenke K, Spitzer RL, Williams JB, et al. Physical symptoms in primary care: predictors of psychiatric disorders and functional impairment. *Arch Fam Med.* 1994;9:774–779.

34. Jensen OK, Nielsen FF, Vosmar L. An open study comparing manual therapy with the use of cold packs in the treatment of posttraumatic headaches. *Cephalgia.* 1990;10:241–250.

35. Ferrari MD. Migraine. *Lancet.* 1998;351:1043–1051.

36. Merikangas KR, Dartigues JF, Whitaker A, Angst J. Diagnostic criteria for migraine: a validity study. *Neurology.* 1994;44(suppl 4):Sll.

37. Smetana GW. The diagnostic value of historical features in primary headache syndromes: a comprehensive review. *Arch Intern Med.* 2000;160:2729–2737.

38. Warner JS. Time required for improvement of an analgesic rebound headache. *Headache.* 1998;38:229–230.

39. Hansson L, Smith DHG, Reeves R, Lapuerta P. Headache in mild-to-moderate hypertension and its reduction by irbesartan therapy. *Arch Intern Med.* 2000; 160:1654–1658.

40. Dalrymple J, Appleby J. Cross sectional study of reporting of epileptic seizures to general practitioners. *BMJ.* 2000;320:94–97.

41. Zaidi A, Clough P, Scheepers B, Fitzpatrick A. Treatment resistant epilepsy or convulsive syncope? *BMJ.* 1998;317:869–870.

42. Whitaker JN. The confluence of quality of care, cost-effectiveness, pragmatism, and medical ethics in the diagnosis of nonepileptic seizures: a provocative situation for neurology. *Arch Neurol.* 2001:58;2066–2067.

Chapter 16

43. Van Ness PC. Therapy for the epilepsies. *Arch Neurol.* 2002;59:732–735.

44. Berg AT, Shinnar S. The risk of seizure recurrence following a first unprovoked seizure: a quantitative review. *Neurology.* 1991;41:965–972.

45. King MA, Newton MR, Jackson GD, et al. Epileptology of the first-seizure presentation: a clinical, electroencephalographic, and magnetic resonance imaging study of 300 consecutive patients. *Lancet.* 1998;352:1007–1011.

46. Aminoff MJ. *Electrodiagnosis in Clinical Neurology.* 2nd ed. New York, NY: Churchill Livingstone; 1986.

47. Spudis EV, Penry JK, Gibson P. Driving impairment caused by episodic brain dysfunction. *Arch Neurol.* 1986;43:558–564.

48. Macciocchi SN, Reid DB, Barth JT. Disability following head injury. *Curr Opin Neurol.* 1993;6:773–777.

49. Martelli MF, Grayson RL, Zasler ND. Posttraumatic headache: neuropsychological and psychological effects and treatment implications. *J Head Trauma Rehabil.* 1999;14:49–69.

50. King N. Mild head injury: neuropathology, sequelae, measurement and recovery. *Br J Clin Psychol.* 1997;36:161–184.

51. Beers SR. Cognitive effects of mild head injury in children and adolescents. *Neuropsychol Rev.* 1992;3:281–320.

52. Capruso DX, Levin HS. Cognitive impairment following closed head injury. *Neurol Clin.* 1992;10:879–893.

53. Bohnen N, Jolles J. Neurobehavioral aspects of postconcussive symptoms after mild head injury. *J Nerv Ment Dis.* 1992;180:683–692.

54. Jacobson RR. The post-concussional syndrome: physiogenesis, psychogenesis and malingering: an integrative model. *J Psychosom Res.* 1995;39:675–693.

55. Anderson SD. Postconcussional disorder and loss of consciousness. *Bull Am Acad Psychiatry Law.* 1996;24:493–504.

56. Katz RT, DeLuca J. Sequelae of minor traumatic brain injury. *Am Fam Physician.* 1992;46:1491–1498.

57. Dikmen SS, Machamer JE, Winn HR, et al. Neuropsychological outcome at 1-year post head injury. *Neuropsychology.* 1995;9:80–90.

58. Thornhill S, Teasdale GM, Murray GD, et al. Disability in young people and adults one year after head injury: prospective cohort study. *BMJ.* 2000;320:1631–1635.

59. Graham DI, Adams JH, Nicoll JA, et al. The nature, distribution and causes of traumatic brain injury. *Brain Pathol.* 1995;5:397–406.

60. van der Naalt J, van Zomeren AH, Sluiter WJ, Minderhoud JM. One year outcome in mild to moderate head injury: the predictive value of acute injury characteristics related to complaints and return to work. *J Neurol Neurosurg Psychiatry.* 1999;66:207–213.

61. Mittenberg W, DiGiulio DV, Perrin S, et al. Symptoms following mild head injury: expectation as aetiology. *J Neurol Neurosurg Psychiatry.* 1992;55(3):200–204.

62. Gasquoine PG. Postconcussion symptoms. *Neuropsychol Rev.* 1997;7:77–85.

63. Satz PS, Alfano MS, Light RF, et al. Persistent post-concussive syndrome: a proposed methodology and literature review to determine the effects, if any, of mild head and other bodily injury. *J Clin Exp Neuropsychol.* 1999;21:620–628.

64. Kurztke JF. Rating neurologic impairment in multiple sclerosis: an Expanded Disability Status Scale (EDSS). *Neurology.* 1983;33:144–152.

65. Riahi F, Zijdenbos A, Narayanan S, et al. Improved correlation between scores on the Expanded Disability Status Scale and the cerebral lesion load in relapsing-remitting multiple sclerosis: results of the application of new imaging methods. *Brain.* 1998;121:1305–1312.

Chapter 17

Working With Common Rheumatologic Disorders

Yvonne Smallwood Sherrer, MD

Rheumatologic disorders are a leading cause of work disability in the United States.[1,2] Of 41 million disabled adults, 7.2 million (17%) report "arthritis and rheumatism" as the cause.[3] These disorders represent a wide array of illnesses. Specific rheumatic disorders may affect individuals differently. Some disorders are regional; others are widespread soft-tissue pain syndromes. The more common osteoarthritis (OA) can be monoarticular, oligoarticular, or generalized. Systemic lupus erythematosus (SLE) and rheumatoid arthritis (RA) are systemic disorders, and as such may affect multiple organs. The specific rheumatic disorder and its particular expression will impact on an individual's ability to work.

There has been no uniform approach to work assessment in the rheumatic disorders. Consideration for work disability has generally centered around perceived impressions of the individual's risk for work or presumed capability rather than on measures of true risks or true capacity. The lack of standardized assessments undoubtedly contributes to the documented discordance among physician evaluators when assessing work disability in rheumatic disorders. Liang et al[4] demonstrated only 67% agreement between Social Security administrative evaluating physicians and rheumatologists in determining work disabilities in patients with RA, SLE, and OA. Chart review assessment of residual functional capacity agreed with observed functional capacity testing only 59% of the time, which was not more than expected by chance. For the most part, physicians, generalists, and specialists alike, have been on their own in making work assessments in the rheumatic diseases.

For the patient with severe systemic disease such as SLE, vasculitis, or RA, the issue of work ability and risk may be intuitive and an easy assessment to make. The difficulty centers on the larger percentage of patients who have mild or moderate disease. Typically, the model for working or returning to work in these instances has been physician driven and based on objective disease criteria coupled with patient and/or physician perception of work capacity. This model may not be the most effective because it may not adequately account for the complex interplay between biology and the nonobjective psychosocial issues that factor greatly into decisions to work, commonly considered tolerance.

Nonobjective Factors in Assessing Work Disability

Several nonobjective factors play a major role in assessing work disability in rheumatic diseases:

- **Pain.** Pain is a major contributor to work disability in the rheumatic disorders, as illustrated by Table 17-1. Yet, pain is poorly explained on the basis of biological disease alone. In osteoarthritis, pain correlates poorly with x-rays. Studies of RA have often shown that social issues rank higher than pain as predictors of disability. The emerging science of psychobiology teaches that the expression of pain is multifactorial and is a factor of psychosocial issues as much as biological ones.
- **Fatigue.** Fatigue is ubiquitous among the systemic disorders and also plays a major role in an individual's perception of his or her ability to work (tolerance). Yet, fatigue cannot be explained on the basis of disease severity alone. In some studies, fatigue correlates more with depression than it does with biological factors. In SLE, fatigue correlates strongly with patient-perceived disability, though not necessarily with physician assessment of objective disease activity.

Table 17-1 Predictors of Work Disability in Rheumatoid Arthritis

- Visual Analog Pain Scale
- Work Type (Moderate/Heavy vs Sedentary/Light)
- Sex
- Rheumatoid Factor
- Educational Level (Years)
- Body Mass Index

Adapted from Wolfe and Hawley.[8]

- **Waxing and Waning Course.** Many of the systemic rheumatic disorders are characterized by periods of flare, punctuated by periods of relative disease quiescence, the so-called waxing and waning disease course. Common patterns of disease include (1) ongoing evidence of disease activity around a stable baseline, (2) periods of major disease activity interspersed between periods of relative disease quiescence, of which the frequency and duration vary, and (3) progressive, increasing disease activity. This characterization of disease course patterns is further complicated by the tendency for some individuals' disease course to change character over time. An individual with frequent substantive disease flare-ups may be incapable of meeting work attendance and performance demands, but may wrongly be deemed capable of work if evaluated during a brief quiescent period.
- **Cognitive Difficulties.** Many of the systemic disorders, particularly SLE, have been associated with cognitive factors such as poor executive functioning and memory loss. These difficulties negatively impact on work performance. They may be subtle and often must be specifically evaluated for. Tools exist for such evaluations.
- **Psychological Issues.** Depression and anxiety are common associations with chronic rheumatologic disorders. They impact on the patient's and physician's perceptions of pain, fatigue, and ability to work. Both pain and depression impact on fatigue and functional scores. Affected individuals do not have to be in the highest disease severity categories to have the highest scores for pain and depression.[5] Psychobiological studies have demonstrated improvement in depression and self-esteem in individuals who work vs those who do not. Often successful management of depression and anxiety can expedite an individual's return to work.
- **Work Instability.** Work instability is defined as a mismatch between an individual's functional abilities and job demands.[6] The consequence of work instability is job loss if issues are not addressed expeditiously. This is further complicated by employers who do not want disabled patients to continue in the workplace. Many employers have fears and concerns regarding their liability and costs, as well as patient capability. Often education of the employer will be helpful and may serve to keep the patient in the workplace. Negative impressions of coworkers can affect the self-esteem of the disabled and negatively impact on their desire to work. Evidence suggests that when patients have no control over work activities, pace, or time, they are less likely to successfully remain in the workplace.
- **Socioeconomic Factors.** Work disability is higher among those with lower incomes and lower educational levels. Professionals are less likely to be work disabled than manual workers. Social Security Administration (SSA) disability applications correlate with the economy. As the economy improves, applications diminish.[7] As the economy deteriorates, applications increase.

Chapter 17

Rheumatoid Arthritis

Rheumatoid arthritis is the most common of the systemic rheumatic disorders. It is estimated to affect approximately 1.2% of the US population. Disability occurs early in the disease course and progresses with disease duration, as outlined in Table 17-2.[9-11] A myriad of studies have documented significant income or work loss related to RA.[8,12-17] While in most of these studies work reduction was attributed to the physical impact of arthritis, detailed reasoning for work loss is less clear. There is little, if any, scientific information that systematically assesses the risk to the RA patient relative to the work environment. It stands to reason that individuals with significant RA will have hampered physical responses because of loss of muscle mass (capacity) and loss of joint mobility (capacity). As such, these individuals may be at risk in handling hazardous equipment or very heavy loads. These situations would usually not be difficult to identify and are usually intuitive.

A more difficult task is to determine whether the "work" of the job is a risk to the patient. Typically it has been thought that working might increase risk of flares. There is no scientific evidence to support this conclusion. Rather, recent scientific studies have documented that exercising arthritic joints is

Table 17-2 Work Disability in Rheumatoid Arthritis: Cross-Sectional and Longitudinal Studies

Reference	Type of Study	No. of Patients	Mean Disease Duration (years) at Start/at Review	% Working at Review
Yelin et al[1]	CS	180	10	40
Pincus et al[10]	LO, 9 years	75	11/20	15
Yelin et al[11]	LO, 4 years	306	10/14	50
Callahan et al[18]	CS	175	11	28
Reisine[19]	LO, 5 years	392	9/14	66
DeRoos and Callahan[20]	CS	705	11	64
Sokka and Pincus[21]	CS	127	2	90

CS indicates cross sectional; LO, longitudinal.
Reproduced with permission from Sokka.[22]

safe and effective.[23-25] Fifield et al[5] demonstrated that work loss by itself is associated with high levels of pain and depression at all levels of disease severity. Thus, those who are not working fare worse than those who continue to work.

In that same study, commonly assessed workplace characteristics such as lifting, climbing, stooping, and reaching did not substantially affect the probability of work disability.[5] Rather, work disability correlated with whether an individual was self-employed (10% vs 54% disabled), whether an individual had control (autonomy) within the workplace (27% vs 62% disabled), and whether the individual had control over other work activities (38% vs 52% disabled). This emphasizes the importance of workplace adaptation in the return to work of individuals with RA and suggests that tolerance plays a larger role than capacity in determining who is more likely to stay at work.

There are three main considerations in determining return to work in individuals with RA:

- **Disease Severity.** Work disability becomes more likely as disease severity worsens. Determinants of disease severity involve assessments of current disease activity and prior damage. Current activity can be measured on the basis of the number of swollen tender joints, morning stiffness, and elevation of inflammatory measures. Damage includes evidence of structural loss, which can be assessed by deformities, range of motion, and radiographs. Functional measures are critical in assessing disease severity and correlate with work disability. Many validated functional measures exist. The Stanford Health Assessment Questionnaire (HAQ) is a simple and widely used measurement tool that is easily adapted to the office.[26] One must be careful, however, in overdependence on functional measures above other assessments of disease impact. The HAQ score has been shown to correlate more with pain (subjective) than with joint swelling (objective).[27] It also correlates significantly with fatigue and depression. Thus, the HAQ and other functional measures must be evaluated in the context of the overall clinical picture. When pain and function are not consistent with objective disease parameters, then consideration should be given to psychosocial factors as contributors. Psychosocial factors can best be assessed via a multidisciplinary approach involving psychology or neuropsychology. Such specialists can be very useful in helping the physician determine nonbiological contributors to pain, fatigue, and functional loss. Functional capacity evaluations and standardized musculoskeletal examinations may also be useful in accurately assessing work ability.[4] In the at-risk patient, early aggressive treatment intervention plays an important role in diminishing functional

Chapter 17

loss and work disability. Recent studies have documented the positive effect of early aggressive RA treatment on work disability.[28-30]

- **Psychosocial Factors.** Chorus et al[31] demonstrated that work factors and behavioral coping were important risk factors for work disability. In their study, those who coped with pain by limiting activity were much less likely to be employed (low tolerance due to "fear avoidance"). Of those individuals who limited activities to cope with pain, only 30.9% were working vs 69% of those who did not limit activities to cope with pain. Yelin et al[1] demonstrated that individuals with mild to moderate RA (stages I and II) who were single continued to work, while 58% of those who were married and 48% of those divorced, widowed, or separated were work disabled. In the more severe disease categories (stages III and IV) there was no significant difference in work disability based on marital status. This suggests that as disease severity worsens, biological factors (capacity) play a greater role than social factors (tolerance) in work disability.
- **Vocational Rehabilitation.** Vocational rehabilitation and/or physician involvement with workplace factors will be instrumental in successfully returning the patient to work. Rehabilitation can effectively promote employment in individuals with musculoskeletal impairments, including RA.[32]

In an Alabama study[33] of individuals with arthritis, 64% of those who received vocational rehabilitation services were employed at the completion of the study vs only 8% of those who did not successfully complete the vocational rehabilitation program. Of those who did not successfully complete the program, 62% did not because of failure to cooperate. In the motivated individual, vocational rehabilitation can be very successful.

Generally, vocational rehabilitation is most successful when instituted before long periods of work loss. Nevertheless, Straaton et al[34] demonstrated that a substantial percentage of persons with arthritis and musculoskeletal disorders can be returned to work even after long absences. In 1971, Robinson and Walters[35] documented that 58% of middle-aged men with RA returned to work after intervention. This occurred at a time when it was thought difficult to return middle-aged men to work and when currently effective therapies for RA were not available.

Disability income benefits play an important negative role in return to work. In one study, receiving Social Security disability income was the strongest factor correlating with successful rehabilitation—and it correlated in an inverse fashion.[36] Those receiving disability benefits may not be motivated to return to work. Even so, 55% of those receiving Social Security disability were successfully returned to work.

Addressing the three issues of disease severity, psychosocial factors, and vocational rehabilitation will help the physician get the patient with RA back to work. Expert intervention can be sought as needed to help with managing these issues.

Systemic Lupus Erythematosus

Systemic lupus erythematosus (SLE) affects 15 to 50 persons per 100,000 in the US.[37] Studies have shown that as many as 40% of patients with SLE quit work completely within 3.4 years of diagnosis.[38] Predictors of disability in Partridge and coworkers' study of 159 SLE patients were (in rank order) high school education or less, low insurance status at diagnosis, greater physical strength required for the job, income below the poverty level, and higher disease activity at diagnosis.[38] Cumulative organ damage, sex, and race were not significant predictors of work disability. Disease activity ranked lowest of the five predictors.

The assessment of disease activity may be more difficult in the SLE patient than the RA patient. Typically organ (joint) involvement is obvious in the RA patient, whereas it may be less apparent in the SLE patient with predominantly renal or vascular disease. A number of disease activity scales have been developed to help assess disease activity.[39] They include the Systemic Lupus Erythematosus Disease Activity Index, the Systemic Lupus Activity Measure, the British Isles Lupus Activity Group, and the European Consensus Lupus Activity Measure. All of these scales are composites of multiple organ system activity in SLE. While they may not be practical for everyday office use, they underscore the need to look at the totality of the disease expression in SLE to determine true disease activity. Expert input may be beneficial in determining severity of disease. It is not uncommon for SLE patients to be overtreated or undertreated, and both impact on ability to work.

Ward et al[40] found that depressive symptoms and anxiety parallel patients' self-assessment of disease activity and that physician global activity scores or standardized disease activity measures did not. Fatigue is common in SLE.[41,42] Zonana-Nacach et al[43] showed that it is one of the most prevalent clinical manifestations of SLE across all ethnic groups. Fatigue is a limiting complaint and factors into patient and physician perceptions of functional ability. Causality of fatigue in SLE is multifactorial. Sorting out the contributors to fatigue can be quite complex. There is controversy among experts regarding the relative role of disease severity and psychosocial issues. Bruce et al[44] found that fatigue in SLE correlated with the presence of fibromyalgia, whereas Tayler et al[45] found that disease status was the only predictor of

Chapter 17

fatigue over time. They did find, however, that there was a significant association between fatigue, depression, and helplessness.[45]

Yen et al[46] demonstrated discordance between the patient's assessment of disease activity and the physician's assessment. Twenty-one of patients scored disease activity higher than their physician did. Only 8% of patients scored lower disease activity than their physician did. Discordance between the patient's perception and the physician's assessment of disease activity and functional ability reflects nonbiological psychosocial issues (tolerance). This discordance can often interfere with the patient-physician relationship. It also impacts on the accuracy of work assessment. The multidisciplinary approach can be effective in sorting out the different components of functional ability and help in preserving the patient-physician relationship.

The risk of work factors in significant SLE has not been studied adequately. Many physicians discourage work for SLE patients because of fear that the physical demand might induce a flare. Yet, a study by Ramsey-Goldman and Isenberg[39] in a small cohort of patients with SLE demonstrated that exercise was associated with improvement in fatigue, functional status, muscle strength, and cardiovascular fitness. Moreover, there were no data to suggest increased disease activity or flare-ups because of exercise. This would suggest that the physical demand of light to medium work might not be harmful in the SLE patient. Larger studies need to be accomplished, but the fear of having SLE patients exercise or work may be unfounded.

As with RA, there are three major areas of consideration in assessing the SLE patient for work:

- **Disease Severity.** The totality of current disease activity must be considered. All organ involvement must be taken into account. Prior damage must be a consideration as well. In the SLE patient, both disease activity and damage are essential to an accurate determination of work ability. For instance, the individual with transient postpartum SLE may, several years later, have no parameters of disease activity, but may have been left with significant cardiac damage that renders her unable to work because of poor cardiac function. Conversely, the individual with prior severe SLE who is left with only mild renal insufficiency, but has no other disease activity, may be able to resume full work. Expert input may be useful at this juncture. Disease pattern must also be considered. The patient with frequent flares may be incapable of meeting the demands of the workplace on an ongoing basis.
- **Psychosocial Factors.** Depression and anxiety can play a major role in fatigue and perception of functional ability in patients with SLE (tolerance). If there is a significant discrepancy between objective disease

activity parameters and the patient's perception of ability, then referral
for neuropsychological evaluation might be appropriate. Such evaluations are also helpful in identifying subtle cognitive deficits that reduce
executive functioning and hinder work ability.
- **Workplace Accommodation.** Physicians should help patients remain
  working by making the appropriate recommendations for adaptations and
  limitations at the workplace. Here, consultation with a vocational rehabilitation specialist can be useful.

Osteoarthritis

Osteoarthritis is the most common chronic disease in the US. It affects
nearly 20 million individuals. Its incidence increases with age. In a study of
Olmsted County (Minnesota) residents, 39,979 adults over age 35 years
were evaluated.[47] The average age of the 7889 individuals with OA was 67.3
years vs 51.5 years in the 25,893 individuals who served as controls.

In this same study, 10.5% of respondents with OA vs 1.7% of nonarthritis
respondents reported a reduction in work hours related to illness. Inability
to work due to illness (capacity) was reported by 9.4% of respondents
with OA vs 5.2% of nonarthritis respondents, and 13.7% of respondents
with OA vs 3.4% of nonarthritis respondents retired early because of pain
(tolerance). Thus, OA has a major impact on the individual's ability and
willingness to work.

Osteoarthritis is heterogeneous. The disease may be oligoarticular, monoarticular, or generalized. Typically, the individual with generalized disease is
most affected. The OA patient complains of pain that worsens with use. The
location of pain will vary depending on the joints affected. The hip, knee,
and small joints of the hands are the most common joints involved in OA.
In advanced disease there is significant cartilage loss leading to joint space
narrowing, osteophytes, loss of joint motion, and associated decreased
muscle mass.

A number of studies have documented a growing association between OA
and occupation. Rossignol et al[48] looked at a cohort of 10,412 patients
with symptomatic OA who were assessed for functional and work limitations. This study showed that the prevalence of OA in men aged 20 to 59
years across all occupations was 0.4 compared to 0.3, 0.7, and 0.4 in the
white collar group, agriculture group, and blue collar group, respectively.
The agricultural group clearly had a trend to more OA. This was even
more striking in women. In the 20- to 59-year age group, the prevalence
of OA in women was 0.3 across all occupations compared to 0.1, 1.0, and
0.2 in the white collar, agricultural, and blue collar occupational groups.

Chapter 17

The prevalence of OA in women who did agricultural work was ten times that of those who did only white collar work. These data clearly suggest that blue collar work does not pose a risk to workers.

Pope et al[49] demonstrated that hip arthritis may be related to cumulative workplace mechanical loads. They demonstrated that hip pain correlated with occupational prolonged standing (longer than two hours) for many years, occupational sitting (longer than two hours) for long periods, lifting more than 50 lb for many years, jumping between different levels, and walking more than two miles per day on rough ground for many years. Since the vast majority of jobs require either standing for more than two hours or sitting for more than two hours, the significance of this association is problematic. Vingard et al[50] also showed an association of work-related physical demand and the development of OA of the hip in women aged 50 to 70 years. High exposure to jumping, significant stairs, heavy lifting, and physically demanding tasks was associated with hip OA, with relative risks of 2.1, 2.1, 1.5, and 2.3, respectively.

Since these studies are observational and not prospective cohort studies, they can only generate hypotheses for testing in prospective studies. They cannot be used as proof of causation. Physicians should remember the epidemiologic "rule of thumb" that if observational studies show a relative risk of 3 or less, prospective controlled studies rarely find a causal association. The apparent risk is usually attributable to biases.[51]

The paradox of OA is that, in general, those who develop it in the hips usually do not develop it in the knees, those who develop it in the knees usually do not develop it in the hips, and neither group develops OA in the ankles, even though all three joints carry the same body weight the same number of steps. Reflecting on this fact and after reviewing multiple scientific studies, Hadler[52] concluded that there probably is a role for joint usage in OA, but it is neither necessary or sufficient, and it is probably minor. While most individuals have OA of either the hip or the knee, 10% to 20% will have both. Many of these individuals have generalized OA, which would support a genetic or hereditary causation but would not preclude an occupational impact. While the associations between occupation and OA of the hip have been weak, they have been consistently positive. Associations have been somewhat stronger for the knee. In men, certain job-related activities may account for as much knee OA as obesity, as discovered in the National Health and Nutrition Examination Survey (NHANES I) Study.[53] Further, there are certain occupations with higher rates of OA of the hip (farmers) and knee (miners). There are other accepted explanations as to why the ankle and other joints seem to be spared high incidences of OA despite physical stresses similar to those of affected joints. One is that spared joints such as the ankle are more resistant to OA-inducing stresses.[54] Therefore, the impact of joint usage for OA is variable, complex, and not currently quantifiable.

The limiting factor in most OA patients' ability to work is pain (tolerance). A number of studies have documented the beneficial impact of exercise in reducing pain and functional limitation in individuals with OA of the knee and hip. Fransen et al[55] documented the ability of land-based exercises to reduce pain and improve function in OA of the knee. Exercise to keep joint mobility and muscle strength is now routinely prescribed by rheumatologists for mild and moderate OA. Work activity may be the major source of exercise for many individuals.

As with other diseases, the causes of pain in OA are multifactorial and not limited to biological factors.[56] There is often discordance between radiologic findings and the severity of pain. In an individual with mild to moderate disease, whose pain seems to be disproportionate to physical and radiographic findings, it may be appropriate to get multidisciplinary input in identifying factors driving pain.

In individuals with end-stage disease, it may be necessary to recommend reconstructive surgery to get them back to work.

Risk

There is no clear scientific literature to indicate that working despite arthritis poses a risk. Exercise is therapeutic and is prescribed as treatment by rheumatologists for patients with arthritis.

Highly repetitive hand work might hasten tendon rupture in patients with active synovitis about forearm and hand tendons (RA or SLE). This might be a reason for physician-imposed work restrictions (based on risk) until more aggressive treatment of the disease "quiets down" the synovitis.

Osteoporosis is common in RA and SLE, but is uncommon in OA. Osteoporosis can be documented objectively (dual photon scans, quantitative computed tomography, and so on). If significant osteoporosis is present from inactivity and corticosteroid treatment, work involving heavy lifting and carrying, jumping, or activities with above-average risk of falls may need to be proscribed by physician-imposed restrictions (based on fracture risk).

Similarly, if lower limb total joint replacement has occurred, the individual should be limited to light or light-moderate work to prevent loosening of prosthetic joints, especially if they are implanted in osteoporotic bone.

Chapter 17

If prolonged knee effusions and articular cartilage loss have combined to produce knee instability on ligamentous testing, physicians usually restrict the individual to sedentary work (work done sitting, with standing and walking limited to one hour or less per day, lifting and carrying limited to 10 lb or less).

If C1-C2 instability is present on cervical spine flexion-extension roentgenograms, major physical activity restrictions or work prohibition may be necessary until surgical stabilization.

Capacity

Patients with RA and SLE may have significant work limitations that need to be documented by physicians. These patients are frequently anemic and deconditioned, and thus have a decreased capacity for aerobic or endurance exercise that can be documented on treadmill testing. As discussed in Chapter 15, a person generally has the capacity to perform sustained work (eight-hour work day with typical breaks) to at least 40% of his or her maximal metabolic equivalent (MET) level. He or she could also be expected to perform for 15-minute intervals, once or twice a day, at 80% of the maximal MET level. Similarly, extra-articular disease (for example, rheumatoid lung disease) may limit exercise capacity.

Loss of motion in joints may limit ability. If shoulder and/or elbow disease prevents the individual from reaching overhead, the use of overhead controls on a factory press is not possible (work limitation). Significant hand synovitis may limit grip strength, pinch strength, hand opening, and/or hand closing to a degree that prevents many hand activities.

Tolerance

Tolerance for the pain and fatigue of arthritis may be the only factors apparently explaining work absence. If a physician cannot postulate an issue of risk or capacity, then the issue is tolerance, which is not scientifically measurable. As long as Western society makes disability decisions by using a strictly biomedical model for disability, patients will be expected to work and physicians will be expected to certify work ability when tolerance for symptoms like pain and fatigue is not accompanied by objective evidence of severe disease. While some physicians may opine that a patient with pain or fatigue and only mild or moderate arthritis is unable to work, other physicians will certify that this patient is able to work. Since both groups of physicians are stating opinion about unmeasurable tolerance, and yet both may be perceived by third parties as giving medical opinions that should be based on sound science, physicians will be perceived as being biased and their testimony "paid for." If physicians certify disability only on the basis of tolerance accompanied by severe disease (the SSA criteria, for example), it is likely that they will usually agree on the work ability of patients.

Summary

Rheumatologic disorders are varied, but they uniformly have a negative impact on work. Emerging data suggest that the majority of patients with rheumatic disease can continue to work within certain parameters. These include aggressive disease activity and pain control. They also include assessing for work instability and making the appropriate adaptations in the work environment or workplace. This assessment should be done early, before long-term work loss occurs. This approach is likely to be successful in keeping most patients with rheumatic disease working.

References

1. Yelin E, Meenan R, Nevitt M, Epstein W. Work disability and rheumatoid arthritis: effects of disease, social and work factors. *Ann Intern Med.* 1980;93:551–556.

2. Straaton KV, Maisiak R, Rigley JM, Johnson P, Fine PR. Variants to return to work among persons unemployed due to arthritis and musculoskeletal disorders. *Arthritis Rheum.* 1996;39:101–109.

3. Prevalence of disabilities and associated health conditions among adults—United States, 1999. *MMWR.* 2001;50:120–125.

4. Liang MH, Daltroy LH, Larson MG, et al. Evaluation of Social Security disability in claimants with rheumatic disease. *Ann Intern Med.* 1991;115:26–31.

5. Fifield J, Reisine ST, Grady K. Work disability and the experience of pain and depression in rheumatoid arthritis. *Soc Sci Med.* 1991;33:579–585.

6. Gilworth G, Chamberlain MA, Harvey A, et al. Development of a work instability scale for rheumatoid arthritis. *Arthritis Care Res.* 2003;49:349–354.

7. Allaire SH. Personal communication, May 2004.

8. Wolfe F, Hawley D. The long-term outcomes of rheumatoid arthritis: work disability: a prospective 18 year study of 823 patients. *J Rheumatol.* 1998;25: 2108–2117.

9. Sherrer YS, Bloch DA, Mitchell DM, Young DY, Fries JF. The development of disability in rheumatoid arthritis. *Arthritis Rheum.* 1986;29:494–500.

10. Pincus T, Callahan L, Sale WG, et al. Severe functional declines, work disability, and increased mortality in 75 rheumatoid arthritis patients studied over 9 years. *Arthritis Rheum.* 1984;27:864–872.

Chapter 17

11. Yelin E, Hinke C, Epstein W. The work dynamics of a person with rheumatoid arthritis. *Arthritis Rheum.* 1987;30:507–512.

12. Mitchell JM, Burkhauser RV, Pincus T. The importance of age, education, and comorbidity and the substantial earnings losses of individuals with symmetric polyarthritis. *Arthritis Rheum.* 1988;31:348–357.

13. Callahan LS. The burden of rheumatoid arthritis: facts and figures. *J Rheumatol.* 1998;25(suppl 53):8–12.

14. Doeglas D, Suurmeijer T, Korol B, Sanderman R, Van Leeuwen M, Van Rijswijk M. Work disability in early rheumatoid arthritis. *Ann Rheum Dis.* 1995;54:455–460.

15. Sokka T, Kautiainen H, Mottonen T, Hannonen T. Work disability in rheumatoid arthritis 10 years after the diagnosis. *J Rheumatol.* 1999;26:1685.

16. Van Jaarsveld CHM, Jacobs JWG, Schrijvers AJP, Van Albada-Kuipers GA, Hofman DM, Bijlsma JWG. The effects of rheumatoid arthritis on employment and social participation during the first years of disease in the Netherlands. *Br J Rheumatol.* 1998;37:848–853.

17. Minaur MJ, Jacoby RK, Cosh JA, Taylor G, Rasker JJ. Outcome after 40 years with rheumatoid arthritis: a perspective study of function, disease activity, and mortality. *J Rheumatol.* 2004;31(suppl 69):3–8.

18. Callahan LF, Bloch DA, Pincus T. Identification of work disability in rheumatoid arthritis: physical, radiographic and laboratory variables do not add explanatory power to demographic and functional variables. *J Clin Epidemiol.* 1992;45:127–138.

19. Reisine S, McQuillan J, Fifield J. Predictors of work disability in rheumatoid arthritis patients. A five-year followup. *Arthritis Rheum.* 1995;38:1630–1637.

20. DeRoos AJ, Callahan LF. Differences by sex in correlates of work status in rheumatoid arthritis patients. *Arthritis Care Res.* 1999;12:381–391.

21. Sokka T, Pincus T. Markers for work disability in rheumatoid arthritis. *J Rheumatol.* 2001;28:1718–1722.

22. Sokka T. Work disability in early rheumatoid arthritis. *Clin Exp Rheumatol.* 2003;21(suppl 31):S71–S74.

23. Hakkinen A, Sokka T, Lietsalmi A, Kautiainen H, Hannonen P. Effects of dynamic strength training on physical function, Valpar 9 work sample test, and working capacity in patients with recent-onset rheumatoid arthritis. *Arthritis Care Res.* 2003;49:71–77.

24. Hakkinen A. Effectiveness and safety of strength training in rheumatoid arthritis. *Curr Opin Rheum.* 2004;16:132–137.

25. de Jong Z, Munneke M, Zwinderman AH, et al. Is a long-term high-intensity exercise program effective and safe in patients with rheumatoid arthritis? Results of a randomized controlled trial. *Arthritis Rheum.* 2003;48:2415–2424.

26. Bruce B, Fries JF. The Stanford Health Assessment Questionnaire: a review of its history, issues, progress and documentation. *J Rheumatol.* 2003;30:167–178.

27. Koh ET, Seow A, Pong LY, et al. Cross cultural adaptation and validation of the Chinese Health Assessment Questionnaire for use in rheumatoid arthritis. *J Rheumatol.* 1998;25:1705–1708.

28. Yelin E, Trupin L, Kats P, Lubeck D, Rush S, Wanke L. Association between Etanercept use and employment outcomes among patients with rheumatoid arthritis. *Arthritis Rheum.* 2003;48:3046–3054.

29. Strand V, Tugwell P, Bombardier C, et al. Function in health related quality of life: results from a randomized controlled trial of Leflunomide v. methotrexate or placebo in patients with active rheumatoid arthritis. *Arthritis Rheum.* 1999; 42:1870–1878.

30. Puolakka K, Kautiainen H, Mottonen T, et al. Impact of initial aggressive drug treatment with a combination of disease-modifying antirheumatic drugs on a development of work disability in rheumatoid arthritis: a five year randomized follow-up trial. *Arthritis Rheum.* 2004;50:55–62.

31. Chorus AMJ, Miedema HS, Wevers CWJ, van der Linden S. Work factors and behavioural coping in relation to withdrawal from the labour force in patients with rheumatoid arthritis. *Ann Rheum Dis.* 2001;60:1025–1032.

32. Schmidt SJ, Ort-Marburger D, Meijman TS. Employment after rehabilitation for musculoskeletal impairments: the impact of vocational rehabilitation and working on a trial basis. *Arch Phys Med Rehabil.* 1995;76:950–954.

33. Straaton KV, Harvey M, Maisiak R. Factors associated with successful vocational rehabilitation in persons with arthritis. *Arthritis Rheum.* 1992;35:503–510.

34. Straaton KV, Maisiak R, Wrigley JM, White MB, Johnson P, Fine PR. Barriers to return to work among persons unemployed due to arthritis and musculoskeletal disorders. *Arthritis Rheum.* 1996;39:101–109.

35. Robinson HS, Walters K. Return to work after treatment of rheumatoid arthritis. *CMAJ.* 1971;105:166–169.

36. Straaton K, Maisiak R, Wrigley MN, Fine PR. Musculoskeletal disability, employment and rehabilitation. *J Rheumatol.* 1995;22:505–513.

37. WebMD Health. Classification of lupus erythematosus. Available at: http://my.webmd.com/hw/health_guide_atoz/tn8151.asp. Accessed November 3, 2004.

38. Partridge AJ, Karlson EW, Daltroy LH, et al. Risk factors for early work disability in systemic lupus erythematosus. *Arthritis Rheum.* 1997;40:2199–2206.

39. Ramsey-Goldman R, Isenberg DA. Systemic lupus erythematosus measures. *Arthritis Care Res.* 2003;49(suppl):S225–S233.

40. Ward MM, Marx AS, Barry NN. Psychological distress and changes in the activity of systemic lupus erythematosus. *Rheumatology.* 2002;41:184–188.

41. Omdal R, Mellgren SI, Koldingsnes W, Jacobsen EA, Husby G. Fatigue in patients with systemic lupus erythematosus: lack of associations to serum cytokines, antiphospholipid antibodies, or other disease characteristics. *J Rheumatol.* 2002;29:482–486.

42. Tench CM, McCurdi I, White PD, D'Cruz DP. The prevalence of fatigue in systemic lupus erythematosus. *Rheumatology.* 2000;39:1249–1254.

43. Zonana-Nacach A, Roseman JM, McGwin G, et al. Systemic lupus erythematosus in three ethnic groups, VI: factors associated with fatigue within 5 years of criteria diagnosis. *Lupus.* 2000;9:101–109.

Chapter 17

44. Bruce IN, Mak VC, Hallett DC, Gladman DD, Urowitz MB. Factors associated with fatigue in patients with systemic lupus erythematosus. *Ann Rheum Dis.* 1999;58:379–381.

45. Tayler WG, Nicassio PM, Weisman MH, Schuman C, Daly J. Disease status predicts fatigue in systemic lupus erythematosus. *J Rheumatol.* 2001; 28:1999–2007.

46. Yen JM, Abrahamowicz M, Dobkin PL, Clarke AE, Battista RN, Fortin PR. Determinants of discordance between patients and physicians in their assessment of lupus disease activity. *J Rheumatol.* 2003;30:1967–1976.

47. Gabriel SE, Crowson CS, O'Fallon WM. Cost of osteoarthritis: estimates from a geographically defined population. *J Rheumatol.* 1995;22(suppl 43):23–25.

48. Rossignol M, Leclerc A, Hilliquin P, et al. Primary osteoarthritis and occupations: a national cross sectional survey of 10,412 symptomatic patients. *Occup Environ Med.* 2003;60:882–886.

49. Pope DP, Hunt IM, Birrell SN, Silman AJ, MacFarland GJ. Hip pain onset in relation to cumulative workplace and leisure time mechanical load: a population based case-control study. *Ann Rheum Dis.* 2003;62:322–326.

50. Vingard E, Alfredsson L, Malchau H. Osteoarthrosis of the hip in women and its relation to physical load at work and in the home. *Ann Rheum Dis.* 1997; 56:293–298.

51. Cocchiarella L, Lord S. *Master the AMA Guides Fifth: A Medical and Legal Transition to the Guides to the Evaluation of Permanent Impairment, Fifth Edition.* Chicago, Ill: AMA Press; 2001.

52. Hadler NM. *Occupational Musculoskeletal Disorders.* 2nd ed. Philadelphia, Pa: Lippincott Williams & Wilkins; 1999.

53. Anderson JJ, Felson DT. Factors associated with osteoarthritis of the knee in the First National Health and Nutrition Examination Survey (NHANES1): evidence for an association with overweight, race, and physical demands of work. *Am J Epidemiol.* 1988;128:179–189.

54. Eger W, Schumacher BL, Mollenhauser J. Human knee and ankle cartilage explants: catabolic differences. *J Orthop Res.* 2002;20:526–534.

55. Fransen M, McConnell, Bell M. Therapeutic exercise for people with osteoarthritis of the hip: a systematic review. *J Rheumatol.* 2002;29:1737–1745.

56. Nahit ES, Hunt IM, Lunt M, Dunn G, Silman AJ, MacFarland GJ. Effects of psychosocial and individual psychological factors on the onset of musculoskeletal pain: common and site specific effects. *Ann Rheum Dis.* 2003;62:755–760.

Chapter 17

Chapter 18

Working With Common Psychiatric Problems

John D. Pro, MD

An employee witnessed a coworker die as a forklift raised him to the ceiling, crushing the worker's skull. Afterward, the employee developed intrusive recollections of the event, frequent dreams of the event, insomnia, depression, withdrawal, and an intense fear of machinery. He also had a history of exposure to violence as a child. When he was unable to perform his duties at work, he was seen by his primary care physician. How does a physician approach this patient, who has post-traumatic stress disorder and cannot function at work? How can a primary care physician decide how long the patient needs to be off work, what treatment he needs, and when he will be ready to return to work? This chapter focuses on the process of making those decisions.

For Further Reference

The primary care physician is referred to the *AMA Guides to the Evaluation of Permanent Impairment, Fifth Edition*,[1] Chapters 1, 2, and 14, to understand the psychiatric impairment rating system and to the *Diagnostic and Statistical Manual of Mental Disorders, Fourth Edition* (DSM-IV),[2] which provides diagnostic criteria for psychiatric illnesses. An excellent basic review of psychiatry is *Psychiatry for Primary Care Physicians*.[3]

The Problem of Mental Illness in the Workplace

Mental illness is a significant cause of disability in the workplace. Individuals who have job-related physical injuries or psychological job stress often develop psychiatric problems necessitating treatment. Violence in the workplace also has become a reason for concern among employers, employees, and providers alike. For all of these reasons, it is important to understand principles of psychiatric diagnosis and how psychiatric illnesses cause functional impairment in the workplace. Often these illnesses require absence from work for evaluation and treatment.

Using depression as an example, the total cost of lost production time due to depressive disorders in the US workforce has been estimated at $21.4 billion for major depression, $12.8 billion for dysthymia (mild chronic depression), and $9.8 billion for partially remitted major depression. The average loss of productive time from major depression is estimated at 8.4 hours per week. This phenomenon, "presenteeism," or lack of productivity while at work, is much more of a problem than absenteeism from work in individuals who are depressed. More than 80% of the lost productive time costs are explained by reduced performance while at work.[4] It has been noted among patients who had major depression during the past 12 months that this group lost 35.2 days compared to an average of 15 days for patients with most chronic medical conditions.[5]

Clearly, depression and other mental illnesses are a frequent cause of inability to work, and it is important for the examining physician to understand how mental illness causes impairment and the inability to work. It is equally important to initiate treatment so that the patient can resume productive work as soon as possible and achieve full remission of the psychiatric illness. For most people, working is a source of self-esteem, structure, and social support. For these patients, working can be therapeutic once the burden of their symptoms is lifted.

Evaluating Mental Impairment

Understanding How Symptoms Interfere With Functioning

The first step in establishing whether someone has a psychological impairment is understanding how the symptoms interfere with functioning. This requires taking a careful psychiatric history. The history should include a thorough assessment of the person's activities of daily living, social functioning, concentration, ability to tolerate stress, and whether the individual has deteriorated psychologically in any sort of work-like setting. Many psychiatric patients, especially those who are depressed, or severely anxious, lose interest in recreation and pleasure, self-care, and reading and other hobbies. Sleep is commonly disturbed in psychiatric patients, and a thorough assessment of a person's sleep pattern is important. Virtually any number of activities of daily living may be affected by psychiatric illness, and it is important to review them all with the patient. Common activities of daily living are listed in Table 18-1.

Assessing the person's social functioning is also important in understanding whether he or she can work. Social functioning includes the ability to interact and communicate with others, to function in social situations, and to be responsive to authority. Many psychiatric patients are unable to initiate or sustain social contact because they are withdrawn, irritable, paranoid, or apathetic.

Reviewing the person's concentration, persistence, ability to keep up a pace, and memory functioning is also an important part of understanding his or her ability to work. Concentration is the ability to sustain attention long enough to complete a task in a work-like setting, and the ability to remember details or instructions long enough to perform a task. A person with severe anxiety, depression, or psychosis can suffer significant impairment in concentration, persistence, and pace.

Finally, assessing stress tolerance determines whether one can adapt to work. Attending meetings or conducting personal business affairs at home are examples of work-like situations. A person who deteriorates in a work-like setting will have an escalation of problems concentrating, maintaining social functioning, and/or maintaining activities of daily living adequately.

This history should also include the date that the person was unable to work and the reasons that he or she stopped working. An assessment of

Table 18-1 Activities of Daily Living

Activity	Example
Self-care, Personal Hygiene	Urinating, defecating, brushing teeth, combing hair, bathing, dressing oneself, eating
Communication	Writing, typing, seeing, hearing, speaking, reading
Physical Activity	Standing, sitting, reclining, walking, climbing stairs
Sensory Function	Hearing, seeing, tactile feeling, tasting, smelling
Nonspecialized Hand Activities	Grasping, lifting, tactile discrimination
Travel	Riding, driving, flying
Sexual Function	Orgasm, ejaculation, lubrication, erection
Sleep	Restful, nocturnal sleep pattern

Chapter 18

Adapted from Cocchiarella and Andersson.[1]

any stressors (work related and non–work related) at the time of the illness or accident and information regarding attempts to return to work, current psychiatric treatment, psychiatric medications, and substance abuse is necessary.

Mental Status Examination

The next step in assessing the psychiatric patient's ability to work includes performing a physical examination and a mental status examination. This should include assessment of vital signs and evaluation for tremors, gait disturbance, dyskinetic movements, or any unilateral sensory loss or weakness. Posture, gait, and speech patterns should also be assessed. Visual field assessment is a good measure of temporal lobe functioning in anyone with complaints of memory loss or concentration. The mental status examination also includes general observations about the patient's dress, grooming, general attitude, and cooperativeness. Any pain behaviors present are noted. Documenting the presence of anger, persecution and obtaining revenge, and homicidal thoughts is important in patients who are blaming others for their problems. Asking about hope for improvement and suicidal thoughts is necessary as well in depressed patients. Determining the presence of delusions and hallucinations establishes the diagnosis of psychosis.

How the person feels subjectively should be assessed, and whether his or her affect is dramatic, despondent, angry, anxious, or flat should be noted. The individual's cognitive status can be evaluated by assessing orientation, recent and past memory, abstractions, calculations, and general fund of knowledge, attention, concentration, and alertness. The Mini Mental State Examination and serial-7 tests are particularly useful bedside tests for cognition and concentration.

After the psychiatric history and mental status examination are performed, the primary care physician can be confident in making a general statement about the person's psychiatric diagnosis, need for treatment, and level of impairment present in activities of daily living, social functioning, concentration, and work stress tolerance. *It is the psychiatric symptoms that influence one's functioning rather than the psychiatric diagnosis alone.* For example, the hallucinations of a schizophrenic patient or the panic attacks of an anxious patient can cause the inability to leave one's house, leading to a significant restriction in the activities of daily living in both patients.

Table 18-2 lists the psychiatric rating system used to determine psychiatric impairment taken from the *Guides to the Evaluation of Permanent Impairment, Fifth Edition*.[1] This system is useful in deciding when to take someone off work and when to return him or her to work.

Table 18-2 Classes of Impairment Due to Mental and Behavioral Disorders

Area or Aspect of Functioning	Class 1: No Impairment	Class 2: Mild Impairment	Class 3: Moderate Impairment	Class 4: Marked Impairment	Class 5: Extreme Impairment
Activities of Daily Living; Social Functioning; Concentration; Adaptation	None noted	Impairment levels are compatible with most useful functioning	Impairment levels are compatible with some but not all useful functioning	Impairment levels significantly impede useful functioning	Impairment levels preclude useful functioning

Adapted from Cocchiarella and Andersson.[1]

Social Security Administration's Criteria for Total Disability

Common to the Social Security Administration's (SSA's) extensive discussion of mental illness and total disability is the requirement that the mental condition persist despite treatment for at least 12 months at a level that produces at least two of the following:

1. marked restriction of activities of daily living,
2. marked difficulties in maintaining social functioning,
3. marked difficulties in maintaining concentration, persistence, or pace, and
4. repeated episodes of decompensation, each of extended duration[6]

If the mental impairment does not meet these severity criteria, the individual is capable of being gainfully employed, but perhaps not in the premorbid occupation.

Moderate or marked impairment in work ability without concomitant at least moderate impairment in other areas of mental function rarely occurs. For example, a patient who becomes more anxious at work because she has to leave her ailing mother during the day is neither impaired nor "sick." Rather this person should apply for Family and Medical Leave Act benefits as opposed to disability benefits. True psychological impairment is never confined exclusively to the boundaries of work, and it affects other areas of the person's life besides work. People whose condition deteriorates in a work-like setting by definition also have dysfunction outside of the workplace.

Chapter 18

Criteria for Disability for Specific Jobs

Certain psychiatric conditions preclude the return to certain jobs for the following reasons:

- **Risk Assessment:** Paranoid schizophrenia and delusional disorders would be rational reasons for permanent disqualification from safety-sensitive jobs like police work or any job that provides access to weapons or classified information. Similarly, commercial driving and airplane piloting would be precluded by the Department of Transportation regulations. Other jobs where other people depend on the performance of the patient, so called safety-sensitive jobs, would also be prohibited with these disorders.

  Individuals expressing homicidal ideation, if directed toward coworkers, should not return to that workplace. These situations may require consideration of psychiatric hospitalization and warning of intended victims. The "Tarasoff duty to warn" preempts patient consent to release medical information. Most states provide for this as an exception to physician-patient and psychiatrist-patient confidentiality.

  Pedophilia and antisocial behavior would usually preclude return to work for teachers, guidance counselors, or coaches. Individuals with these disorders can work, but they require supervised structured jobs and ongoing treatment.

- **Capacity Assessment:** Individuals with psychotic disorders may have permanent moderate or severe impairment of mental functioning as defined by the AMA *Guides* (mentioned above). If this level of impairment persists despite treatment, employment options are still possible but limited to structured, supervised work. This would be an example of work limitation base on impaired capacity.

- **Tolerance Assessment:** Many psychiatric patients with severe symptoms cannot tolerate the stress of work. Other patients with only mild symptoms, however, may complain that they are "not able" to do their job, but simply because they do not like their job. Dislike of one's job is not a legitimate reason for disability. In these cases, a physician may decline to certify the patient's disability by saying:

  You do not appear to meet the Social Security Administration's criteria for total disability. Because there is no medical evidence that you are at high risk of significant harm by working, I cannot certify that you are disabled for this job. There is no basis for work restrictions based on risk. Whether the rewards of working are sufficient for you to choose to remain at work, or whether the [fill in symptoms] you feel are sufficient for you to choose a different type of work, or not to work at all, is a question only you can answer.

I can record what you feel to be your current activity intolerances, but these are not work restrictions or work limitations. Your intolerances are not scientifically measurable and they may change in the future, depending on how actively you participate in your treatment.

Major Depression

Major depression is one of the most common illnesses in individuals who present with psychiatric impairment, and who may need to be taken off of work temporarily. Major depression is often a complication of physical illness or injury and is comorbid with a wide variety of other psychiatric illnesses, particularly anxiety disorders and substance abuse.

Major depression imposes a heavy disability burden, and the loss of function caused by depression is often much greater than the dysfunction caused by physical illnesses, including hypertension, diabetes, and arthritis. Depression is also comorbid with a number of general medical conditions, including dementia and other neurodegenerative diseases, coronary artery disease, cancer, diabetes, fibromyalgia, chronic fatigue syndrome, rheumatoid arthritis, and migraine headaches, as well as human immunodeficiency virus infection. A careful workup for underlying medical illnesses is important. It is important to diagnose and treat depression promptly and aggressively because approximately 2% to 9% of patients with depression commit suicide,[7] and a large number have premature mortality and increased morbidity from their depression. Central to the diagnosis is depressed mood, lack of pleasure, or loss of interest. Other symptoms include fatigue, withdrawal, pain, poor concentration and memory, appetite and sleep disturbance, and irritability. All of these symptoms can cause impairment in activities of daily living, social functioning, concentration, persistence, and pace. If this dysfunction is great enough, then the person may need to be taken off work temporarily.

Risk

If a patient is seriously suicidal, and if work is thought to be a psychosocial stressor, work restriction based on risk is indicated. Serious suicidal ideation usually requires inpatient treatment.

Capacity

When major depression produces moderate or severe impairment, the patient may well lack the capacity to be productive at work. Impaired cognition and judgment, psychomotor retardation, and sleep deprivation all impair productivity. When antidepressant medication is started, these patients need to be monitored closely as the dose is increased. If major improvement does not occur in 3 to 4 weeks or there are significant side effects, and a depressed

Chapter 18

patient is still at least moderately impaired, referral to a psychiatrist is usually indicated.

Tolerance

Depression is common, and most individuals with mild impairment from depression can work without difficulty. A brief time out of work, generally no longer than 1 week, may be appropriate to permit adaptation to the side effects of initiating antidepressant medication. For those who do not wish to work and who have only mild impairment, physicians should decline to certify disability, saying:

> You do not appear to meet the Social Security Administration's criteria for total disability. Because there is no medical evidence that you are at high risk of significant harm by working, I cannot certify that you are disabled for this job. There is no basis for work restrictions based on risk. Whether the rewards of working are sufficient for you to choose to remain at work, or whether the [fill in symptoms] you feel are sufficient for you to choose a different type of work, or not to work at all, is a question only you can answer. I can record what you feel to be your current activity intolerances, but these are not work restrictions or work limitations. Your intolerances are not scientifically measurable and they may change in the future, depending on how actively you participate in your treatment.

Pain Syndrome With Medical and Psychological Factors

Many patients have severe pain in the absence of objective findings to explain the pain. These patients are well known to physicians. They present with chronic back and/or neck pain, headaches, temporomandibular joint pain, atypical facial pain, chronic pelvic pain, and other nonspecific pain syndromes.[3] There is often some basis for pain, for example, age-appropriate degenerative changes on imaging studies, but these findings are insufficient to explain the degree of dysfunction.[3]

Many of these patients suffer from a pain syndrome with medical and psychological factors. This syndrome is the most common somatoform disorder, and it occurs when pain becomes the predominant focus for clinical attention and is severe enough to warrant clinical treatment and attention. Psychological factors are judged to have an important role in the onset and maintenance of the pain. Patients with pain disorder have enhanced pain perception and lower pain tolerance. As mentioned above, if they have tissue damage, the pain experienced is disproportionate to the tissue damage based on the experience of the examiners. Many pain patients often have distorted beliefs about their pain and have a disability conviction that often makes it difficult to return them to work. These individuals often have other comorbid psychiatric problems, especially major depression, and often have a history of sexual or physical abuse or neglect in childhood or adolescence. Many have been working since childhood and/or have been given adult responsibilities prematurely.

Fatigue, pain intensity, sleep disorders, self-preoccupation and anxiety, and medication side effects can affect the person's activities of daily living, social functioning, concentration, and ability to keep up the pace at work. The decision to take a patient with chronic pain syndrome out of work temporarily follows a diagnosis and thorough assessment of how the patient's symptoms create impairment on the job.

Risk
Patients with this diagnosis have a medical condition that is painful (eg, osteoarthritis) and yet the pain seems to medical providers to be out of proportion to the objective findings. Psychologic factors are felt to explain the apparent pain amplification. Patients with pain disorder with both medical and psychologic factors may develop suicidal ideation. If present, and if work is a psychosocial stressor, time out of the workplace may be necessary while comorbid depression and pain are treated.

Capacity
These patients may be deconditioned from inactivity, but deconditioning can improve with activity. Capacity is not usually affected, and although these patients may dislike an activity because it hurts, they can often perform the activities they dislike because there is no severe tissue pathology. By definition these cases involve pain out of proportion to the objective findings. Consistent with the advice given in other chapters in this book, pain is an issue of tolerance, *not* capacity.

Tolerance
For patients with chronic pain disorder, tolerance for the pain accompanying activity is *the* issue. However, tolerance is *not* an issue for physician-imposed work restrictions (those are based on risk) or for physician-prescribed work limitations (those are based on capacity). The treatment of pain disorder includes setting goals and emphasizing rehabilitation. Treating comorbid depression may be a reason to suspend working temporarily. On the other hand, declining to certify disability in some of these patients may be appropriate. The discussion as to why a physician

will not certify disability in such a case may include the previously suggested comments:

> You do not appear to meet the Social Security Administration's criteria for total disability. Because there is no medical evidence that you are at high risk of significant harm by working, I cannot certify that you are disabled for this job. There is no basis for work restrictions based on risk. Whether the rewards of working are sufficient for you to choose to remain at work, or whether the [fill in symptoms] you feel are sufficient for you to choose a different type of work, or not to work at all, is a question only you can answer. I can record what you feel to be your current activity intolerances, but these are not work restrictions or work limitations. Your intolerances are not scientifically measurable and they may change in the future, depending on how actively you participate in your treatment.

Posttraumatic Stress Disorder

Posttraumatic stress disorder (PTSD) is also a common psychiatric disorder that is increasingly important in the workplace and often accounts for absenteeism. Victims of bank robberies, assaults, or serious accidents at work often develop PTSD. Posttraumatic stress disorder is classified as an anxiety disorder along with panic disorder, agoraphobia, social phobia, obsessive-compulsive disorder, generalized anxiety, and anxiety disorder due to a medical condition or a substance. All of the anxiety disorders can cause psychological impairment, but PTSD very frequently causes significant impairment.

Posttraumatic stress disorder is a severe reaction to witnessing or experiencing a traumatic horrifying event, such as assault, rape, accidents, or military combat. The event involves actual or threatened death or serious injury to self or others, and a person's response involves fear, helplessness, and horror.

The symptoms of PTSD appear in three clusters: reexperiencing, avoidance, and hyperarousal clusters. Patients who reexperience trauma do so with recollections of the events, frequent dreams of the event, or feeling that the event is actually recurring. When these patients experience cues resembling the event, they often experience physical or psychological distress. The avoidance cluster includes the presence of avoidance of any thoughts, feelings, or conversations about the trauma, or any activities, places, or people associated with the trauma, which reignite the symptoms. Often avoidance includes amnesia for part of the trauma. The avoidance cluster also includes depressive symptoms. Finally, the hyperarousal cluster includes difficulty sleeping, anger outbursts, poor concentration, hypervigilance, and exaggerated startle response. Posttraumatic stress disorder is more common in women and leads to significant impairment in the quality of life of individuals. Suicidal behavior is more frequent than in other anxiety disorders as well. Half of PTSD cases resolved in three months.[3] More than 80% are comorbid with other mental disorders, most frequently panic disorder, agoraphobia, and major depression and substance abuse.

The treatment of PTSD generally requires selective serotonin reuptake inhibitors (SSRIs) and cognitive and behavioral therapy. If mild cases are responding to treatment, primary care physicians can manage them. A subset of these patients develop severe lifelong symptoms with exacerbations and remissions that make employment and interpersonal relationships difficult to maintain.[8] Thus, cases with severe symptoms and cases without improvement within a month should be referred to a psychiatrist.

Risk
If significant suicidal ideation is present, work absence during intensive (usually inpatient) treatment is appropriate. If the PTSD occurs because of a workplace incident (robbery, rape, witnessing a death at work) and if the symptoms are moderate or severe, psychiatric referral and work absence are appropriate.

Capacity
Any of the symptoms of PTSD may be severe enough to interfere with capacity to work. For example, poor concentration from intrusive recollections may preclude ability to follow instructions or to keep up a work pace. Thus, work tasks may require modification or accommodations.

Tolerance
If the PTSD symptoms are severe and unimproving (as mentioned earlier under "Risk"), a psychiatric referral is indicated.[9] If the PTSD arises from a workplace injury and if intolerance for the symptoms delays return to work past the time off required for the physical injury, a psychiatric referral is clearly indicated. Overcoming a patient's avoidance of work may require gradual job reentry and desensitization by a therapist working with the employer and the patient.

Adjustment Disorder

Adjustment disorder implies that symptoms of depression or anxiety are related to stressful events. Once the stress is removed, the symptoms usually resolve. Adjustment disorders are common in work settings and also in personal stress, such as divorce or family problems. Common causes of work stress that may result in an adjustment disorder include changes in management, stress with coworkers or supervisors, budget cuts, hiring freezes, fear of losing one's job, seeing a colleague terminated, and having a high-stress job.[10,11] Once again, in making the decision to take someone who has an adjustment disorder off work, the primary care physician needs to thoroughly understand how the symptoms are impairing work performance.

Risk

In adjustment disorder with depressed mood and in adjustment disorder with anxious mood, risk is not usually a problem. These disorders describe depressive and anxiety symptoms that develop in response to specific stressors. Some reaction to stress is expected in all people, but these diagnoses indicate an excessive reaction to a stressful stimulus that may cause significant impairment.

If the "stressor" is a conflict with a person at work or a situation at work, the physician may be justified in restricting work until a solution to the stressor is implemented. The analogy of occupational asthma or occupational contact dermatitis may be helpful. In these diseases, the physician will impose work restrictions preventing exposure to the specific chemical to which the patient has developed an allergy. Physicians do not consider these patients totally disabled and unable to work because they react to a specific chemical. In adjustment disorder, physicians may restrict patients from exposure to a stressor in a particular workplace, but this does not always mean these patients are totally disabled. A small number of patients may be quite impaired from an adjustment disorder.

Capacity

Capacity is not usually the issue with adjustment disorders. Although the mental symptoms may decrease work performance (productivity), people may be able to continue working. In other cases, however, capacity may be so impaired that the person needs to be off work.

Tolerance

Many patients choose to change employers or change careers when they find the symptoms experienced at a particular work site exceed their tolerance. This is an issue of patient choice (tolerance) and not an issue for physician-imposed work restriction (risk) or physician-described work limitation (capacity). A sobering reminder for physicians is the following scenario. A patient complains about stress at work and is considered to have adjustment disorder. Meaning well, her physician certifies that she is temporarily unable to work in this job. Medical treatment is not effective. The patient returns to her physician requesting a "full work release" because the employer decided to promote her. She will be paid more, but she will have the same supervisor, with *more* stress and responsibility. She now is willing to tolerate the same stressors because she will be paid more. Keeping the issues of risk, capacity, and tolerance separate helps primary care physicians think through return-to-work decisions.

Excusing the Patient From Work

Regardless of their diagnosis, most patients should have at least a moderate psychological impairment to be off work. A moderate rating means that their function is compatible with some but not all useful functioning. It is important to understand that a moderate rating is an average rating derived from an impairment determination in each of the following categories: activities of daily living, social functioning, concentration, and work stress tolerance. *Moderate or marked impairment in work ability without concomitant at least moderate impairment in other areas of mental function does not occur.* If a patient complains only of work intolerance that does not affect concentration, activities of daily living, or social functioning outside of work, this is not a reason for disability.

A few people with mild impairment, because of their job description, might still need to be taken off work. For example, an air traffic controller with mild anxiety might need to be excused from work. Patients with marked or extreme psychological impairment, regardless of their job description, should not be working.

Understanding the patient's risk, tolerance, and capacity to do work is also a vital part of the evaluation for absence from work.

Initiating Treatment Planning

Most psychiatric patients with a moderate impairment rating will need to be off work for at least three to four weeks. Many of these patients will need antidepressant medications, which require at least 3 weeks for response. With the patient's written consent, the treatment plan should also include involvement of the patient's family, the case manager, other medical specialists, and in some cases the patient's supervisor. All of these people can provide corroboration, support, and continuity of care, and can facilitate reentry into the workplace. The patient should agree with the need to be off work, agree to treatment, and demonstrate compliance. Treatment planning should also include assessment and initiation of treatment of comorbidities, especially substance abuse. All psychotropic medications need to be closely monitored by the primary care physician.

Chapter 18

As coordinator of the patient's treatment, the primary care physician may initiate referrals to appropriate specialties, such as physical therapy or pain clinics for patients with chronic pain and psychotherapists for patients with adjustment disorders, depression, and PTSD. Referral to an employee assistance program (EAP) may also be helpful for these patients. Referral to a psychiatrist may be necessary for difficult cases, as described throughout this chapter. Table 18-3 outlines the indications for a psychiatric referral. For difficult cases, *early referral* to the psychiatrist can minimize treatment complications and prolonged disability.

Returning the Patient to Work

To return to work, the patient should have regained the ability to perform most activities of daily living and should have regained adequate social functioning, concentration, persistence, and pace. He or she should also demonstrate stress tolerance in a work-like setting. All of these functions should be no greater than *mildly* impaired for at least one week before returning to work. In particular, these patients should be able to relate to others, concentrate, drive, enjoy some pleasurable activities, and sleep. These people should also be in control of their anger. Although most patients can return even though they are not yet in full remission, the treatment established during their absence from work should continue after they return in order to achieve full remission of symptoms. Without full remission, they may relapse and have a more complex course in the future.

Table 18-3 Common Reasons for a Referral to a Psychiatrist

- Poor response to initial treatment
- Poor motivation to return to work
- Diagnostic uncertainty
- Multiple comorbid problems
- Presence of psychosis
- Violence, violent threats, or suicidal thoughts
- Problems with anger control
- Complicated medical-psychiatric problems
- Secondary gain (symptom magnification)
- Question of malingering
- Poor social support

In addition, upon returning to work, the patient should not have any significant side effects from medications that may impair their concentration or coordination. Substance abuse should be under control and other comorbidities should be stabilized. If job restrictions, limitations, or accommodations are required (eg, low stress, weight restrictions, part time), the primary care physician should discuss these needs with the case manager and/or the supervisor or human resources manager with the proper authorization from the patient. Arranging discussions between the patient and his or her supervisor can dramatically improve work stress tolerance. After a patient returns to work, efforts should be made to follow up the patient closely to achieve remission of symptoms, minimize the possibility of relapse, ensure continuity of care, and monitor medications. Patients should agree that they are ready to return to work. For those patients who seem psychiatrically ready to return to work, but who do not agree that they are ready, referral to a psychiatrist is indicated.

Summary

The primary care physician often makes the decision to take someone off work and then later decides when he or she is fit to return to duty. The foundation of these decisions is laid by conducting a comprehensive history and examination. Formulating a psychiatric diagnosis and understanding how the person's symptoms are causing impairment in activities of daily living, social function, concentration, persistence and pace, and work tolerance are vital to this process. Additionally, the primary care physician needs to have a thorough understanding of the person's job description and the ways in which the impairment impedes or interferes with job performance. Once this is done, a treatment plan can be initiated. After improvement with treatment, the decision to return the person to work can be made rationally. Having a treatment alliance with the patient, family, and the employer will greatly facilitate an earlier return to work and more productive work. Ongoing treatment after return is usually necessary to achieve full remission of symptoms.

Chapter 18

References

1. Cocchiarella L, Andersson G. *Guides to the Evaluation of Permanent Impairment*. 5th ed. Chicago, Ill: AMA Press; 2001:4, 363.

2. American Psychiatric Association. *Diagnostic and Statistical Manual of Mental Disorders, Fourth Edition*. Washington, DC: American Psychiatric Association; 1994.

3. Goldman LS, Wise TN, Brody DS. *Psychiatry for Primary Care Physicians.* 2nd ed. Chicago, Ill: AMA Press; 2004.

4. Stewart W, Ricci J, Chee E, Hahn S, Morganstein D. Cost of lost productive work time among US workers with depression. *JAMA.* 2003;289:3135–3144.

5. Kessler R, Berglund P, Demler O, et al. The epidemiology of major depressive disorder. *JAMA.* 2003;289:3104.

6. *Disability Evaluation Under Social Security.* Baltimore, Md: Social Security Administration; January 2003. SSA publication 64-039.

7. Bostwick J, Pankratz V. Affective disorders and suicide risk: a reexamination. *Am J Psychiatry.* 2000;157:1925–1932.

8. Reed P. *The Medical Disability Advisor: Workplace Guidelines for Disability Duration.* 5th ed. Westminster, Colo: Reed Group Ltd; 2005.

9. Colledge AL, Johnson HI. S.P.I.C.E: a model for reducing the incidence and costs of occupationally entitled claims. *Occup Med.* 2000;15:695–722.

10. Baron R, Neuman J. Workplace violence and workplace aggression: evidence on their relative frequency and potential causes. *Aggress Behav.* 1996;22:161–173.

11. Baron R, Neuman J, Geddes D. Social and personal determinants of workplace aggression: evidence for the impact of perceived injustice and the type A behavior pattern. *Aggress Behav.* 1999;25:281–296.

Chapter 18

Chapter 19

Working With Common Functional Syndromes: Fibromyalgia and Chronic Fatigue Syndrome

James B. Talmage, MD

Fibromyalgia and chronic fatigue syndrome are *syndromes*. As syndromes, they are labels for collections of symptoms. There is no currently proven pathophysiology for these syndromes. The diagnosis of many clinical conditions is similarly based on subjective criteria established by consensus of experienced physicians. Migraine headache, irritable bowel syndrome, and major depression are examples.

Fibromyalgia is a syndrome of widespread chronic pain (above and below the diaphragm, and on the left and right sides of the body), usually accompanied by some combination of stiffness, fatigue, headaches, bowel and/or bladder complaints, sleep disturbance, paresthesias, and cognitive difficulties. This diagnosis is generally verified by determining the presence of "tender points."[1,2]

Chronic fatigue syndrome is characterized by new-onset significant fatigue that does not resolve with rest, that reduces the premorbid activity level, and that persists without obvious explanation by systemic disease for at least six months.[3,4]

While these syndromes are discussed separately in many texts and articles, this chapter follows the example of other authors, and discusses these as a single entity. The overlap in symptoms between these conditions is extensive, and the label given to a particular patient may depend more on the specialty of the physician making the diagnosis than on the features of the disease.[2,5] This chapter discusses these conditions when they are present in isolation, and not when they accompany other conditions like rheumatoid arthritis, systemic lupus erythematosus, and so on. For those more complex cases with comorbidity, primary care physicians should consult with appropriate specialists.

Social Security Administration's Criteria for Total Disability

Fibromyalgia syndrome and chronic fatigue syndrome are not discussed in the Social Security Administration's (SSA's) guide for physicians.[6] Because the US Social Security system is based on the biomedical model, in which severe objective impairment is the criterion for disability, and since these syndromes have no objective findings on physical examination, laboratory tests, electromyography, muscle biopsy, and routine imaging studies, these conditions are not mentioned in the text for physician evaluators of disability for the SSA.

Countries differ in their approach to disability for functional syndromes. In Norway, for example, 11% of the female population met the criteria for a diagnosis of fibromyalgia, and it became the single most frequent diagnosis for disability.[7] In Iceland, when claims for government-funded disability began to be filed for patients with fibromyalgia, these claims were rejected by the system. In many cases the patients' physicians filed amended applications for disability listing a secondary psychiatric diagnosis.[8] In Iceland the psychiatric comorbidity may be a basis for state-funded disability.

While most patients with fibromyalgia do not have a current psychiatric illness, patients with fibromyalgia have a higher rate of current or past psychiatric illness than normal controls. In addition, the presence of a comorbid psychiatric illness makes fibromyalgia patients more likely to seek health care and to seek disability certification.[2]

Risk

Risk is not an issue. These conditions are not associated with the criteria of the Americans With Disabilities Act of 1990 of "significant risk" of "substantial harm" that is "imminent." (See Chapter 8.) These patients experience symptoms, like pain and fatigue, with activity; however, the increase in subjective symptoms without any detectable objective correlate is *not* significant harm. If these patients are willing job applicants, there is no basis for a pre-placement examining physician to recommend against the hiring and placement of these individuals because these syndromes have been diagnosed and are still present. Fibromyalgia has been shown to improve with aerobic exercise,[1] and progressive exercise is recommended as treatment. Work may involve exercise, and thus be therapeutic, in addition to its psychosocial benefits, as discussed in Chapter 1.

Capacity

Capacity in fibromyalgia is not usually an issue. Patients dislike doing what they *can do* because it hurts. Both fibromyalgia and chronic fatigue syndrome patients complain of fatigue. Both groups may have a decreased exercise capacity documented on treadmill testing. Both conditions frequently result in patients adopting a sedentary lifestyle, so cardiovascular deconditioning is to be expected. For heavy and very heavy jobs, aerobic exercise capacity may be an issue and may be a basis for physician-described work limitations. However, the result of treadmill exercise testing in chronic fatigue syndrome may change on a day-to-day basis, so the result of a single test may not be a valid test of disability.[9] This is especially true if the test is stopped by "fatigue" (tolerance) long before the predicted maximal heart rate is reached (exercise testing) or the anaerobic threshold is crossed (cardiopulmonary exercise testing).

If cognitive complaints affect job performance in intellectually demanding jobs, formal neuropsychological testing by a neuropsychologist may document a problem with intellectual capacity that would be a basis for physician-described work limitations. If psychiatric comorbidity is suspected, psychiatric referral is indicated for diagnosis and treatment. Psychiatric comorbidity may be a basis for work limitations.

Because these are chronic conditions that do not generally respond dramatically to treatment, there is no logical basis for temporary work modification. Physicians would not be able to state that temporary work modifications would permit time for effective treatment that would result in expected prompt return to full duty.

Tolerance

Tolerance for subjective symptoms is generally the issue in these conditions. As long as Western society is using a biomedical model for disability, in which severe impairment is expected to be present to justify physician certification of disability, these functional syndromes with no objective findings would *not* qualify for work restrictions (risk) or work limitations (capacity).

Chapter 19

The fibromyalgia patient's inability to tolerate symptoms (especially pain) may well be due to "central sensitization" or enhanced symptom perception.[2] The pain and fatigue may be "real," but physicians have yet to discover a way to measure either pain or fatigue. These patients' plight is similar to that of the patients with nonspecific regional arm pain (Chapter 13) or mechanical low back pain (Chapter 12), where significant symptoms exist without confirmatory objective findings.

Chapter 2 stated that when tolerance in the Western biomedical model is "believable" on the basis of the presence of severe objective pathology, physicians will probably agree on supporting a patient's disability application. In these cases there is no basis for physician-imposed work restrictions or physician-described work limitations. This disability application must be supported by noting on disability certification forms under "comments" that the patient has problems with activity that are proportionate to the severe objective pathology present.

In cases where the symptoms are dramatic but there is no objective impairment or pathology, as is the case in these functional syndromes, physicians will disagree as to whether patients should choose to limit activity. Since work tolerance is *not* an area of medical science, physicians will disagree according to their perspectives and biases. It is sobering to remember that in a study to determine whether experienced pain clinic physicians could correctly distinguish individuals with fibromyalgia from paid volunteers simulating fibromyalgia, simulators were misidentified as fibromyalgia patients in one third of the judgments, and fibromyalgia patients were misidentified as simulators in one fifth of the judgments.[10] Thus, the best course for physicians is to agree that there is no contraindication to work activity, and the decision of whether or not the rewards of work outweigh the symptoms experienced is the *patient's choice*. It is *not the physician's decision* to certify or not certify disability. It is the patient's decision to work or not to work.

Summary

Fibromyalgia and chronic fatigue syndrome are syndromes, with symptoms, but no objective findings. In the Western biomedical model of disability, there is usually no basis for physician-imposed work restrictions (risk) or physician-described work limitations (capacity). Tolerance for the symptoms experienced during activity the patient can do is the issue. Whether or not the rewards of work outweigh the symptoms is the patient's choice, and physicians should not certify disability in these syndromes based only on tolerance.

References

1. Simms RW. Fibromyalgia syndrome: current concepts in pathophysiology, clinical features, and management. *Arthritis Care Res*. 1996;9:315–328.

2. Goldenberg DL. Fibromyalgia syndrome a decade later: what have we learned? *Arch Intern Med*. 1999;159:777–785.

3. Holmes GP, Kaplan JE, Gantz NM. Chronic fatigue syndrome: a working case definition. *Ann Intern Med*. 1988;108:387–389.

4. Komaroff AL, Buchwald D. Symptoms and signs in chronic fatigue syndrome. *Rev Infect Dis*. 1991;13(suppl):S12–S18.

5. Buchwald D, Garrity D. Comparison of patients with chronic fatigue syndrome, fibromyalgia, and multiple chemical sensitivities. *Arch Intern Med*. 1994;154:2049–2053.

6. *Disability Under Social Security*. Baltimore, Md: Social Security Administration; January 2003. SSA publication 64-039.

7. Brusgaard D, Evensen AR, Bjerkedal T. Fibromyalgia: a new cause for disability pension. *Scand J Soc Med*. 1993;21:116.

8. Thoriacius S. Fibromyalgia and chronic fatigue syndrome. *Disability Med*. 2001;1:14–15.

9. Alpern HL, Ranavaya MI, Govindan S. *Chronic Fatigue Syndrome: Impairment and Disability Issues*. Chicago, Ill: American Academy of Disability Evaluating Physicians; 1999.

10. Khostanteen I, Tunks ER, Goldsmith GH. Fibromyalgia: can one distinguish it from simulation? *J Rheumatol*. 2000;27:2671–2676.

Chapter 20

The Social Security Administration Disability System

Edward B. Holmes, MD, MPH

Primary care physicians are frequently asked to complete disability paperwork or otherwise assist in a disability claim for their patients. There are several different types of disability programs that compensate individuals for the loss of function caused by physical or mental impairments. These include workers' compensation, the Social Security Administration (SSA) disability system, state and local government disability programs, and private disability insurance policies.

Clarifying Misunderstanding of the Social Security Administration Disability System

This chapter is designed to explain to primary care providers how the SSA disability system works and to assist them in their dealings with patients applying for disability under the SSA system. Other chapters in this book may refer to the Social Security "listings of impairments" or the "Blue Book" and cite specific wording from those listings. Many words in the SSA listings of impairments have specific and legally defined meanings, and presenting these listings to the public and practitioners can lead to confusion and misunderstanding. For example, SSA has a listing that allows disability to individuals with major weight-bearing joint abnormalities and "inability to ambulate effectively."[1] At first glance, one not familiar with the SSA program may think that because a patient has a "bad knee" and a significant "limp," he or she is not able to ambulate effectively. One might conclude that because a patient has a significant limp, cannot run and jump, and must rest after walking extensively, that patient has an "inability to ambulate effectively." However, the SSA has extensive written policy interpretation and rule application guidance used by adjudicators, with specific examples of what this phrase means. In this instance, some SSA policy examples of "inability to ambulate effectively" are "The inability to walk without the use of a walker, two crutches, or two canes." One can easily see how the written wording in the listing could be misinterpreted by well-meaning claimants or treating physicians who feel their patients qualify for "disability," yet when reviewed by the adjudicators, following written policy and examples, a person with a limp would not necessarily meet listed criteria. These types of specifically and legally defined meanings are found throughout the complex SSA listings of impairments, and therefore they should be interpreted with caution.

Another unusual and often misunderstood aspect of the SSA disability system is the built-in "discrimination" between older individuals and younger individuals as well as between educated and uneducated individuals. The SSA has a vocational profiling process that allows benefits to older individuals, those with less education, and those with poor English-speaking skills much more frequently than to younger, educated, and fluent English-speaking individuals with transferable work skills who have the same impairments. This often leads to frustration and confusion among the medical community and claimants because people have heard tales of others with relatively "minor" impairments being allowed full SSA disability benefits and yet those with seemingly "more severe" impairments are denied. This is not random decision making but rather a complex set of legally defined words and vocational profiling that leads to the ultimate determination of allowance vs denial of benefits.

The SSA disability program is essentially designed to determine whether adults are incapable of performing substantial gainful activity because of a severe physical or mental impairment(s). The program also allows for disability benefits to children with severe impairments that seriously interfere with the performance of age-appropriate activities. However, the distinction between disability and impairment is often misunderstood in the medical community, the public, and the scientific literature. This chapter helps define the differences between disability and impairment and describes the current SSA disability process. Further, the ever-increasing number of people alleging disability and impairment necessitates a professional understanding of these terms and the most effective means to deal with these issues in a medical practice.

The Differences Between Impairment and Disability

The SSA defines a medically determinable *impairment* as:

An impairment that results from anatomical, physiological, or psychological abnormalities which can be shown by medically acceptable clinical and laboratory diagnostic techniques. A physical or mental impairment must be established by medical evidence consisting of signs, symptoms, and laboratory findings—not only by the individual's statement of symptoms.[1]

The SSA defines *disability* as:

the inability to engage in any substantial, gainful activity by reason of any medically determinable physical or mental impairment(s), which can be expected to result in death or which has lasted or can be expected to last for a continuous period of not less than 12 months.[1]

Distinguishing impairment and disability is critical for physicians in making appropriate statements in records and in assisting patients. One patient can be impaired significantly and have no disability, and someone else can be quite disabled with only limited impairment. For example, a paraplegic who is wheelchair bound may be employed full time quite successfully and therefore not meet the definition of "disabled" for the SSA. On the other hand, a professional pianist might have a relatively minor injury to a finger tendon that severely limits her ability to perform her usual and customary basic work activities (playing piano) and in some systems she might meet the definition of "disabled," even though she can do other work. Because of this difference between impairment and disability, physicians are encouraged to rate impairment on the basis of the level of impact of the condition on performance of daily activities other than work. The American Medical Association's *Guides to the Evaluation of Permanent Impairment, Fifth Edition (Guides)*, states that impairment ratings derived from the *Guides* are "not intended for use as direct determinants of work disability."[2]

Disability involves several different factors. Disability can be temporary or permanent. Also, disability is usually described as complete (total) or partial.

Different programs have various categories of disability. An individual can be temporarily unable to carry on work activity for remuneration or profit

Chapter 20

(eg, after trauma, surgery, and intensive care) and be "disabled" under some disability programs, but if recovery occurs within 12 months, the individual would likely not be disabled under the SSA permanent disability program. Many workers' compensation systems allow for partial disability, hence the need for the *Guides* to measure the extent of the impairment to normal functional capacity as a percentage of whole-person impairment. However, SSA disability is essentially an "all or none" type of disability program; the claimant is either entirely disabled or not disabled.

Overview of the Social Security Administration Disability System

The SSA disability system is composed of two main programs: the Title II program, which provides benefits to individuals who are "insured" under the system to receive benefit by virtue of their contributions to the Social Security system through taxes, and the Title XVI program, which provides supplemental security income (SSI) payments to children and those with limited income and resources. The medical and psychiatric criteria for determining disability are essentially the same between the two programs.

An individual who feels he or she has a physical and/or mental impairment that prevents him or her from working can apply for disability on the Internet at www.SSA.gov, over the telephone with a SSA field office, or in person at a local SSA office. The field office consists of mainly clerical and administrative personnel, but generally not medical personnel.

When the application is made, the claimant will be asked to list the conditions causing impairment, the onset of these conditions, when he or she became unable to work because of the conditions, and the names and addresses of all treating physicians and facilities, among other things.

This claims file is then forwarded to a state disability determination services (DDS) office. Each state has a contractual arrangement with the federal government to administer the SSA disability program for its residents. All states use the same rules, regulations, and forms, with a few circuit court–mandated differences between the regions. The DDS employees are state workers and contractors who consist of physicians, psychologists, psychiatrists, claims examiners, clerical personnel, and administrators. The claim files are assigned to a disability claims examiner, trained in the evaluation of medical evidence under the SSA disability program. The file is developed, with medical sources contacted and records obtained. If insufficient medical evidence has been obtained to establish the existence of the alleged impairments, the DDS may purchase consultative examinations from community physicians, trained and contracted for such purposes.

Unlike many other disability programs, under SSA programs the claimant is either allowed full disability benefits or denied; there is no partial disability.

Once the claim file is complete, the DDS adjudicators follow a defined sequence of evaluation in determining whether each claimant meets disability criteria, considering his or her impairments, residual functional capacity, education, English-speaking skills, and age.

The first step in evaluation involves a determination of whether the individual is currently working at "substantial gainful activity" (SGA), which has a legally defined earnings limit. If he or she is working at this level, he or she is denied benefits. Thus, an individual who is gradually getting worse but applies for benefits while still working at SGA levels, to determine whether he or she qualifies, will likely be denied benefits by the SSA. If the person is not working at SGA levels, the next step in the sequential evaluation is to determine whether he or she has an impairment that meets the SSA definition of "severe." Essentially what this means is that there is an objective, diagnosable condition (physical or mental) that limits the ability to perform basic work activities. If so, then the third step in sequential evaluation is to determine whether the individual has an impairment that meets or is medically equivalent to the very specific criteria listed in the SSA blue book listings of impairments. If the claimant does not meet the criteria on a word-for-word basis, as defined by SSA policy, then the fourth step involves an assessment of the individual's residual physical and mental functional capacity. This residual capacity is then compared, by a disability claims examiner, to past work performed by the individual and/or other work in the national economy to determine whether the individual (considering age, education, and English-speaking skills) can return to work. If he or she cannot return to work, then SSA disability benefits are allowed. After allowance of benefits and depending on the type of claim, the individual will likely be eligible for either Medicaid or Medicare through the SSA.

What the Physician Needs to Know

The SSA disability process discourages the treating physician from attempting to make a determination of whether the claimant is disabled. This is a decision reserved under the rules to the commissioner of the SSA or his/her agents. What is much more useful to the claimant, the SSA, and DDS is for

Chapter 20

the treating physician to provide objective and subjective information about the specific conditions leading to impairment. Furthermore, it is very useful for the physician to provide to the SSA, via well-documented progress notes, discharge summaries, or letters, the extent of objective functional limitation, *not just a repetition of the alleged limitations subjectively provided by the claimant to the physician.* What DDS really needs to know about the patient is how he or she looks objectively, how well he or she functions (for example, motor strength, sensation, range of motion, concentration ability, and so on), what deficits the physician can actually observe, and then *the physician's professional, expert opinion* as an examining or treating professional about residual capacity with regard to lifting, carrying, standing, walking, bending, seeing, hearing, concentrating, interacting, and so on.

Since treating physicians generally are quite unaware of SSA rules on disability determination and are not generally qualified or expected to interpret the SSA blue book (since there are so many policies in place to define the meaning of specific terms and words in the blue book), it is really unfair to expect a treating physician to comment on whether a claimant meets or medically equals a particular level of impairment listed in the blue book. It is much more logical and procedurally more efficient for the physician who knows the patient best to define for DDS the extent of the objective physical or mental impairment and provide a professional opinion about function with regard to basic work activities. This allows the DDS and SSA to make an informed decision based on the physician's professional observations and opinion while at the same time allowing the physician to stay out of the disability determination business for the patient.

The DDS physician and psychologist consultants do not have the luxury of examining and evaluating the patient in person. The DDS consultants and claims examiners simply review written medical evidence from the physician and other providers to make their functional determinations regarding whether the patient has the capacity to return to gainful employment. Without good, reasoned medical opinions about function from the providers who know the patient best, innocent errors can be made.

Under SSA rules and regulations, the commissioner or her agents must decide whether a particular claimant is disabled. The treating physician, although given great weight, cannot make this determination, so writing a note stating "this patient is totally disabled" does not ensure that the patient will be given benefits. Instead, the physician should thoughtfully prepare an objective report of the patient's residual functional capacity, addressing those areas in question. Some of the specific types of work capacities SSA adjudicators must assess are listed in Table 20-1. It would be helpful if the

Table 20-1 SSA and DDS Disability Requirements

Physical Capacity	Mental Capacity
Maximum occasional lift (very little up to one third of a work day)	Understanding and memory
Maximum frequent lift (one third to two thirds of a work day)	Concentration and persistence
Cumulative sitting time in an 8-hour work day (in hours)	Social interaction
Cumulative stand/walk time in an 8-hour work day (in hours)	Adaptation
Ability to reach, push, pull, finger, handle, feel	
Ability to bend, stoop, squat, kneel, climb	
Ability to see, hear, speak, and work around hazards, cold, heat, or other environmental conditions	

Table 20-2 SSA and DDS Disability Do's and Don'ts

Do's	Don'ts
Send copies of your records	Get angry if your patient is denied disability benefits
Carefully record objective findings for each applicable impairment in all your notes	Expect brief statements that the patient is disabled, without substantive evidence, to win an award of benefits
Respond to inquiries from DDS or SSA in a timely fashion	Ignore DDS requests for information; they will likely keep trying
Bill SSA or DDS for copies of records, evaluations, or reports where appropriate in your state	Document for free if your state has a method of compensating you for your time
Document *your opinion* about residual functional capacity (Table 20-1)	Just reiterate the patient's allegations of limitations
	Make a statement about "disabled" or "not disabled"

physician addressed the applicable areas of function that are impaired in the particular patient. Hints for dealing with the SSA and the DDS on behalf of patients applying for disability are noted in Table 20-2.

Chapter 20

The types of observations that are useful to adjudicators of a disability claim include the physician's observation about function in the examination room, in the hall, in the waiting room, and sometimes in the parking lot of the office. These types of observations are frequently quite revealing. For example, a recent disability claim involved a case where the individual was applying for disability for "total blindness." The ophthalmologist noted that the claimant had driven to the appointment in a van. The claimant had a driver's license. The claimant had read magazines in the waiting room, walked down the hall, grabbed the doorknob without assistance, and then proceeded to present on examination as being completely incapable of seeing. Incidentally, the results of ophthalmologic examination, with the exception of the subjective visual acuity and visual field testing, were normal.

Another example is a claimant who applied for disability because of inability to walk from a spinal cord injury. After his visit to the physician, the claimant was observed to wheel out to a truck in his wheelchair, stand up, pick up the wheelchair and throw it in the back of the truck, and then proceed to drive away.

In other cases, the observations can prove useful in finding limitations not verbalized by the patient. For example, a claimant may present at the office showing great difficulty with the paperwork, forms, and so forth. There may be difficulties in understanding, memory, cognition, writing, fingering, reading, etc. Some claimants are so impaired that family and friends are required to complete paperwork, answer questions, and make decisions. When observed, these things become evident, but unless they are recorded, they can be missed by a paper review of the file by DDS.

Having the patient pick up coins in the office from the examination table or counter can be very revealing about fine fingering and dexterity. Observing a claimant as she is bending to pick up a purse off the floor can be quite revealing, especially when the patient does not realize that she is being observed. Making notes about how the patient performs when moving from chair to examination table and back and while walking in the office can be very useful to adjudicators in helping to determine true function.

Writing a Medical Source Opinion About Function

The SSA publishes a guide for health professionals who prepare consultative examinations for SSA claimants.[3] This guide is designed for practitioners specifically contracted to SSA to provide needed examinations where evidence is insufficient in the file. However, the guide can also provide clues to the treating physician on the scope, content, and reporting requirements that SSA prefers. Essentially what the SSA wants is good, objective documentation of the impairing conditions with objective measurements (range of motion, circumference, test results, etc), and then the physician's professional opinion about residual functional capacity in the areas noted earlier in this chapter. *It is very important to have the physician's true, reasoned opinion about function and not just a reiteration of the claimant's alleged limitations.* The SSA and DDS already likely know and have likely received extensive written documentation regarding the claimant's alleged limitations; what DDS needs to fairly adjudicate the claim is objective professional documentation of the true level of impairment to function.

Weighing of Source Opinions About Function by the Social Security Administration

The SSA has rules for DDS to follow with regard to evaluating the opinions about function present in a claim file. There are several types of medical source opinions in many files:

1. Opinion reserved for the commissioner
2. Opinion from the reviewing source about function
3. Opinion from the examining source about function
4. Opinion from the treating source about function.

Opinions of "disabled" or "meets an SSA listing" are reserved for the commissioner of the SSA or her agents. These opinions are not to be ignored by DDS but are much less useful in adjudicating a claim according to SSA rules than a true opinion about function. Opinions from reviewing physicians such as insurance company reviewers who do not examine the claimant are not ignored but generally carry less weight than opinions from sources who have actually examined the claimant.

Examining sources, contracted specifically to examine claimants for their disability claim, or other one-time consultants not involved in treatment are likely to get a different overall presentation than a treating source when it comes to level of impairment, symptoms, and so forth. Examining-source opinions can be given great weight in adjudication depending on the specialty of the physician, the consistency of the evaluation with the other evidence in the file, and the level of detail and justification for any opinion about function offered in the report. *The potentially most valuable source of*

information about a claimant's true functioning is from the treating source.
This physician likely knows the patient well, has a longitudinal relationship,
and can offer unique, professional insight. Unfortunately, the physician-
patient relationship can occasionally cloud the judgment and presentation of
functioning by treating sources. Nevertheless, SSA and DDS value the well-
supported, consistent opinions of treating sources above all other sources in
the file.

Providing good documentation with complete physical examination, history,
and test result reporting, combined with a well-reasoned opinion about the
patient's actual residual functional ability (not whether he or she is disabled), will likely be the most useful thing the physician can do to assist the
patient in traveling through the complex SSA disability process.

Summary

Treating physicians are often asked to assist in completing disability paperwork for their patients. Requirements vary to qualify for compensation, but
usually include loss of function caused by physical or mental impairment.
These include workers' compensation, the Social Security Administration
disability system, state and local government disability programs, and private disability insurance policies.

References

1. Social Security Administration. *Disability Evaluation Under Social Security.*
Baltimore, Md: Social Security Administration; January 2003. SSA publication
64–039.

2. Cocchiarella L, Andersson G, eds. *The Guides to the Evaluation of Permanent
Impairment.* 5th ed. Chicago, Ill: AMA Press; 2001.

3. Social Security Administration. *Consultative Examinations: A Guide for Health
Professionals.* Baltimore, Md: Social Security Administration; November 1999.
SSA publication 64-025.

Index

Best Selling Books

By Rene Cailliet, MD

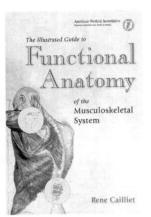

The Illustrated Guide to Functional Anatomy of the Musculoskeletal System

Ground your impairment evaluations in the right foundation.
While clinicians today are trained in gross musculoskeletal anatomy, solid clinical evaluations demand a thorough knowledge of functional anatomy as well.

The Illustrated Guide to Functional Anatomy of the Musculoskeletal System provides the groundwork you need to truly understand musculoskeletal function, the basis of all biomechanics. This outstanding guide will give you an important base knowledge of normal musculoskeletal function and how deviations are caused, helping you determine the most appropriate clinical diagnoses and treatments for your patients.

Combining easy-to-read text with numerous quick-reference tables and clear illustrations, *The Illustrated Guide to Functional Anatomy of the Musculoskeletal System* logically covers both regional and systemic function. Chapters are organized by each segment of the musculoskeletal system for easy reference, presenting anatomical material that analyzes everyday activities and associated movements. Informative illustrations further deepen your knowledge of each musculoskeletal segment?s function and how to clinically diagnose impairment.

This is an outstanding primer for medical clinicians, medical students, residents, reimbursement coding staff, and other musculoskeletal allied health disciplines.

Softbound, 7 x 10", 320 pages
Order #: OP857003
Price: $69.95
AMA Member Price: $59.95

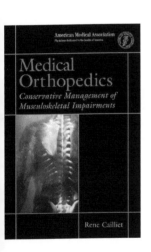

Medical Orthopedics:
Conservative Management of Musculoskeletal Impairments

Treat orthopedic impairments with confidence.
Medical Orthopedics provides an important primer to help medical clinicians provide accurate diagnoses of orthopedic problems and outline appropriate treatments and therapies.

This thorough guide lays the groundwork for understanding how impaired function is clinically diagnosed and managed, helping you to recognize and effectively treat problems that respond to non-surgical interventions. *Medical Orthopedics* outlines a systematic approach to conservative orthopedic management as it addresses the impairments encountered most frequently in primary care practice.

Thirteen chapters encompass every aspect of the musculoskeletal system, discussing how to improve function for specific problems while decreasing pain and impairment. This outstanding resource contains more than 80 visual aids, including clear illustrations to help you recognize abnormal function, enhance visual and manual examinations, and convey information to your patients.

Covering musculoskeletal impairments for all joints as well as the spine, *Medical Orthopedics* also devotes two additional chapters to pain including reflex sympathetic dystrophy, areas often neglected in the diagnosis and treatment of musculoskeletal impairments.

Softbound, 6 x 9", 210 pages
Order #: OP857103
Price: $69.95
AMA Member Price: $59.95

Call 800-621-8335 or order online at www.amapress.com

American Medical Association
Physicians dedicated to the health of America

The Practical Guide to
Range of Motion Assessment

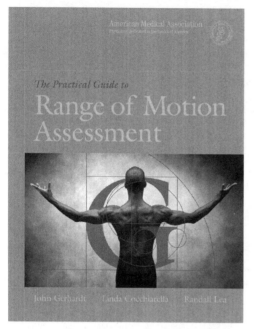

Anyone who wants to effectively diagnose, document, or treat musculoskeletal conditions must be able to accurately measure joint ROM by a standardized method that can be referenced and reproduced. Includes detailed instruction and photographs to demonstrate use of a standardized methodology to measure ROM.

* Select and apply appropriate instrumentation
* Prepare patient psychologically, physiologically, and physically
* Learn how to help the patient warm-up with standardized exercises
* Recognize and evaluate the factors that affect range of motion
* Have the ability to look for factors that affect ROM
* Learn how to cite your methodology and efficiently record findings
* Overall helps to lessen differences in measurements between examiners

Call 800-621-8335 or order online at www.amapress.com

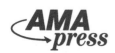

American Medical Association
Physicians dedicated to the health of America

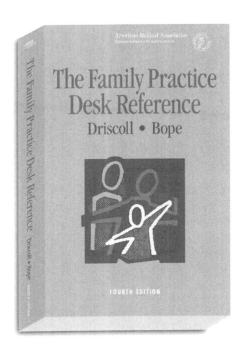

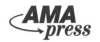

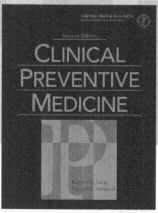
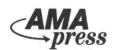

Guides Fifth Essentials!

The Guides Casebook
2nd Edition

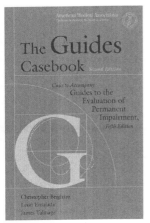

Over 68 case studies help to further understand the appropriate usage of the *Guides Fifth*.

Organized to further explain how to compare the results of analysis with the impairment criteria to correctly determine whole person impairment. Arranged to follow the chapter order of the Guides 5th. All 11 systems are covered in the Casebook in addition to ear, nose, throat and related structures and mental and behavioral disorders. Also compares and contrasts the 4th against the 5th edition. Valuable to anyone who wants to explain values, how to convert them and have the ability to discuss critical issues that are relevant to the proper use of Guides 5th.

Softbound, 6 x 9", 384 pages
Order #: OP210002
Price: $62.95
AMA Member Price: $57.95

Master the AMA
Guides Fifth

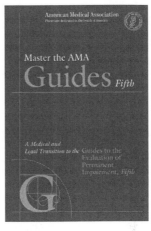

This valuable tool helps to make a seamless transition to Guide 5th.

Offers a comprehensive, chapter-by-chapter comparison of the content changes between Fourth and Fifth Editions. Includes practical applications by giving state-by-state breakdowns of workers compensation systems, provides a how-to on incorporating changes into medical and legal practices. Aids in helping to fully understand impairment ratings, records and reports. A valuable must-have for any impairment library.

Softbound, 6 x 9", 400 pages
Order #: OP721600
Price: $79.95
AMA Member Price: $69.95

Buy both and save 10%!
Master the AMA Guides Fifth and
The Guides Casebook, Second Edition
Order #: OP722904
Price: $128.00
AMA Member Price: $115.00

Call 800-621-8335
or order online at
www.amapress.com

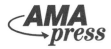

American Medical Association
Physicians dedicated to the health of America

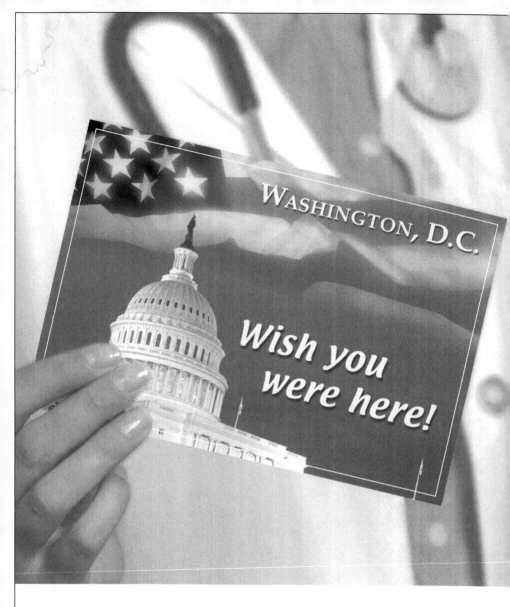

The most effective way you can influence the most important public health and professional issues facing medicine today is through your involvement in the AMA.

The AMA is recognized as one of the most effective lobbying forces on Capitol Hill. Washington's *Roll Call* magazine calls the AMA *"one of the most powerful advocacy organizations in the nation."*

More than a quarter of a million physicians from every state and specialty are marshaling their passion for medicine into meaningful action on medical issues.

American Medical Association
Physicians dedicated to the health of America

800 262-3211
www.ama-assn.org

Be a member of the AMA.